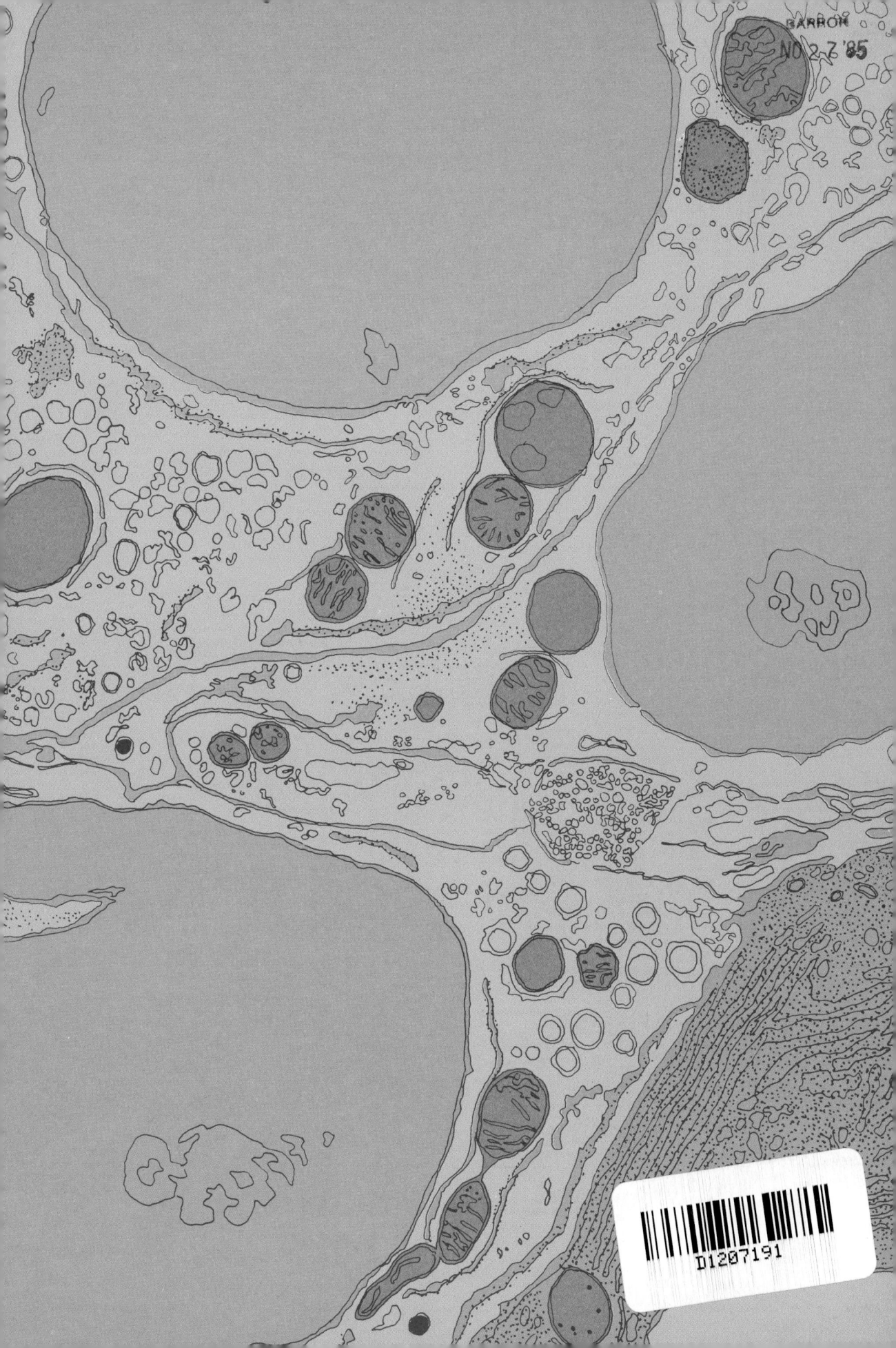

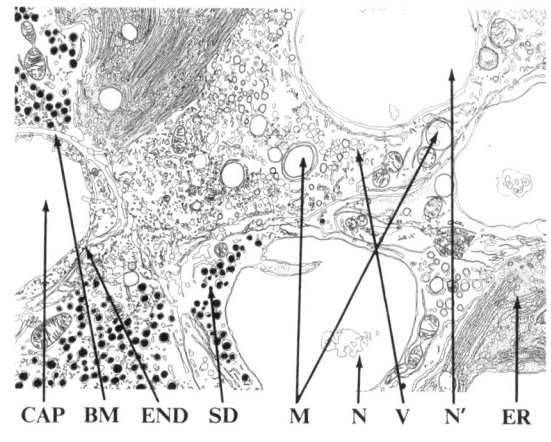

CAP BM END SD   M   N V   N'   ER

Artist's Concept of an Islet of Langerhans
(Electron Micrograph, 10,000×)

The hormone insulin is a product of beta cells. Alpha cells contain dense secretion droplets in a membrane-bound vacuole. The alpha cells may secrete glucagon, the glycogenolytic hormone.

CAP	Capillary	**V**	Vesicles
BM	Basement membrane	**N'**	Nucleus of beta cell
END	Endothelium	**ER**	Endoplasmic reticulum; intra-cellular membrane systems and asso-ciated ribosomes of acinar cells
SD	Secretion droplets		
M	Mitochondria		
N	Nucleus of alpha cell		

DIABETES MELLITUS

Eighth Edition
(First Revision)

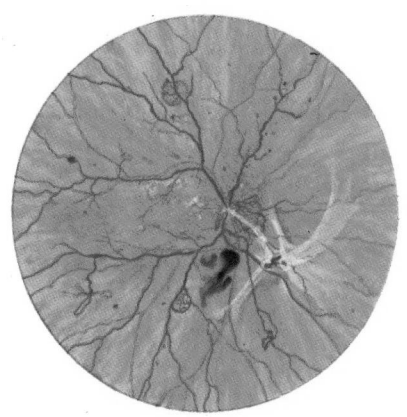

Published for the Medical Profession

by the Lilly Research Laboratories

Indianapolis, Indiana

Foreword

The rapidity of advances in diabetes has made a revision of the eighth edition of DIABETES MELLITUS (1979) necessary.

The seventh edition of DIABETES MELLITUS was published in 1966. Over the past years, it has undergone three revisions, and over 400,000 copies have been distributed. The wide acceptance of the book and the recent important advances in our knowledge of Insulin have necessitated a new edition. For instance, in 1966, the clinical significance of differences among the chemical structures of beef, pork, and human Insulins was beginning to be understood. Now, the existence of insulin precursors and their amino acid sequences is established, and the technology that promoted these discoveries has led to marked improvements in the purity of Insulin preparations. These are discussed in Chapters 4 and 7. The ability to determine the chemical structure of these Insulin-related proteins has led in part to the incredible achievement of synthesizing DNA for human Insulin "A" and "B" chains and their production in bacteria.

In the seventh edition, data resulting from the immunoassay of Insulin were still novel, and the significant differences between adult-onset and juvenile diabetes were just beginning to be appreciated. Now, diabetes is being viewed as a highly heterogeneous syndrome that encompasses a number of metabolic disorders.

Furthermore, in 1966, oral therapy in adult-onset diabetes was virtually unquestioned. However, as a consequence of the University Group Diabetes Program, some doubts have been raised about both the safety of the oral agents and the ability of large-scale clinical research to answer pressing clinical questions. As a result, there has been a renewed interest in effective *dietary* therapy and an acknowledgement of the critical role of the patient's responsibility in the management of diabetes.

Recent advances in our knowledge of hereditary factors and in blood glucose regulation have led to extensive revisions of appropriate chapters.

The goals of this volume, as before, are twofold. First, Eli Lilly and Company wishes to make available to the medical profession information, developed in its research laboratories and clinical units, which emphasizes those topics most often included in inquiries from physicians. Second, we hope to provide our readers with a concise manual for the management of diabetes mellitus. Thus, an attempt has been made to stress the points that seem to be of greatest practical use.

The published works of many investigators have been consulted freely, but, owing to the vast bibliography, references to some publications may have been omitted inadvertently.

This volume has been prepared by John A. Galloway, M.D., F.A.C.P., Senior Clinical Pharmacologist, Lilly Laboratory for Clinical Research, Eli Lilly and Company, with the assistance of Peg Kimberlin, R.D., M.S., Dietitian, Lilly Laboratory for Clinical Research, who prepared the diets in Chapter 6. Also, numerous individuals within and outside Eli Lilly and Company reviewed the manuscript and offered comments.

S. O. WAIFE, M.D., F.A.C.P.
Editor and Director
Medical Services Division

Contents

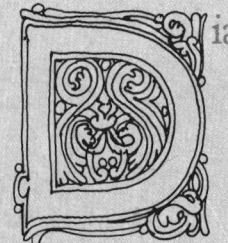

Diabetes is a wonderful affection, not very frequent among men, being a melting down of the flesh and limbs into urine. Its cause is of a cold and humid nature, as in dropsy. The course is the common one, namely, the kidneys and bladder; for the patients never stop making water, but the flow is incessant, as if from the opening of aqueducts. The nature of the disease, then, is chronic, and it takes a long period to form; but the patient is short-lived, if the constitution of the disease be completely established; for the melting is rapid, the death speedy. Moreover, life is disgusting and painful; thirst unquenchable; excessive drinking, which, however, is disproportionate to the large quantity of urine, for more urine is passed; and one cannot stop them either from drinking or making water. Or if for a time they abstain from drinking, their mouths become parched and their bodies dry; the viscera seem as if scorched up; they are affected with nausea, restlessness, and a burning thirst; and at no distant term they expire.

ARETAEUS THE CAPPADOCIAN, A.D. 81-138

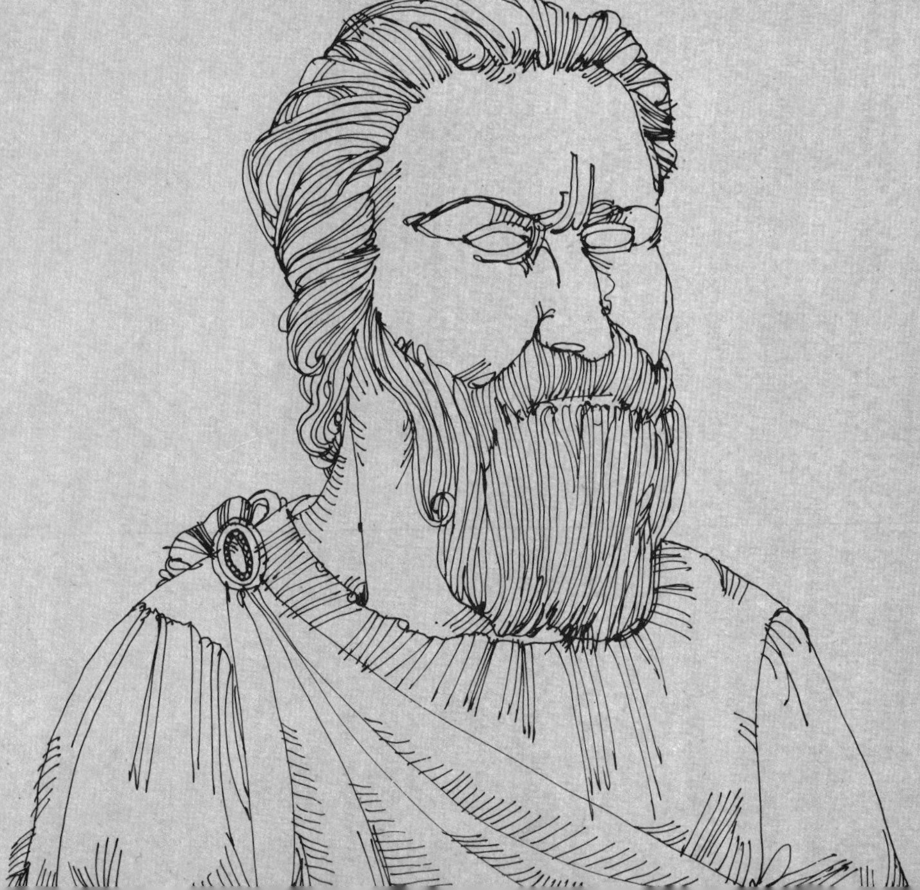

Definition and Diagnosis of Diabetes

1

DEFINITION

Diabetes mellitus is a chronic systemic disease characterized by disorders in (1) metabolism of insulin and of carbohydrate, fat, and protein and (2) the structure and function of blood vessels. The principal early symptoms and signs are usually related to the metabolic defects; findings late in the disease are linked with complications resulting from vascular defects.

Diabetes mellitus ordinarily appears as one of two recognized clinical pictures—the juvenile (or growth-onset, ketosis-prone) type (Type I) or the more common adult-onset, ketosis-resistant type (Type II). The incidence of these two kinds of diabetes is shown in Figure 1, and their characteristics are listed and compared in Table 1.

The essential abnormalities in growth-onset (ketosis-prone) diabetes are related to absolute insulin deficiency, whereas those of adult-onset diabetes are more often the result of a delayed release of endogenous insulin in relation to carbohydrate challenge. However, some patients with adult-onset, ketosis-resistant diabetes may have a subnormal capacity for insulin synthesis and release.

The vascular abnormalities associated with diabetes are often referred to as the "complications of diabetes." They consist in microangiopathic changes which give rise to characteristic lesions in the retina and the kidney. These are described in the chapter on "Chronic Complications of Diabetes." There is a third member in the diabetic triad—neuropathy. It is thought by some to be due to the metabolic defect[1] and by others to be the result of vascular disease.[2]

CARBOHYDRATE TOLERANCE TESTS

Although a number of tests may be utilized in the diagnosis of diabetes, the most commonly accepted one is an oral glucose tolerance test. This may consist merely in determining the blood sugar in a fasting state and two hours after a meal containing approximately 100 Gm. of carbohydrate. (In a nondiabetic, the blood sugar returns to normal level within two hours after glucose loading.) A more satisfactory method is the *standard glucose tolerance test*, in which 100 Gm. of carbohydrate (or 1.75 Gm. per Kg. of

Figure 1. The Incidence of Various Types of Diabetes

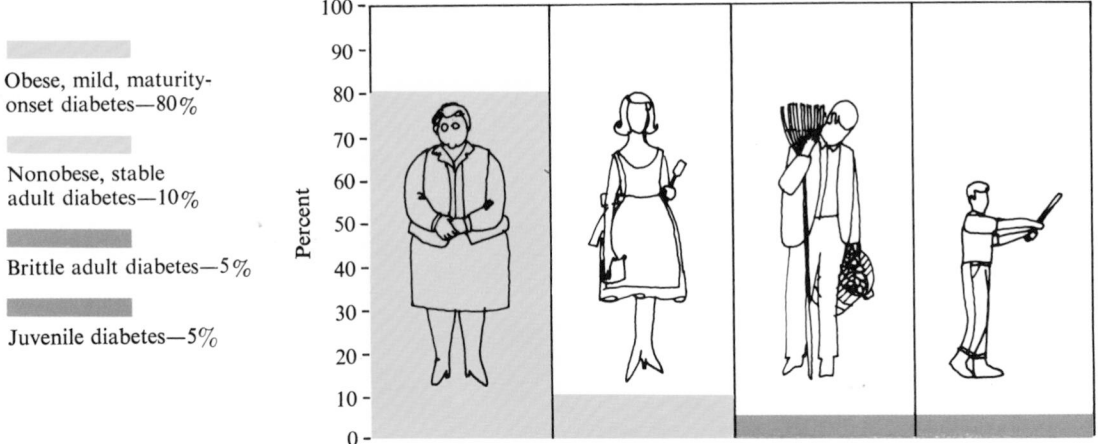

Obese, mild, maturity-onset diabetes—80%

Nonobese, stable adult diabetes—10%

Brittle adult diabetes—5%

Juvenile diabetes—5%

Table 1. A Comparison of the Essential Features of Type I and Type II Diabetes

	TYPE I	TYPE II
Other Names	Juvenile, growth-onset, ketosis-prone	Adult-onset, maturity-onset, ketosis-resistant
Age of Onset	Usually under 35	Usually over 35
Type of Onset	Abrupt (days to weeks)	Usually gradual (weeks to months)
Nutritional Status at Onset	Usually undernourished	Usually obese
Symptoms	Polydipsia, polyphagia, and polyuria	Frequently none
Ketosis	Frequent, unless diet, Insulin, and exercise are properly coordinated	Infrequent except in the presence of infection or stress
Endogenous Insulin	Negligible to absent	Present; may be in excess but relatively ineffective because of obesity
Associated Lipid Abnormalities	Hypercholesterolemia frequent, particularly when control is suboptimal. All lipid fractions elevated in ketoacidosis	Cholesterol and triglycerides frequently elevated and related to obesity. Carbohydrate-induced hypertriglyceridemia common
Insulin	Needed for all patients	Necessary in only 20 to 30 percent of patients
Oral Agents	Rarely efficacious, should not be used	Efficacious
Diet	Mandatory along with Insulin for blood glucose control	Diet alone frequently sufficient to control blood glucose

body weight) are given and the blood sugar is determined at 30, 60, 90, 120, and 180 minutes and, in selected cases, at four, five, and six hours.

Because it is less expensive and more convenient than the standard oral glucose tolerance test, the *two-hour postprandial blood sugar determination* is commonly used as a screening procedure. It places less stress on patients whose diabetes is moderate to markedly severe. However, when carbohydrate intolerance is mild (i.e., the fasting blood glucose levels are normal and/or the postprandial levels are under 200 mg. per 100 ml.), the standard oral glucose tolerance test is used. In approximately 75 percent of the patients observed[3] in one study, the two-hour value of the standard glucose tolerance test was found to be lower than that of the two-hour postprandial blood sugar test.

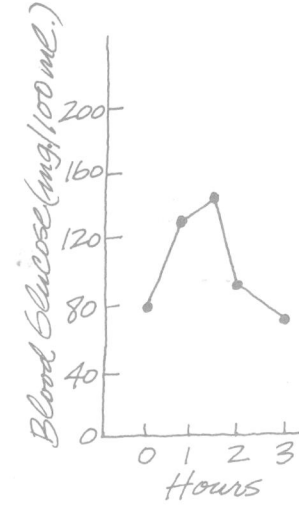

The criteria for diagnosing diabetes by means of the standard oral glucose tolerance test differ from clinic to clinic and author to author.[4-8] The critical blood sugar levels used by various authorities are compared in Table 2 and Figure 2.[9, 9A] Four factors must be considered in the interpretation of these results. First, when a diagnosis of true diabetes mellitus is made, a number of conditions and situations which also may result in diminished carbohydrate tolerance must be excluded (Table 3).

Diagnosis

Second, it must be recognized that the criteria in Table 2 may have diminishing value in older patients. The Tecumseh[10] and other studies have shown that the incidence of "abnormal" carbohydrate tolerance ranges from 53[11,12] to 100 percent[13] in older patients. The work of Streeten *et al.*[14] has demonstrated that carbohydrate intolerance occurs in 77 percent of elderly subjects. The latter workers assert that this abnormal tolerance of the elderly is related neither to delayed absorption of administered glucose nor to impairment in the secretion of insulin but rather to a higher level of a circulating insulin antagonist or some other form of peripheral defect in the glucose uptake from the blood.

Age

Andres,[15] who has serially tested men of all ages, constructed a nomogram for interpreting the effect of age on glucose tolerance, using the concentration of the blood glucose two hours after a glucose load of 1.75 Gm. per Kg. (Figure 3). Although it is not known what percentage of any age group is abnormal, the establishment of a percentile ranking of responses to the glucose tolerance test makes it easier to assess the possible importance of any given response.

A third point to be considered in interpreting the results of a given glucose tolerance test is the lack of their reproducibility in both normal and diabetic subjects. McDonald *et al.*,[16] using the modified criteria of Fajans and Conn,[17] found an incidence of 1 percent of abnormal tests on at least one of six tests given over a one-year period to 334 normal subjects. In diabetes, also, the degree of carbohydrate intolerance may fluctuate; a test may be normal one time, but marked intolerance may be noted at another.[16] This phenomenon is demonstrated in Table 4 (page 9), which presents the degree of variability of carbohydrate tolerance in the various

Reproducibility

Table 2. Criteria* for an Abnormal Oral Glucose Tolerance Test (Whole Blood, True Glucose in mg. per 100 ml.)† [9A]

	FAJANS-CONN	USPHS‡	SIPERSTEIN
Fasting	110 (125)†	110 (125) [1]	125 (140)
1 hour	160 (185)	170 (195) [½]	225 (260)
1½ hours	145 (165)	—	—
2 hours	120 (140)	120 (140) [½]	200 (230)
3 hours	—	110 (125) [1]	—

*For patients over age fifty, add 10 mg. per 100 ml. per decade to the post-oral-glucose values. All post-glucose values are to be equaled or exceeded for diagnosis.

†Add 15 percent to whole blood glucose levels if glucose is measured in plasma. Plasma glucose criteria are in parentheses.

‡Points credited are in brackets; two points mean diabetes.

Figure 2. Criteria Used for Interpretation of Glucose Tolerance Tests

Diabetes

Probable diabetes

No diabetes

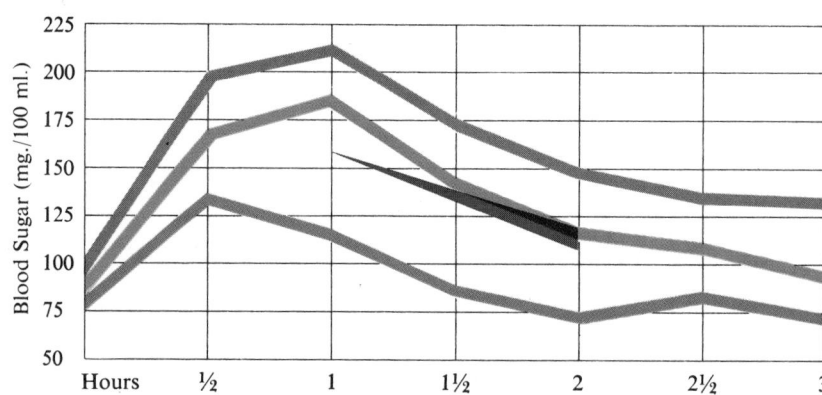

The wedge-shaped area marks the border line between "normal" and "abnormal" results.

Table 3. Clinical Conditions Which May Lead to an Abnormal Oral Glucose Tolerance Test

Diabetes mellitus
Improper feeding before the test
Malnutrition
Obesity
Infection and/or fever
Bed rest
Endocrine abnormalities
  Hypothyroidism and
    hyperthyroidism
  Pituitary disorders
  Acromegaly
  Adrenal cortical hyperfunction
  Pheochromocytoma
Renal disease
Intracranial tumors
Advanced age

Neoplastic disease
Medications such as thiazide diuretics,
  steroids, epinephrine, and morphine
Oral contraceptive therapy
Nonhereditary conditions associated
  with diabetes
  Hemochromatosis
  Pancreatitis
  Carcinoma of the pancreas
  Pancreatic trauma
Postgastrectomy syndrome
Islet-cell tumors
Lipid disorders, including
  lipoatrophic diabetes
Burns and surgery
Psychological factors*

*In view of the fact that these represent stress, a resulting abnormal glucose tolerance test probably indicates the presence of true diabetes.

stages of diabetes. The extreme situation is represented by occasional reports of the total remission of severe diabetes.[18-20] The occurrence of these variations indicates that a single glucose tolerance test may not necessarily rule out the presence or absence of diabetes. However, in most instances, three or four additional tests at intervals of two to three months will usually settle the question.

A fourth factor is related to the source of the blood sample and the method of analysis employed to determine its glucose content. For instance, when the Folin-Wu method (which measures all reducing substances) is used, about 20 mg. per 100 ml. should be subtracted in order to convert the value obtained to the "true glucose"* level. Furthermore, there are differences in the sugar content of capillary and venous blood. Therefore, when a specimen (capillary blood) is collected by a finger prick, 30 mg. per 100 ml. should be deducted to convert the value to a true glucose level.[8] Glucose values determined from plasma or serum will be about 15 percent higher than those determined from whole blood. With this information, standards for glucose tolerance based on whole-blood determinations can be converted to results from serum or plasma.

Capillary
versus
venous blood

*The only method that measures glucose per se is one which utilizes the enzyme glucose oxidase. However, extensive studies have shown a marked similarity between the levels obtained when this enzyme is used and those obtained with analysis of sugar filtrates by means of the Somogyi-Nelson and Autoanalyzer® methods.

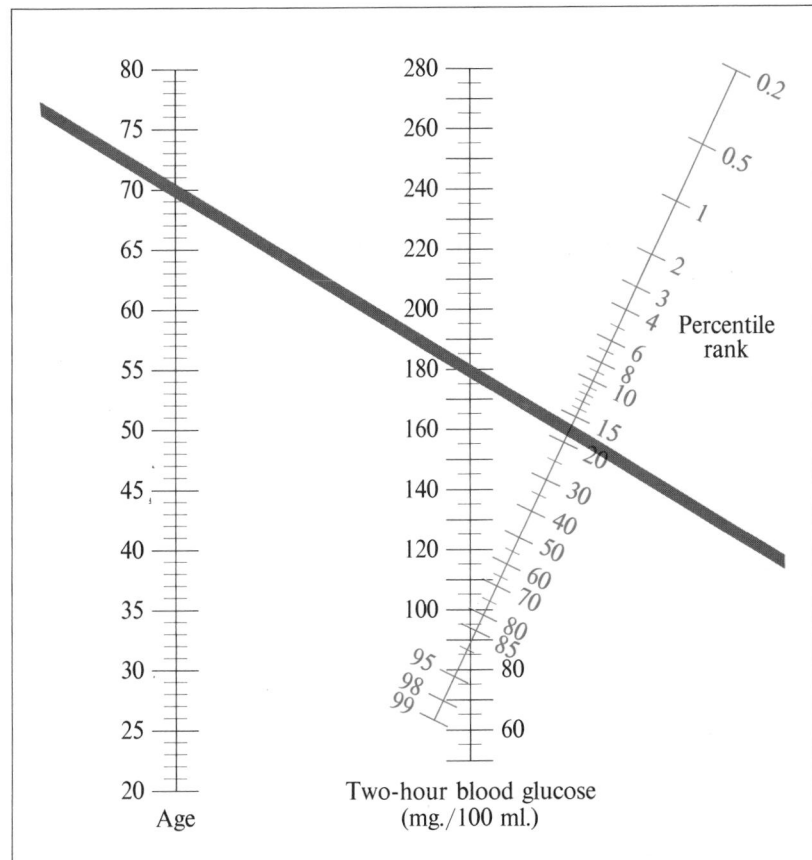

Figure 3. Nomogram for Oral Glucose Tolerance Responses (After Andres[15])

A line is drawn from the patient's age through the value obtained at two hours for the oral glucose tolerance test (see text) and is extended to the percentile rank line. The example shown indicates that a seventy-year-old person with a two-hour value of 180 mg. per 100 ml. has a percentile rank of 18 percent—that is, 82 percent of his age group outperform him.

In addition, since the glucose concentration is considerably higher in plasma than in red cells, the hematocrit of the samples being tested must be taken into consideration.[21, 22] It has been reported[21] that a 10 percent variation in the hematocrit will result in a blood sugar change of 3.6 mg. per 100 ml. in the opposite direction. Hence, mild abnormalities in glucose tolerance observed in anemia may be apparent and not real.

Other tests

Other tests used in the diagnosis of diabetes are the intravenous glucose tolerance test, the cortisone tolerance test, and the oral and intravenous tolbutamide tolerance tests. The *intravenous glucose tolerance test* is used in such situations as disorders of the small bowel, hyperthyroidism, and certain research when it is desirable to avoid variations in glucose absorption that may occur with the oral tests. The technic of the intravenous glucose tolerance test varies. The dose of glucose is usually 0.5 Gm. per Kg. This may be administered as a 20 percent solution over a twenty-minute period or as a 50 percent solution over a three-minute period. In both methods, multiple venous or capillary blood specimens are taken for average periods of one to two hours. The interpretation of results depends upon the method used but is based principally on the rate of fall of the glucose level from the peak obtained after infusion of the glucose. The details of this test have been reviewed by Soeldner.[23]

The *cortisone tolerance test* as used by Fajans[23A] and the *tolbutamide tolerance test*[24-26] have been proposed as procedures to resolve borderline glucose tolerance tests. However, in recent years, with the appreciation of the numerous factors affecting tests of carbohydrate tolerance as well as concern about employment, insurance, and other implications of "tagging" a patient with intermittent hyperglycemia as a diabetic, the vigor with which many clinicians pursue an "abnormal" glucose tolerance test has declined. Moreover, the criteria for the diagnosis of diabetes have been liberalized.[26A]

A middle-of-the-road approach to abnormal glucose tolerance tests has been proposed by Whitehouse.[9A] It consists in telling the patient he has an abnormal glucose tolerance test, explaining that the significance of the finding is not known, de-emphasizing use of the word "diabetes," correcting factors that are known to diminish carbohydrate tolerance (e.g., weight reduction if appropriate, increasing physical activity, and avoiding diabetogenic drugs), and having the patient undergo random blood glucose determinations every three to twelve months to detect any deterioration of carbohydrate tolerance.

STEROID DIABETES

"Steroid diabetes" is the name given to an impairment in carbohydrate metabolism resulting from the use of the various adrenal corticosteroids. Although this side-effect is most often observed when the agents are used systemically, in rare instances it may occur following the topical application of steroids in the treatment of dermatologic disorders.[27] Those glucocorticoids apparently associated with the greatest impairment of carbohydrate metabolism are characterized by the presence of an 11-oxy group.

The diminished carbohydrate tolerance is the result of several mechanisms. The principal one is the increase of glucose production by the liver as a result of gluconeogenesis. There is no evidence that the diabetogenic effect of steroids is due to destruction or more accelerated degradation of insulin. Another mechanism responsible for decreased glucose tolerance is the mobilization of fatty acids from tissue stores. There is no evidence, however, that the glucocorticoids have an effect on the intermediary metabolism of lipids. Other mechanisms that have been postulated include an antagonism to insulin action by the growth hormone and decreased utilization of glucose by the tissues.

Diminished carbohydrate tolerance

Steroid diabetes has been reported in 14 percent of patients treated with glucocorticoids for more than three days.[28] This form of diabetes may have several features, including (1) glycosuria with hyperglycemia of varying degree, (2) normal or diminished glucose tolerance, (3) absence of acidosis and acetonuria even when hyperglycemia is marked, and (4) elevated serum pyruvate levels.

In most instances, steroid diabetes is reversed when the drug is discontinued. According to Fajans and Conn[29] and others, however, hyperglycemia and glycosuria in a patient whose pretreatment carbohydrate tolerance was normal may be indicative of true early diabetes mellitus.

The diabetogenic effects of oral contraceptives have been the subject of intensive research; Spellacy[30] has reviewed much of the information. At this time, however, a definitive statement cannot be made.

THIAZIDE DIABETES

"Thiazide diabetes" is the name applied to a form of impaired carbohydrate metabolism resulting from the administration of the various thiazide diuretics. The incidence of this side-effect is variable, and the hyperglycemic response may be inconsistent. In some known diabetics, it apparently has occurred immediately upon initiation of thiazide therapy, whereas it has remained mild or is totally absent in others. Ordinarily, the increased hyperglycemia that develops in these diabetics can be counteracted by raising the dose of the hypoglycemic agent the patient is receiving, i.e., a sulfonylurea compound or Insulin.* Although this impairment in carbohydrate tolerance rarely causes serious consequences, diabetic acidosis was found in two pregnant women after diuretic treatment,[31] pancreatitis occurred in four patients after long-term treatment with the thiazides,[32] and a fatal case of thiazide-induced diabetes has been reported.[33]

*In this book, "Insulin" with a capital letter refers to the commercial product to distinguish it from "insulin," the natural hormone.

Despite considerable research, the mechanism by which this type of carbohydrate intolerance is produced has not been fully defined. The difficulty has been associated with relative hypokalemia, and some patients treated with thiazides show improved glucose tolerance following the administration of substantial doses of potassium.[34] Reduction in the serum insulin-like activity (ILA) was found to be precipitated or worsened by the use of thiazide diuretics in diabetics.[35] This value rose only partially after discontinuation of the drug.

On the other hand, the diabetogenic effect of these agents may be attributed to increased gluconeogenesis associated with heightened adrenal function, as indicated by a rise in 17-ketosteroid and hydroxycorticosteroid levels after the use of thiazide diuretics.[36]

No abnormality was demonstrable in the serum ILA response to glucose, the insulin tolerance test, urinary steroid excretion, serum potassium, serum nonesterified fatty acids, or serum amylase after administration of thiazide diuretics.[37] However, a reduction of glutathione in whole blood was reported in six of seven patients.

On the basis of available information, added impairment of carbohydrate tolerance among diabetic subjects or mild impairment among nondiabetics should be anticipated when thiazides are used. In most diabetics, the diminished carbohydrate tolerance is reversed when the dosage of the hypoglycemic agent—Insulin or sulfonylurea—is increased. The occurrence of this side-effect does not defeat the usefulness of the thiazides.

STAGES OF DIABETES

The natural history of diabetes, particularly in its early course when the abnormality in carbohydrate metabolism is mild or absent, is becoming an increasingly important field. Diabetes is like a drama, in which the individual's genetic makeup is the stage; his ability to resist the onset of the disease, the hero; and such life stresses as obesity, pregnancy, infection, surgery, aging, illness, or certain endocrinopathies, the villains.

The first act of the drama is called "*prediabetes*"[38] or, by some, "diabetes pre-mellitus." Strictly speaking, these terms denote the presence of some finding or findings that generally are associated with the eventual development of frank clinical diabetes. Notably absent, however, is evidence of diminished carbohydrate tolerance as indicated by the standard glucose or cortisone tolerance tests (Table 4).

Since the concept of prediabetes is relatively recent and the specificity of most of the features has not been firmly established, this diagnosis is usually made after patients develop frank clinical diabetes.

Findings indicative of prediabetes in a given patient include diabetes in an identical twin or, less likely, diabetes in both parents or close relatives; obesity; diabetes-like vascular manifestations; and, in the female, a history of miscarriages or large babies, toxemia of pregnancy, and other more controversial obstetric associations.[39] The most significant physical change appears to be an increase in the venular-arteriolar ratio in the conjunctiva.[40] Electron microscopy of needle biopsy specimens taken from the earlobe shows venular dilatation with leakage. In addition, thickening of the glomerular basement membrane has been found in a large percentage of patients with a genetic predisposition toward diabetes. Also, biochemical studies indicate that prediabetic patients have increased ILA in their blood.[41]

Development of diabetes

The next step in the progression of the disease is *subclinical diabetes*. At this point, glucose tolerance ordinarily is normal, but carbohydrate intolerance can be demonstrated by means of the cortisone tolerance test. Also, the standard glucose tolerance test may show abnormal results during pregnancy or stress. Subclinical diabetes is the first stage in which islet-cell decompensation can be said to occur.

When the standard glucose tolerance test becomes abnormal yet the fasting blood glucose levels remain normal, *latent diabetes* is considered to be present. (The Joslin Clinic group does not differentiate between sub-clinical and latent diabetes. These workers combine subclinical and latent diabetes in a category they call "chemical diabetes.") Finally, when the fasting blood glucose levels are consistently abnormal, the term "*overt diabetes*" is used. All four stages are summarized in Table 4.[38]

Treatment of the early stages of diabetes consists in maintaining normal body weight by means of a reasonable diet, daily exercise, and avoidance of infection and factors known to cause metabolic stress. No specific treatment is recommended for prediabetes and subclinical dia-betes;[42] however, sulfonylurea therapy is used in the management of non-obese young patients with subclinical diabetes.[43] Present results indicate

Table 4. Metabolic and Vascular Changes in Various Stages of Diabetes

DIABETIC STAGE	CARBOHYDRATE TOLERANCE			INSULIN-LIKE ACTIVITY	VASCULAR CHANGES
	FASTING BLOOD SUGAR	GLUCOSE TOLERANCE	CORTISONE TOLERANCE		
Prediabetes	Normal	Normal	Normal	May be increased	+
Subclinical	Normal	Normal (abnormal during pregnancy)	Abnormal	Increased	+
Latent	Normal or increased	Abnormal	Test not necessary	Increased	+ +
Overt	Increased	Test not necessary	Test not necessary	Increased	+ + +

improvement in carbohydrate tolerance in the majority of these patients. Overt diabetics, of course, should have their diets adjusted, whether they are receiving hypoglycemic therapy or not.

PREVALENCE OF DIABETES

Of great importance to the physician is the growing prevalence of clinical diabetes. In the years between 1950 and 1965, the number of known diabetics almost doubled.[44] The U. S. Public Health Service[45] estimates that there are 4.4 million diabetics, 1.6 million of whom are not aware that they have the disease. Approximately 5.6 million are potential diabetics.[46] Similar findings were given in the 1973 Report of the National Diabetes Commission to the Congress regarding the prevalence of diabetes by age, sex, and race in the United States (Table 5).

Information received from several sources by Eli Lilly and Company suggests that, of the 4 to 5 million diabetics in the United States at the present time, approximately a fourth are being treated with Insulin, a third with oral agents, and the remainder with diet alone. The National Diabetes Commission Report indicates an incidence of new cases of about 600,000 per year. If one assumes that 50,000 to 100,000 persons with diabetes die each year, there is a net gain of 450,000 to 500,000 diabetics every year. Data received by the Insulin Study Group of the National Diabetes Advisory Board suggest that by the year 2000, there will be about 15 million diabetics in the United States, a third to a fourth of whom will be receiving Insulin therapy.

Table 5. Reported Prevalence* of Diabetes in the United States by Sex and Race

SEX	NUMBER	RATE/1,000
Total	4,191,000	20.4
Male	1,620,000	16.3
Female	2,571,000	24.1
RACE		
Caucasian	3,570,000	19.9
Other	622,000	23.9

*Approximately 86,000 cases are under seventeen years of age.
Source: 1973 Report of the National Diabetes Commission to Congress.

BIBLIOGRAPHY

1. Pirart, J.: Diabetic Neuropathy: A Metabolic or a Vascular Disease?, Diabetes, *14:*1, 1965.

2. Fagerberg, S.-E.: Diabetic Neuropathy. A Clinical and Histological Study on the Significance of Vascular Affections, Acta med. scandinav., *164* (Supplement No. 345):1, 1959.

3. Rush, T., and Tupper, C. J.: Two-Hour Postprandial Glucose Determinations in a Periodic Health Appraisal Program, Geriatrics, *15:*630, 1960.

4. Joslin, E. P., Root, H. F., White, P., and Marble, A.: The Treatment of Diabetes Mellitus, Ed. 10, p. 243. Philadelphia: Lea & Febiger, 1959.

5. Fajans, S. S.: Diagnostic Tests for Diabetes Mellitus, in Diabetes (edited by R. H. Williams), p. 397. New York: Paul B. Hoeber, Inc., 1960.

6. Forsham, P. H., Renold, A. E., and Thorn, G. W.: Diabetes Mellitus, in Principles of Internal Medicine, Ed. 4 (edited by T. R. Harrison), p. 635. New York: McGraw-Hill Book Company, Inc., 1962.

7. Duncan, G. G.: Diseases of Metabolism, Ed. 5, p. 921. Philadelphia: W. B. Saunders Company, 1964.

8. Fabrykant, M.: Laboratory Aids in Diagnosis, in Clinical Diabetes Mellitus (edited by M. Ellenberg and H. Rifkin), p. 137. New York: The Blakiston Division, McGraw-Hill Book Company, Inc., 1962.

9. Conn, J. W.: The Prediabetic State in Man. Definition, Interpretation and Implications, Diabetes, 7:347, 1958.

9A. Whitehouse, F. W.: The Diagnosis of Diabetes, Med. Clin. North Am., 62:627, 1978.

10. Hayner, N. S., Kjelsberg, M. O., Epstein, F. H., and Francis, T., Jr.: Carbohydrate Tolerance and Diabetes in a Total Community, Tecumseh, Michigan. I. Effects of Age, Sex, and Test Conditions on One-Hour Glucose Tolerance in Adults, Diabetes, 14:413, 1965.

11. Chesrow, E. J., and Bleyer, J. M.: The Glucose Tolerance Test of the Aged, Geriatrics, 9:276, 1954.

12. Marshall, F. W.: The Sugar-Content of the Blood in Elderly People, Quart. J. Med., 24:257, 1930-1931.

13. Gottfried, S. P., Pelz, K. S., and Clifford, R. C.: Carbohydrate Metabolism in Men and Healthy Old Women over 70 Years of Age, Am. J. M. Sc., 242:475, 1961.

14. Streeten, D. H. P., Gerstein, M. M., Marmor, B. M., and Doisy, R. J.: Reduced Glucose Tolerance in Elderly Human Subjects, Diabetes, 14:579, 1965.

15. Andres, R.: Relation of Physiologic Changes in Aging to Medical Changes of Disease in the Aged, Mayo Clin. Proc., 42:674, 1967.

16. McDonald, G. W., Fisher, G. F., and Burnham, C.: Reproducibility of the Oral Glucose Tolerance Test, Diabetes, 14:473, 1965.

17. Fajans, S. S., and Conn, J. W.: The Early Recognition of Diabetes Mellitus, Ann. New York Acad. Sc., 82:208, 1959.

18. Harwood, R.: Severe Diabetes with Remission. Report of a Case and Review of the Literature, New England J. Med., 257:257, 1957.

19. Peck, F. B., Jr., Kirtley, W. R., and Peck, F. B., Sr.: Complete Remission of Severe Diabetes, Diabetes, 7:93, 1958.

20. Stutman, L. J., and Hayes, J. D.: Severe Diabetes with Remission. Report of a Case, Diabetes, 8:189, 1959.

21. Zalme, E., and Knowles, H. C., Jr.: A Plea for Plasma Sugar, Diabetes, 14:165, 1965.

22. Dillon, R. S.: Importance of the Hematocrit in Interpretation of Blood Sugar, Diabetes, 14:672, 1965.

23. Soeldner, J. S.: The Intravenous Glucose Tolerance Test, in Diabetes Mellitus: Diagnosis and Treatment (edited by S. S. Fajans and K. E. Sussman), III:107. New York: American Diabetes Association, Inc., 1971.

23A. Fajans, S. S.: Cortisone Glucose Tolerance Test, J.A.M.A., 186:279, 1963.

24. Unger, R. H., and Madison, L. L.: A New Diagnostic Procedure for Mild Diabetes Mellitus. Evaluation of an Intravenous Tolbutamide Response Test, Diabetes, 7:455, 1958.

25. Vecchio, T. J., Smith, D. L., Oster, H. L., and Brill, R.: Oral Sodium Tolbutamide in the Diagnosis of Diabetes Mellitus, Diabetes, 13:30, 1964.

26. Vecchio, T. J., Oster, H. L., and Smith, D. L.: Oral Sodium Tolbutamide and Glucose Tolerance Tests, Arch. Int. Med., 115:161, 1965.

26A. Siperstein, M. D.: The Glucose Tolerance Test: A Pitfall in the Diagnosis of Diabetes Mellitus, Adv. Intern. Med., 20:297, 1975.

27. Kershbaum, A.: Diabetogenic Effect of Fluorine-Containing Steroids, Brit. M. J., 2:253, 1963.

28. Schubert, G. E., and Schulte, H. D.: Steroid Diabetes, German M. Month., 8:309, 1963.

29. Fajans, S. S., and Conn, J. W.: An Approach to the Prediction of Diabetes Mellitus by Modification of the Glucose Tolerance Test with Cortisone, Diabetes, 3:296, 1954.

30. Spellacy, W. N.: A Review of Carbohydrate Metabolism and the Oral Contraceptives, Am. J. Obst. & Gynec., 104:448, 1969.

31. Sugar, S. J. N.: Diabetic Acidosis during Chlorothiazide Therapy, J.A.M.A., 175:618, 1961.

32. Johnston, D. H., and Cornish, A. L.: Acute Pancreatitis in Patients Receiving Chlorothiazide, J.A.M.A., 170:2054, 1959.

33. Editorial: Diuretics and Diabetes, Brit. M. J., 2:1422, 1963.

34. Rapoport, M. I., and Hurd, H. F.: Thiazide-Induced Glucose Intolerance Treated with Potassium, Arch. Int. Med., 113:405, 1964.

35. Samaan, N., Dollery, C. T., and Fraser, R.: Diabetogenic Action of Benzothiadiazines. Serum-Insulin-Like Activity in Diabetes Worsened or Precipitated by Thiazide Diuretics, Lancet, 2:1244, 1963.

36. Green, S.: The Metabolic Effects of Chlorthalidone in the Diabetic, paper presented at the Fifth Congress of the International Diabetes Federation, Toronto, Canada, July 20-24, 1964 (abstr. in Excerpta Med., International Congress Series No. 74:81, 1964).

37. Chazan, J. A., and Boshell, B. R.: Etiological Factors in Thiazide-Induced or Aggravated Diabetes Mellitus, Diabetes, 14:132, 1965.

38. Conn, J. W., and Fajans, S. S.: The Prediabetic State. A Concept of Dynamic Resistance to a Genetic Diabetogenic Influence, Am. J. Med., 31:839, 1961.

39. Camerini-Dávalos, R. A.: Prevention of Diabetes Mellitus, M. Clin. North America, 49:865, 1965.

40. Lozano-Castaneda, O., Camerini-Dávalos, R. A., Caulfield, J. B., Rees, S. B., Cervantes-Amezcus, A., Catellier, R. C., Krauthammer, J. P., and Marble, A.: Early Diabetes. Chemical Diabetes—A Progress Report, paper presented at the Twenty-Third Annual Meeting of the American Diabetes Association, Atlantic City, New Jersey, June 15-16, 1963.

41. Steinke, J., Soeldner, J. S., Camerini-Dávalos, R. A., and Renold, A. E.: Studies on Serum Insulin-Like Activity (ILA) in Prediabetes and Early Overt Diabetes, Diabetes, 12:502, 1963.

42. Stowers, J. M., Bewsher, P. D., and Brackenridge, R. G.: Trial of Chlorpropamide in Subclinical Diabetes, Diabetes, 11 (Supplement):127, 1962.

43. Fajans, S. S., and Conn, J. W.: The Use of Tolbutamide in the Treatment of Young People with Mild Diabetes Mellitus. A Progress Report, Diabetes, 11 (Supplement):123, 1962.

44. Fact Sheet on Diabetes, p. 2. New York: American Diabetes Association, Inc., 1970.

45. Diabetes Source Book, Public Health Service Publication No. 1168, p. 7. Washington, D. C.: U. S. Dept. of Health, Education, and Welfare, 1968.

46. Facts about Diabetes, p. 1. New York: American Diabetes Association, Inc., 1966.

Heredity and Other Factors in the Development of Diabetes

2

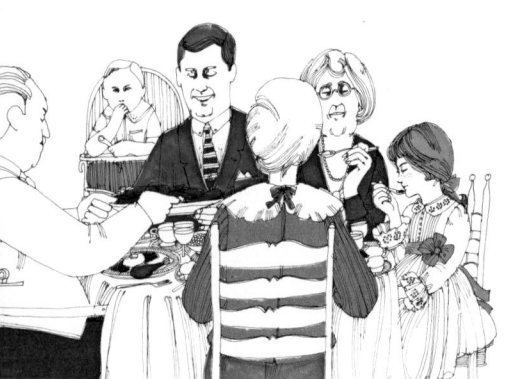

Heredity has long been recognized as an important factor in the development of diabetes, as suggested by the clustering of diabetics in families. However, several limitations have drastically impeded progress in understanding the mode(s) of transmission of diabetes. For instance, rather than being a single disease, diabetes is a heterogeneous group of diseases having in common only the cardinal sign of hyperglycemia. Thus, Goldstein and Podolsky[1] were able to cite thirty-six familial and nonfamilial disorders associated with glucose intolerance and/or Insulin resistance. Among the familial disorders are cystic fibrosis, Friedreich's ataxia, gout, hemochromatosis, Huntington's chorea, Laurence-Moon-Biedl syndrome, muscular dystrophy, and pheochromocytoma. Nonfamilial, or chromosomal, disorders include Down's, Klinefelter's, and Turner's syndromes. Moreover (see Table 1, Chapter 1), both Type I (juvenile, or growth-onset)[2] and Type II (adult-onset, or maturity-onset) diabetes[3] are being viewed as consisting of several separate disease types.[2,3] This being the case, it is unlikely that a single specific genetic "marker," an objective finding uniformly present in patients with diabetes and absent in those without the disorder, ever will be identifiable. Genetic studies of diabetes are also hampered by the fact that environmental influences may be crucial in the development or avoidance of the disease. To offset the problems of understanding the inheritance of diabetes, new tools have been developed that provide vital information. Some examples of these are typing of human leukocyte antigens (HLA), use of animal models, and islet-cell antibody studies. This chapter will briefly summarize some of the new knowledge regarding the genetics of human diabetes.

FAMILY STUDIES OF DIABETES

One of the most useful means of studying the inheritance of disease is the examination of transmission patterns in twins. In their review, Ganda and Soeldner[4] report that the concordance rate (the occurrence of diabetes in both individuals) of monozygotic (identical) twins who developed the disorder was nearly 100 percent when the onset in the index twin was at age forty or older; curiously, however, the rate was less than 50 percent when the index twin developed diabetes before age forty. Juvenile diabetes (Type I) is not inevitable in the twin of a growth-onset diabetic, as noted in a study of a set of monozygotic male triplets.[5] In the initial case (proband), diabetes developed at age thirteen and in the second brother at age twenty-five, but the third triplet was still nondiabetic at age twenty-five. The brothers lived together until they were twenty-one, and there was no previous family history of diabetes.

Patterns of incidence

Studies of the frequency of diabetes in the offspring of two diabetics (conjugal diabetics) indicate a surprisingly low prevalence of the disorder —6 to 10 percent.[6] (In the groups studied, both the parents and the offspring had mild diabetes.) Because marriage between two juvenile diabetics is quite unusual, data on the prevalence of the disorder in the offspring of this group are scanty. However, the frequency of overt diabetes in the offspring of one juvenile diabetic is similar to that when both parents have mild adult-onset diabetes.

When a parent has juvenile diabetes, the likelihood that an offspring will also have this type of diabetes increases. In addition, 25 to 40 percent of offspring of conjugal juvenile diabetics have chemical diabetes. (With successive glucose tolerance testing, the frequency of diabetes increases to 55 to 60 percent.) Ganda and Soeldner observed that, in the sibs of juvenile diabetics, the disease became manifest at a younger age and was more severe than in the sibs of adult-onset diabetics. The frequency of

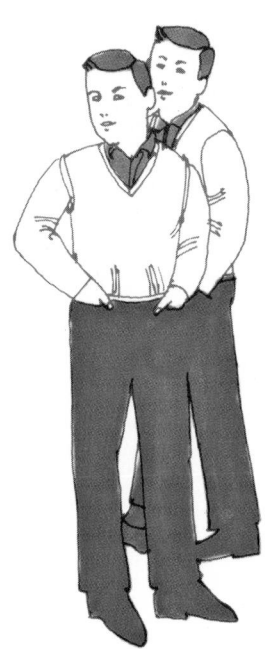

diabetes in the parent or grandparent of a juvenile diabetic is the same as that for an adult-onset diabetic.

In reviewing factors that could explain discordance between monozygotic twins, Pyke and Nelson[6] found a family history of diabetes in 45 percent of concordant twins but in only 17 percent of discordant twins. Analysis of the prevalence of retinopathy and neuropathy disclosed that, in nineteen of twenty-five pairs among whom both had vascular complications of diabetes, the patients had lived apart during their diabetic lives, which suggests strong genetic rather than environmental influences on the course of their disease.

MATURITY-ONSET DIABETES OF THE YOUNG

There is a newly recognized entity, a maturity-onset-type diabetes of youth, "MODY," which is more akin to the classical maturity-onset diabetes of middle age than to the juvenile type. Symptoms are mild, stimulated insulin output is retained although delayed and diminished, and ketonuria and hyperglycemia can be controlled without Insulin.[7]

Most patients with maturity-onset diabetes of youth have little or no progression over the course of two or even four decades of follow-up. A strong family history of diabetes always exists, and the clinical features comprise a nearly identical benign phenotype in all members of the family such that virtually all of the patients can be managed successfully with oral hypoglycemic agents. In addition, both microvascular and macrovascular complications seem to be rare.

TISSUE ANTIGENS

With advancing knowledge of genetics, attempts are being made to study specific genetic "markers" in the maze of human heredity. A useful approach is the study of human leukocyte antigens (HLA). These are classified as the histocompatibility loci (genes) and are present on the surfaces of most human cell membranes. Their composition is determined by four pairs of genetic material (DNA) on the short arm of the sixth chromosome. Their clinical importance is becoming widely recognized. For example, acute anterior uveitis, Reiter's syndrome, and ankylosing spondylitis occur with increased frequency among patients carrying an antigen identified as HLA-A27. Diseases associated with other related HLA antigens include psoriasis and gluten-sensitive enteropathy.

Just why HLA antigens appear to be associated with certain disease states is not known. Conceivably, the antigens may be related to an infecting organism, or they may have a relationship to specific immunoresponsive genes. At any rate, more work needs to be done.

Thus far, there is evidence that adult-onset diabetes (Type II) is *not* correlated with any human leukocyte antigen. However, Insulin-dependent diabetes (Type I) is. For example, Cudworth and Woodrow[8] studied 288 Type I diabetics whose disorder had appeared before age thirty and in whom increased frequencies for the subgroups HLA-B8 and BW15 were confirmed. Patients who have both these antigens also develop diabetes at an earlier age and have reduced secretion of endogenous insulin.[9] Concordant twins were found to have HLA-B8 more frequently than did discordant twins.[10] That racial or ethnic factors are involved (again suggestive of genetic influences) is evidenced by the fact that the HLA association differs among Japanese diabetics, in whom the most positive association is with subgroup BW22.

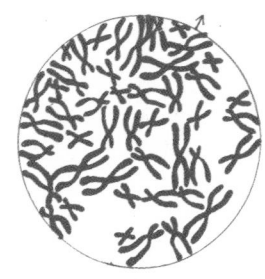

AUTOIMMUNITY

Does a diabetic "self-destruct" his islet cells and thus produce his condition?

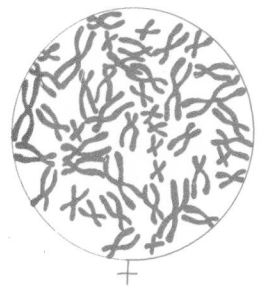

Antibodies against pancreatic islet cells (ICA) have been found in about half of young, recently diagnosed Type I diabetics.[11,12] In one study,[12] for example, antibodies (measured by immunofluorescence methods) were detected in 38 percent of Insulin-dependent but in only 5.3 percent of non-Insulin-dependent patients. Antibodies were detected in 8 percent of diabetics controlled by oral hypoglycemic agents but not in those managed by diet alone. The incidence in over 400 control subjects was 0.5 percent. It is significant that the prevalence declined with increasing duration of the disease.

There are other autoantibodies, that is, antibodies to such organs as the thyroid and the stomach. ICA's appear to have a different prevalence pattern than do other tissue autoantibodies and seem to be a different phenomenon. No correlation was found between ICA's and the presence of human leukocyte antigens in asymptomatic individuals and in those with early forms of diabetes.[13]

VIRUS DISEASE AND DIABETES

The fact that the occurrence of diabetes in one identical twin does not uniformly predict the disorder in the other indicates that nongenetic, or environmental, factors are important in the development of diabetes. Viruses are currently the most actively investigated of these. The possibility of a virus etiology has evolved from epidemiologic studies of patients in whom the onset of diabetes has followed an infection, often after a considerable time interval. Consequently, mumps, Coxsackie virus B, and rubella have been implicated in man. Although an association between virus illness and diabetes in man is suggested by the data, a cause-and-effect relationship has not been established.

With animal models, however, it has been possible to demonstrate clearly the cytotoxic effects of certain viruses on pancreatic beta cells. For instance, Notkins[14] has shown that, during an acute infection with an encephalomyocarditis virus, the beta (but not the alpha and delta) cells of the islands of Langerhans are selectively attacked. Glucose intolerance follows and continues for varying periods of time. Genetic studies of inbred strains of mice have disclosed that the diabetogenic response to the virus is transmitted by a single gene as an autosomal-recessive trait. Moreover, studies with isolated beta-cell cultures suggest that the effect of the diabetogenic gene may be mediated via a surface receptor on the beta cell. These phenomena are independent of the histocompatibility locus of the mouse.

A view of diabetes

The foregoing information suggests that clinical diabetes mellitus is probably a heterogeneous group of diseases resulting from a number of etiologic factors. A tentative hypothesis for relating hereditary factors, human leukocyte antigens, autoimmunity, virus disease, and islet-cell antigens would postulate that, when a genetically susceptible individual with leukocytes of a certain pattern (HLA type) is rendered sufficiently prone to infection with certain agents (viruses?), Insulin-dependent diabetes develops. These events may be causally associated with the production of autoantibodies by the beta cells. Alternatively, an interaction between a virus and a membrane receptor may result in formation of a new antigen to which an antibody (ICA) forms and destroys beta cells.[8] For a genetically susceptible individual not to develop diabetes, one or more of the above events in the pathogenic sequence must be absent.

GENETIC COUNSELING

The clinician is so frequently asked about the "inheritance" of diabetes that he must be prepared to comment. It would seem prudent, in view of the preceding brief survey, to indicate that the mode of inheritance in most families is essentially impossible to determine. Clear and definite counseling is simply not possible at this time, because there are so many factors involved and because our present state of ignorance, in the absence of specific genetic markers, prevents our being predictive.

We can, however, make use of empiric figures that give some idea of the risk potential. Assuming a careful and reliable family history, we can use data such as those derived by Darlow, Smith, and Duncan,[15] which are based on more than 25,000 relatives of 1,367 living diabetics (Table 6). On the basis of age of onset of the disease among family members, the offspring of a diabetic may be advised of the relative increased risk of affliction.

The authors of one review[1] conclude that ". . . it remains difficult to provide sound genetic counselling and perhaps immoral to impose eugenic judgments. Prospective parents should be informed of the risks and, as responsible adults, asked to decide on their own progeny."

Table 6. Probable Ranges of Empiric Risks in Relatives[15]

	RISK (%) OF BEING AFFECTED BY		
	AGE 25	AGE 45	AGE 65
Population at large	0.2-0.3	0.5-0.9	1.8-3.8
1st-degree relative affected			
Age at onset			
0-24	5-8	5-13	5-17
24-44	1-2	2-3	6-10
45-64	0.2-0.5	0.5-1.5	8-10
65-84	0.2-0.5	1.5-2.0	6-8
2d or 3d-degree relative affected	Divide above risks by 2		
Two 1st-degree relatives affected			
Age at onset			
0-44, 0-44	Multiply above risks by 2-4		
0-44, 45-84	Multiply above risks by 1.5-3		
45-84, 45-84	Multiply above risks by 1.5-2		
1st, 2d, or 3d-degree relative affected	Multiply above risks by 1.5-2		

BIBLIOGRAPHY

1. Goldstein, S., and Podolsky, S.: The Genetics of Diabetes Mellitus, Med. Clin. North Am., 62:639, 1978.

2. Rotter, J. I., and Rimoin, D. L.: Heterogeneity in Diabetes Mellitus—Update, 1978, Evidence for Further Genetic Heterogeneity within Juvenile-Onset Insulin-Dependent Diabetes Mellitus, Diabetes, 27:599, 1978.

3. Fajans, S. S.: Etiological and Clinical Heterogeneity of Idiopathic Diabetes Mellitus, Banting Memorial Lecture, 38th Annual Meeting, American Diabetes Association, Boston, Massachusetts, June, 1978.

4. Ganda, O. P., and Soeldner, J. S.: Genetic, Acquired, and Related Factors in the Etiology of Diabetes Mellitus, Arch. Intern. Med., 137:461, 1977.

5. Ganda, O. P., Soeldner, J. S., Gleason, R. E., et al.: Monozygotic Triplets with Discordance for Diabetic Microangiopathy, Diabetes, 26:469, 1977.

6. Pyke, D. A., and Nelson, P. G.: Diabetes Mellitus in Identical Twins, in The Genetics of Diabetes Mellitus (edited by W. Creutzfeldt, J. Kobberling, and J. V. Neel), p. 194. New York: Springer-Verlag, 1976.

7. Barbosa, J., Ramsay, R., and Goetz, C.: Plasma Glucose, Insulin, Glucagon, and Growth Hormone in Kindreds with Maturity-Onset Type of Hyperglycemia in Young People, Ann. Intern. Med., 88:595, 1978.

8. Cudworth, A. G., and Woodrow, J. C.: Genetic Susceptibility in Diabetes Mellitus: Analysis of the HLA Association, Br. Med. J., 2:846, 1976.

9. Ludvigsson, J., Safwenberg, J., and Heding, L. G.: HLA-Types, C-Peptide and Insulin Antibodies in Juvenile Diabetes, Diabetologia, 13:13, 1977.

10. Nelson, P. G., Pyke, D. A., Cudworth, A. G., Woodrow, J. C., and Batchelor, J. R.: Histocompatibility Antigens in Diabetic Identical Twins, Lancet, 2:193, 1975.

11. Irvine, W. J., McCallum, C. J., Gray, R. S., Campbell, C. J., Duncan, L. J. P., Farquhar, J. W., Vaughan, H., and Morris, P. J.: Pancreatic Islet Cell Antibodies in Diabetes Mellitus Correlated with Duration and Type of Diabetes, Coexistent Autoimmune Disease and HLA Type, Diabetes, 26:138, 1977.

12. Lendrum, R., Walker, G., Cudworth, A. G., Theophanides, C., Pyke, D. A., Bloom, A., and Gamble, D. R.: Islet Cell Antibodies in Diabetes Mellitus, Lancet, 2:1273, 1976.

13. Irvine, W. J., Gray, R. S., and McCallum, C. J.: Pancreatic Islet Cell Antibody as a Marker for Asymptomatic and Latent Diabetes and Prediabetes, Lancet, 2:1097, 1976.

14. Notkins, A. L.: Virus-Induced Diabetes Mellitus, Arch. Virol., 54:1, 1977.

15. Darlow, J. M., Smith, C., and Duncan, L. J. P.: A Statistical and Genetical Study of Diabetes. III. Empiric Risks to Relatives, Ann. Hum. Genet., 38:157, 1973.

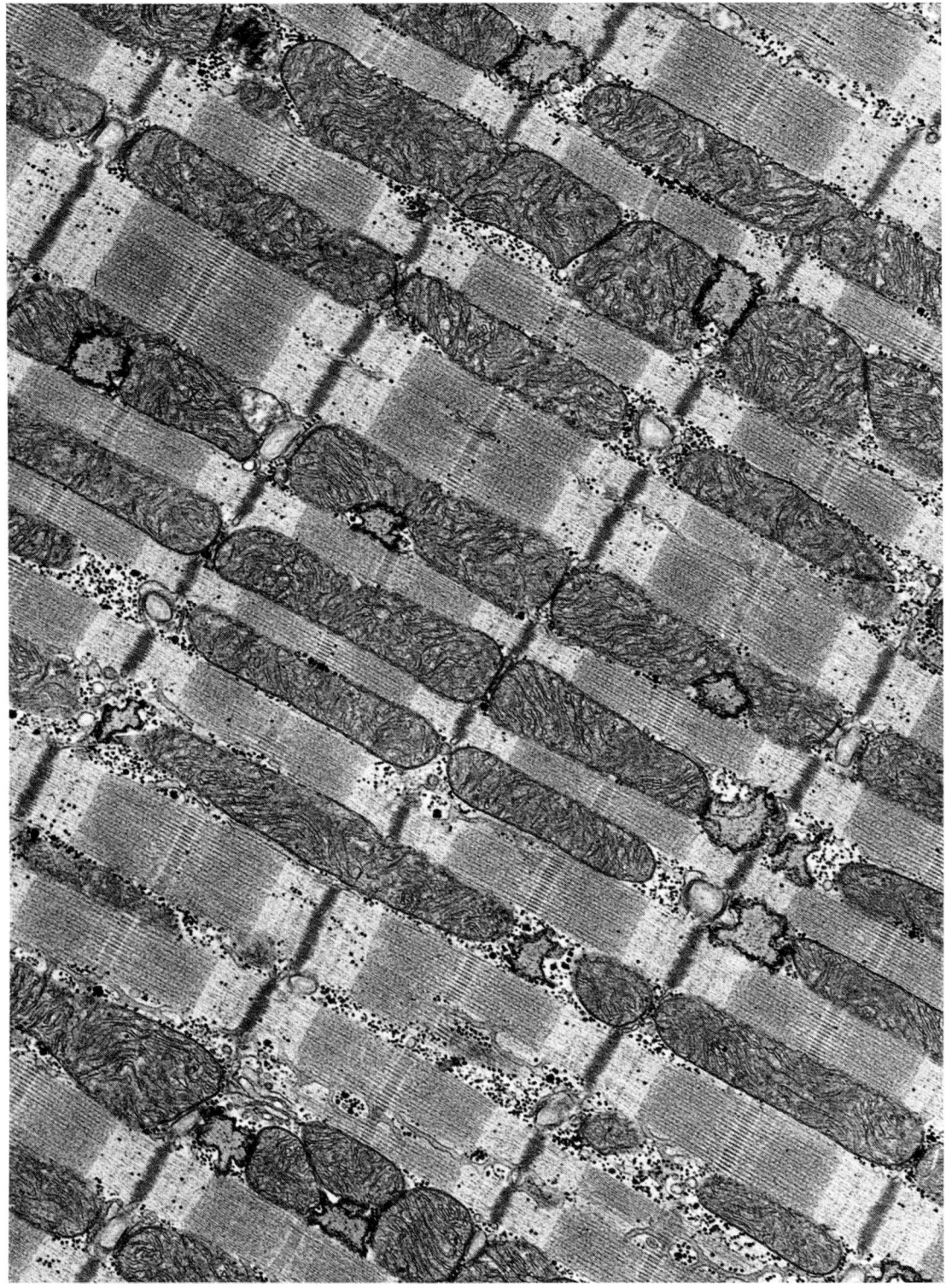

Figure 4. Mitochondria often appear to be random in their intracellular distribution, but in some types of cells they are located in close proximity to other organelles that require ATP to carry out their normal function. This electron micrograph shows numerous mitochondria aligned in rows in the narrow clefts between the myofibrils of cardiac muscle. The contraction of muscle depends upon ATP generated by mitochondria. The intimate association of mitochondria with the myofilaments minimizes diffusion distance and facilitates conversion of chemical energy to mechanical work. Magnification, 14,000×.

(Figures 4, 6, and 7 from The Cell, *by D. W. Fawcett, M.D., W. B. Saunders Company, Philadelphia, 1966, courtesy of the author and publisher)*

Metabolism in the Normal and the Diabetic Subject[*]

3

Man's vulnerability to derangement of glucose metabolism is appreciated when it is considered how essential glucose is to body function and how small an amount there is in the body in relation to the total quantities of protein and fat. Thus, although only 350 to 400 Gm. of glucose are present as such, or as glycogen, it is a major fuel or source of energy for all cells and the *only* fuel for brain and nerve tissue. Glucose (carbohydrate) is readily converted to fat, may supply the carbon atoms for certain amino acids, is the most likely precursor of the pentose of nucleic acids (deoxyribonucleic acid and ribonucleic acid, or DNA and RNA), and is a major source of glycerol (alpha-glycerophosphate) required for esterification of fatty acids in adipose tissue.

Glucose (Haworth formula)

ENERGY AND FUEL SYSTEMS IN BODY FUNCTION

It is necessary to understand the mechanism by which ingested foods, especially glucose, are used as fuel. When any carbon-containing substance is burned in in-vitro experiments (e.g., in a combustion calorimeter), varying amounts of energy are released as heat, depending upon the completeness of the combustion.

[*]The metabolism of carbohydrate, fat, and protein is reviewed and discussed in depth in many texts and articles.[1-9] The information which follows is an attempt to condense and summarize some of the salient points in these publications.

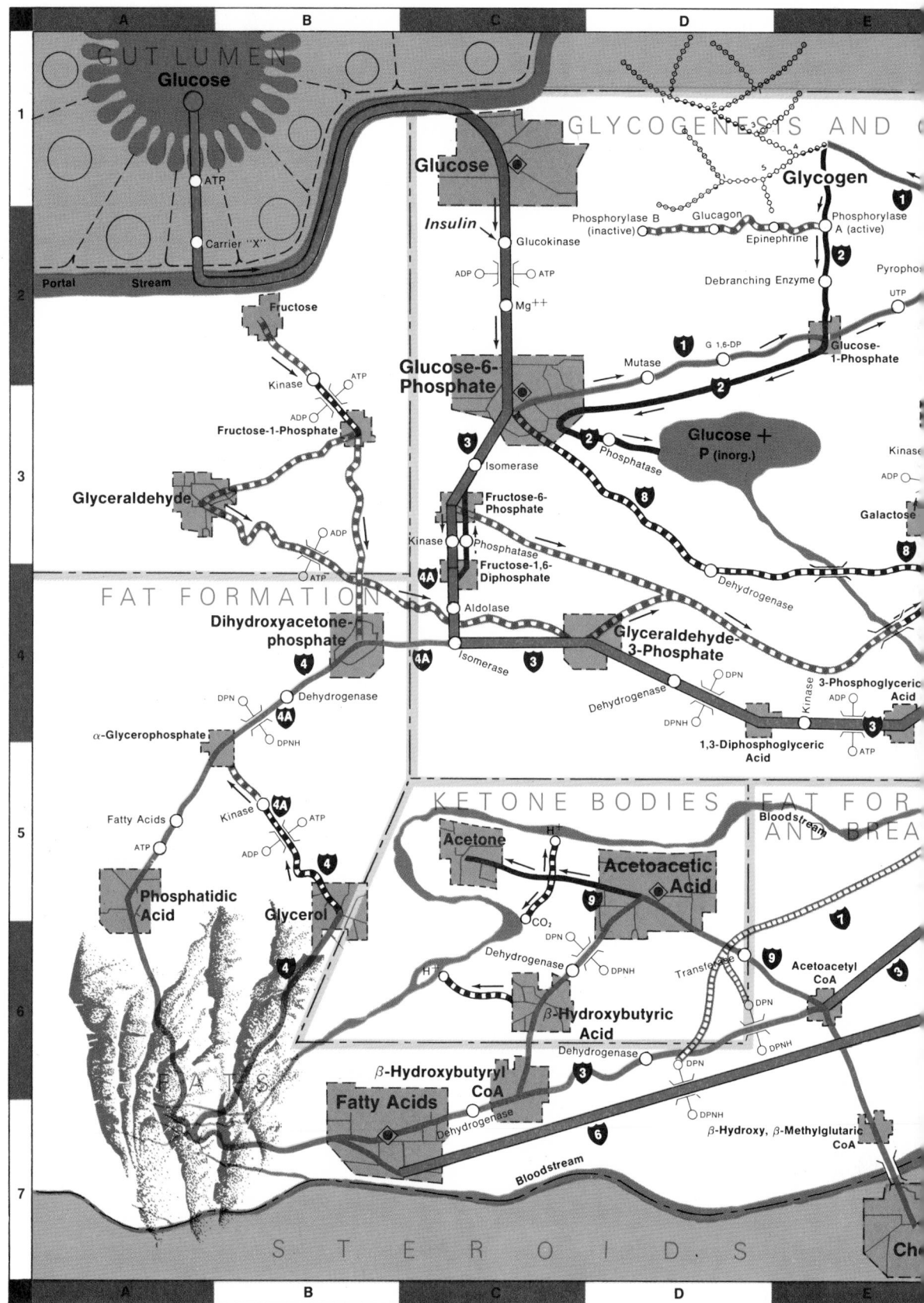

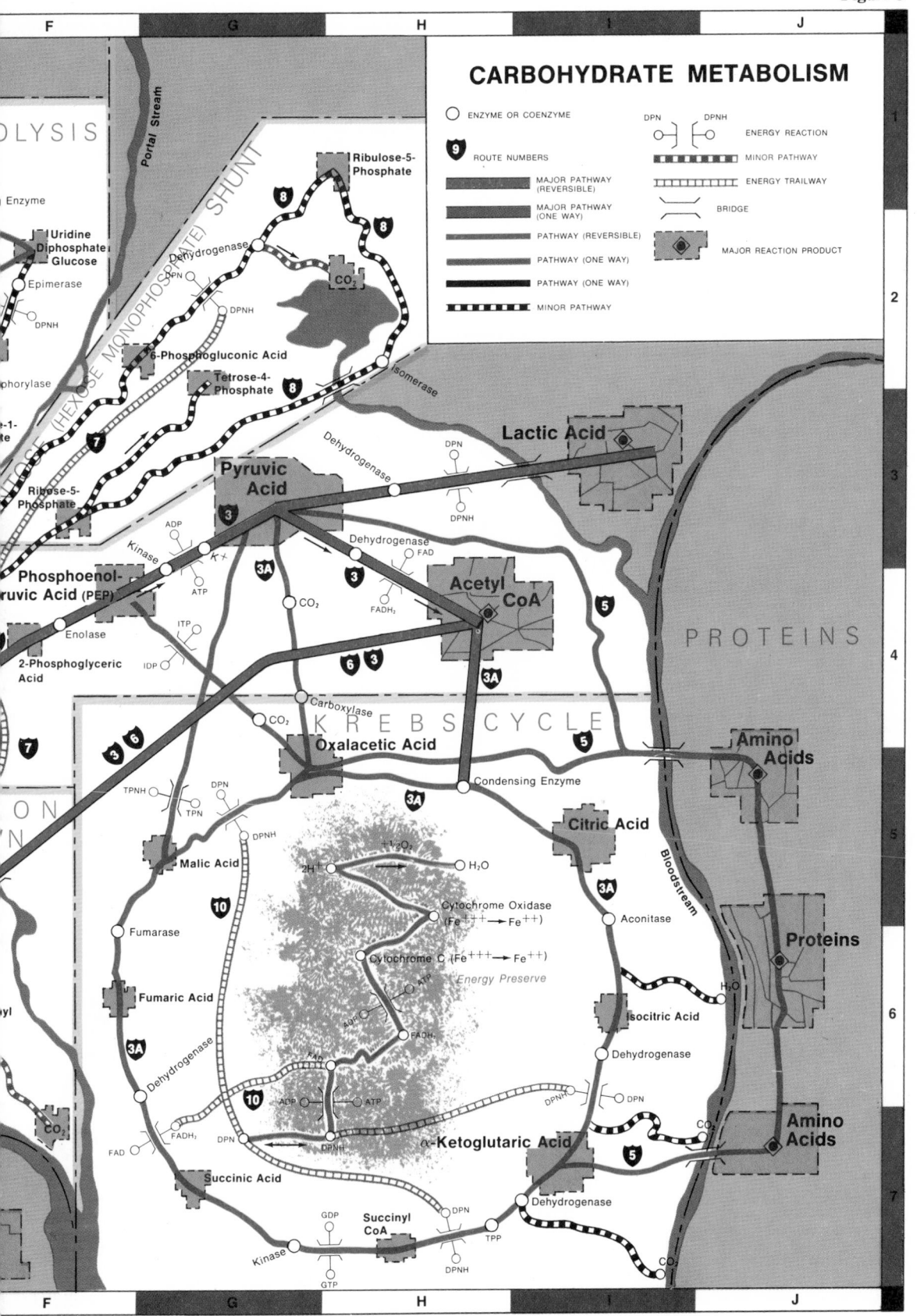

Figure 5

21

The original source of the heat in these substances is, of course, the sun, the thermal energy of which has been converted to chemical energy. Instead of directly releasing energy as heat, however, the body is capable of retaining the chemical energy of the substances being burned by transforming them into other compounds. That is the function of electron transfer mechanisms which occur in conjunction with respiratory enzyme systems in the mitochondria. Such systems are the cytochromes and the flavoproteins, which are in continuously changing states of oxidation and reduction. The precise means, of course, by which chemical energy is retained as such and not immediately freed as heat energy is one of the principal mysteries of life.

Energy at the cellular level

In the body, the metabolism of glucose is accomplished chemically through a high-energy substance called "adenosine triphosphate" (ATP), which provides the energy for the conversion of glucose to glucose-6-phosphate and thence to lactic acid and to carbon dioxide (Figures 4 and 5). This is a process which results in the phosphorylation of glucose and in the conversion of adenosine triphosphate (ATP) to adenosine diphosphate (ADP). The usefulness of these remarkable phosphate groups to the body resides in their inherent high-energy content and the fact that they can be restored as follows:

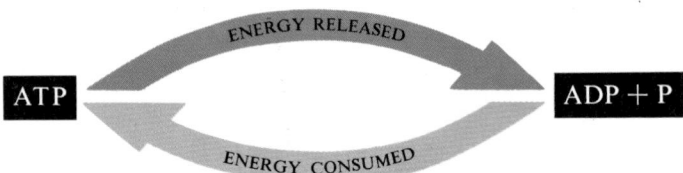

One of the reservoirs for the high-energy phosphate groups in muscle, for instance, is creatine phosphate. During exercise, when ATP is being utilized, creatine phosphate is broken down to yield high-energy phosphate groups as follows:

$$\text{creatine} \sim P + ADP \rightleftharpoons \text{creatine} + ATP$$

In addition to these energy sources, the directions and rates of the various chemical reactions which occur in normal and abnormal metabolism are influenced by the amount of substrate and by a number of hormones, such as insulin (see C1 in Figure 5), growth hormone, cortisol, thyroxine, and glucagon (D2). Body chemistry is in a state of dynamic flux. Depending upon body needs, some chemical reactions release energy as heat, whereas others replenish depleted energy sources chemically through the various electron and energy transfer systems (H6) **10**.

The carbohydrate we eat is converted into its constituent monosaccharides by the action of pancreatic and salivary enzymes. The fundamental unit of all carbohydrates (starch, polysaccharides) is the monosaccharide, a sugar structure containing five, six, or seven carbon atoms.

$$HC\!=\!O$$
$$|$$
$$HCOH$$
$$|$$
$$HOCH$$
$$|$$
$$HCOH$$
$$|$$
$$HCOH$$
$$|$$
$$H_2COH$$

Glucose

The most common monosaccharides are glucose, fructose, and galactose. When two of these units are combined, the result is a disaccharide, such as lactose (glucose and galactose), sucrose (glucose and fructose), or maltose (two glucose molecules). Carbohydrate enters the circulation almost entirely in the monosaccharide form. Transport across the cells of the intestinal lumen (the duodenum in particular and, to a lesser extent, the jejunum and ileum) to the portal vein is accomplished at the rate of 1 Gm. per Kg. per hour after a carbohydrate load (A1). Elevation of blood glucose directly or indirectly stimulates the beta cells of the pancreas (page 51) to produce insulin, the presence of which is a *sine qua non* for normal carbohydrate metabolism.

Digestion

An important function of insulin is to provide molecules of glucose in the bloodstream with a passageway through cell barriers which otherwise are essentially impervious to them. The exact mechanism by which this is accomplished is unknown. However, available information suggests that molecules of insulin somehow interact with key molecules of unknown identity at the surface of certain cells and thus enhance the transport of glucose into some cells but not into others. For instance, skeletal and diaphragm muscle and the muscle of the heart require insulin for efficient sugar transfer. Adipose tissue is also in this category. On the other hand, red blood cells, brain cells, and cells of the intestine, liver, and kidney tubules all permit the passage of glucose across their barriers without the help of insulin. The sensitivity of the various tissues to insulin is summarized in Table 7.

Following their transport to the liver via the portal vein, the various monosaccharides enter the hepatic cell, where they are phosphorylated; that is, a phosphate group is added to the number 6 carbon atom to produce glucose-6-phosphate (C3).

The phosphorylation of glucose is accomplished by the action of an enzyme called "glucokinase" (C2), the activity of which is enhanced by insulin. The phosphorylation step "locks" glucose in the cell and prepares it for its participation in the reactions which ensue; as a result of phosphorylation, glucose (now glucose-6-phosphate) (C2) stands at the hub of several pathways.

Glucose 6-phosphate

Phosphorylation

Table 7. Sensitivity of Different Tissues to Insulin

Insulin Sensitive (require insulin for transfer of glucose)

Muscle	Mammary gland
Skeletal	Anterior pituitary
Cardiac	Lens of the eye
Fibroblast	Aorta

Not Insulin Sensitive (do not require insulin for the transfer of glucose)

Nerve tissues	Kidney tubules
Erythrocytes	Liver
Intestinal mucosa cells	

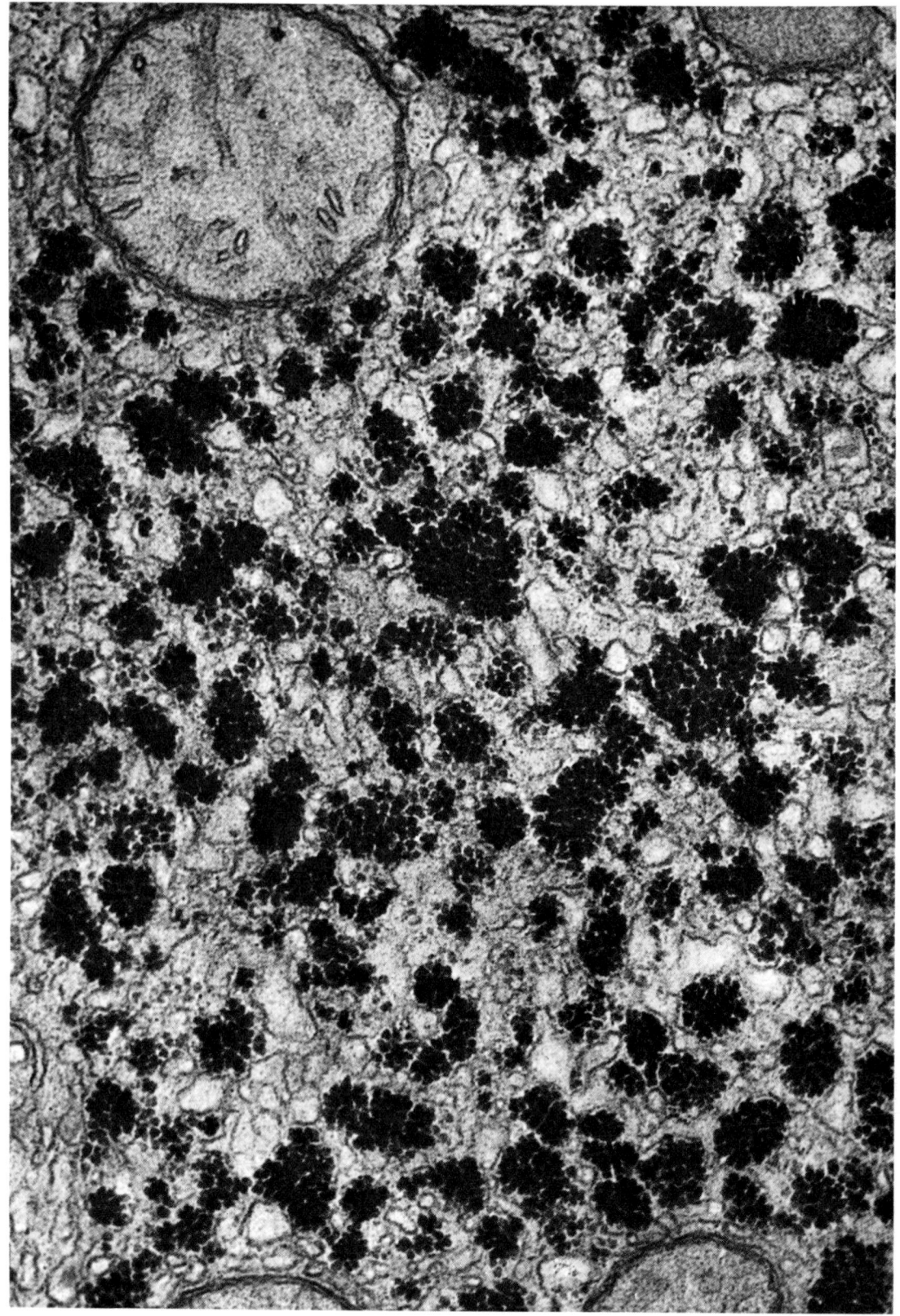

Figure 6. Glycogen in the liver usually appears as conspicuous rosettes of various sizes as seen in this electron micrograph.

In the liver in the fed state (after carbohydrate loading as a result of the action of insulin), glucose is converted to glycogen (Figure 6) **1** . In the fasting state, glycogen is broken down **2** . This results in the re-formation of glucose-6-phosphate molecules; these, in turn, are acted upon by glucose-6-phosphatase (D3), which removes the phosphorus and thus permits glucose to leave the cell. From here it may travel via the systemic circulation to other parts of the body where it is needed, i.e., muscle or fat cells. The chemical events which have been discussed here for the liver cell are depicted in C1 and 2 to E1, 2, and 3.

There are other important pathways for the metabolism of glucose in the fed state; for example, the synthesis of fatty acids occurs in the liver cell and also in adipose tissue. This is accomplished by the conversion of glucose into two molecules of pyruvic acid (G3) and then to acetyl coenzyme A (H4); the latter subsequently goes through several steps of condensation, and eventually fatty acids are formed (B6) **3** . Fatty acids are conjugated to glycerol (B6) **4** , which has been produced from dihydroxyacetonephosphate (B4). The resulting triglycerides are joined to lipoproteins for transport in the blood to sites where they are needed (A5 to E5).

Carbon atoms of glucose can be incorporated into amino acids (J5 and 7). Conversely, amino acids can enter the Krebs cycle (I7) and lead to glucose formation (I5, I7) **5** .

In the fed state, a portion of glucose is released from the liver by the action of the phosphatase mentioned above and is available for metabolism by muscle and fat cells as well as the central nervous system, etc. As a result of the action of insulin, glucose traverses the cellular membrane of muscle and is converted immediately to glucose-6-phosphate (C2). Depending upon the needs of the cell, glycogen may be formed, or the glucose may be metabolized to pyruvic acid (G3) **3** and ultimately to carbon dioxide and water by way of the Krebs cycle (G5) **3A** .

In adipose tissue during the fed state, insulin accelerates the transport of sugar to the intracellular space. Here, the metabolic pathways serve to convert glucose to fatty acids by chemical reactions similar to those in the liver, i.e., transformation of glucose to glucose-6-phosphate and thence to pyruvate (G3) and acetyl coenzyme A (H4) **3** . The two carbon units of acetyl coenzyme A form an intermediate malonyl coenzyme A (F6), which is polymerized to form long-chain fatty acids **6** . Thus, glucose provides the carbon atoms and, by another pathway called the "pentose shunt" (G1) **8** , the hydrogen for the reduction of malonyl coenzyme A to fatty acids **7** . Following their synthesis, the fatty acids are esterified with glycerol, which is formed from alpha-glycerophosphate (A5) **4** .

Carbohydrate stores in the body are limited. Consequently, after a fast of twelve to twenty hours and if no glucose is ingested, the reactions of body metabolism described for the fed state are increasingly changed to supply glucose and other fuels necessary for metabolism. Glucose is pro-

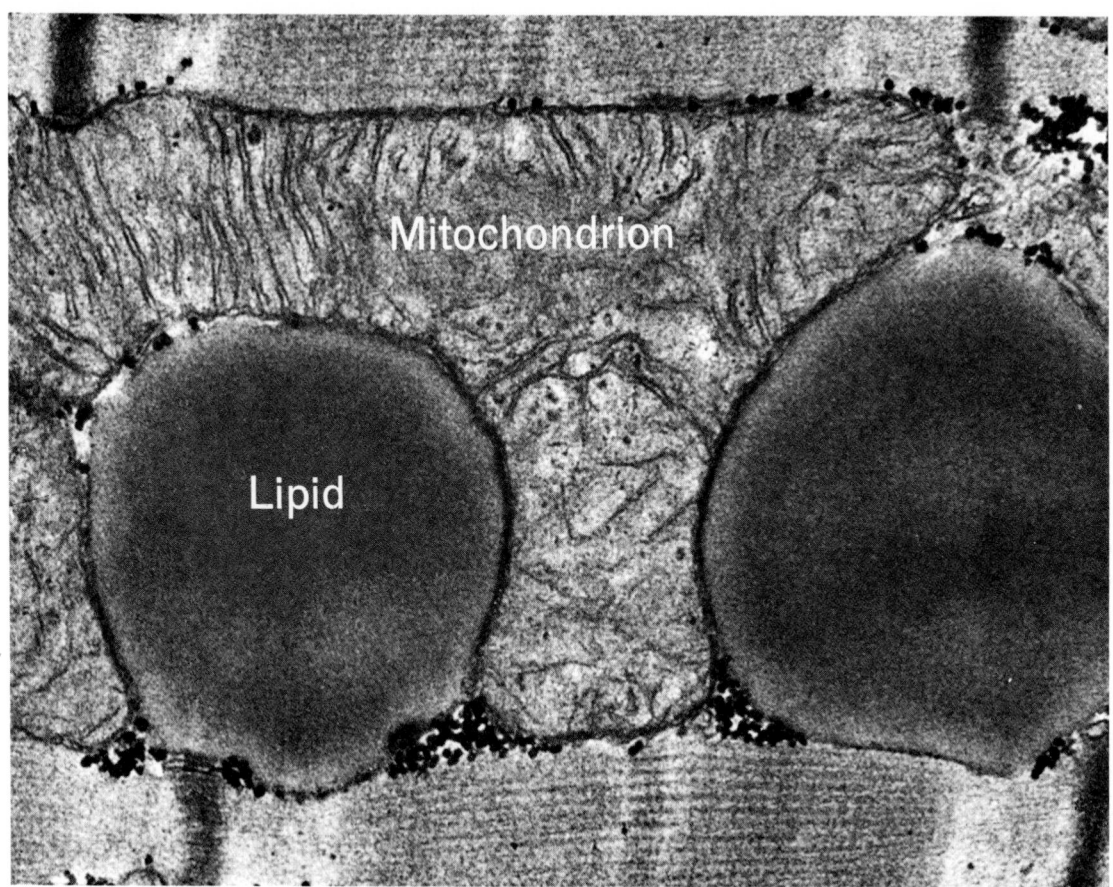

Figure 7. Not infrequently, mitochondria are found in close relation to lipid droplets in the cytoplasm. This is illustrated in the above electron micrograph of the sarcoplasm of cardiac muscle, where numerous lipid droplets are located among the mitochondria that are aligned in the clefts between myofibrils. The mitochondria may almost completely encircle a lipid droplet.

The principal enzymes involved in the metabolism of triglycerides reside in the mitochondria, and the proximity of the latter to the lipid droplets in cardiac muscle is consistent with the interpretation that the mitochondria play an important role in the utilization of lipid as a source of energy for muscular contraction. Magnification, 47,000×.

duced from noncarbohydrate sources (a process called "gluconeogenesis"), and fatty acids are utilized as the major metabolic fuel. The principal substrates for gluconeogenesis are the amino acids (J5 and 7) and glycerol (B6). Glycerol is converted through a series of reactions to fructose-1,6-diphosphate and eventually to glucose **4A**. Depending upon their chemical structure, the various amino acids may enter the Krebs cycle by one of three means **5** and be converted to phosphoenolpyruvic acid (F4). From this compound, as the result of several transformations, glucose is formed.

When glucose is not available from extracellular sources, muscle glycogen is mobilized and metabolized. As glycogen is depleted, the energy for muscular contraction must come increasingly from the combustion of fatty acids (Figure 7).

Since very little insulin is secreted during the fasting state, there is only minimal entry of glucose into the cells of fat or muscle tissue. Fatty acids then leave fat tissue and are metabolized in other types of cells (liver, muscle, etc.). Excessive mobilization of fatty acids from adipose tissue results in their increased conversion in the liver to ketone bodies and thus in metabolic acidosis [9].

The biochemistry of the fasting state is manifested most acutely in ketoacidosis. As a result of insulin deficiencies, the following events ensue:

1. Glucose entry into insulin-sensitive cells (i.e., muscle and fat) is drastically reduced.

2. Liver glycogen is broken down to glucose.

3. A lack of insulin results in the mobilization of free fatty acids from peripheral stores. These circulate to the liver, where they are oxidized to acetoacetyl CoA and acetyl CoA[10] (routes 3 and 9 in southwest corner of Figure 5), both of which are converted to the ketone bodies, chiefly β-hydroxybutyric acid and acetoacetate.

The above events are associated with the elaboration of a number of diabetogenic hormones, particularly epinephrine, glucagon, ACTH, and cortisol, the net effects of which are further mobilization of free fatty acids and gluconeogenesis and resistance to therapeutic Insulin.

The combination of hyperosmolarity (resulting from hyperglycemia) and acidosis (due to the production of excess ketone bodies) leads to progressive dehydration and depression of the sensorium. The reversal of these events can occur only with correction of fluid and electrolyte deficits in association with the administration of both Insulin and glucose. The specific methods for treating ketoacidosis are outlined in Chapter 13.

CH_3
$C=O$
CH_2
$COO-$
acetoacetate

CH_3
$C-O$
CH_3
acetone

CH_3
$HC-OH$
CH_2
$COO-$
β-hydroxybutyrate

BIBLIOGRAPHY

1. Harper, H. A.: Review of Physiological Chemistry, Ed. 9. Los Altos, California: Lange Medical Publications, 1963.

2. Goodner, C. J.: Newer Concepts in Diabetes Mellitus, Including Management, in Disease-a-Month (edited by H. F. Dowling). Chicago: Year Book Medical Publishers, Inc., September, 1965.

3. Levine, R.: On Some Biochemical Aspects of Diabetes Mellitus, Am. J. Med., *31*:901, 1961.

4. Stetten, D., Jr., and Mortimore, G. E.: Carbohydrate Metabolism, in Diabetes (edited by R. H. Williams), p. 89. New York: Paul B. Hoeber, Inc., 1960.

5. Gordon, E. S.: Lipid Metabolism, Diabetes Mellitus, and Obesity, in Advances in Internal Medicine (edited by W. Dock and I. Snapper), Vol. 12, p. 66. Chicago: Year Book Medical Publishers, Inc., 1964.

6. Williams, R. H. (Editor): Textbook of Endrocrinology, Ed. 3. Philadelphia: W. B. Saunders Company, 1965.

7. West, E. S., and Todd, W. R.: Textbook of Biochemistry, Ed. 3. New York: The Macmillan Company, 1961.

8. White, A., Handler, P., and Smith, E. L.: Principles of Biochemistry, Ed. 3. New York: McGraw-Hill Book Company, Inc., 1964.

9. Duncan, G. G.: Diseases of Metabolism, Ed. 5, p. 921. Philadelphia: W. B. Saunders Company, 1964.

10. Sherwin, R., and Felig, P.: Pathophysiology of Diabetes Mellitus, Med. Clin. North Am., *62*:695, 1978.

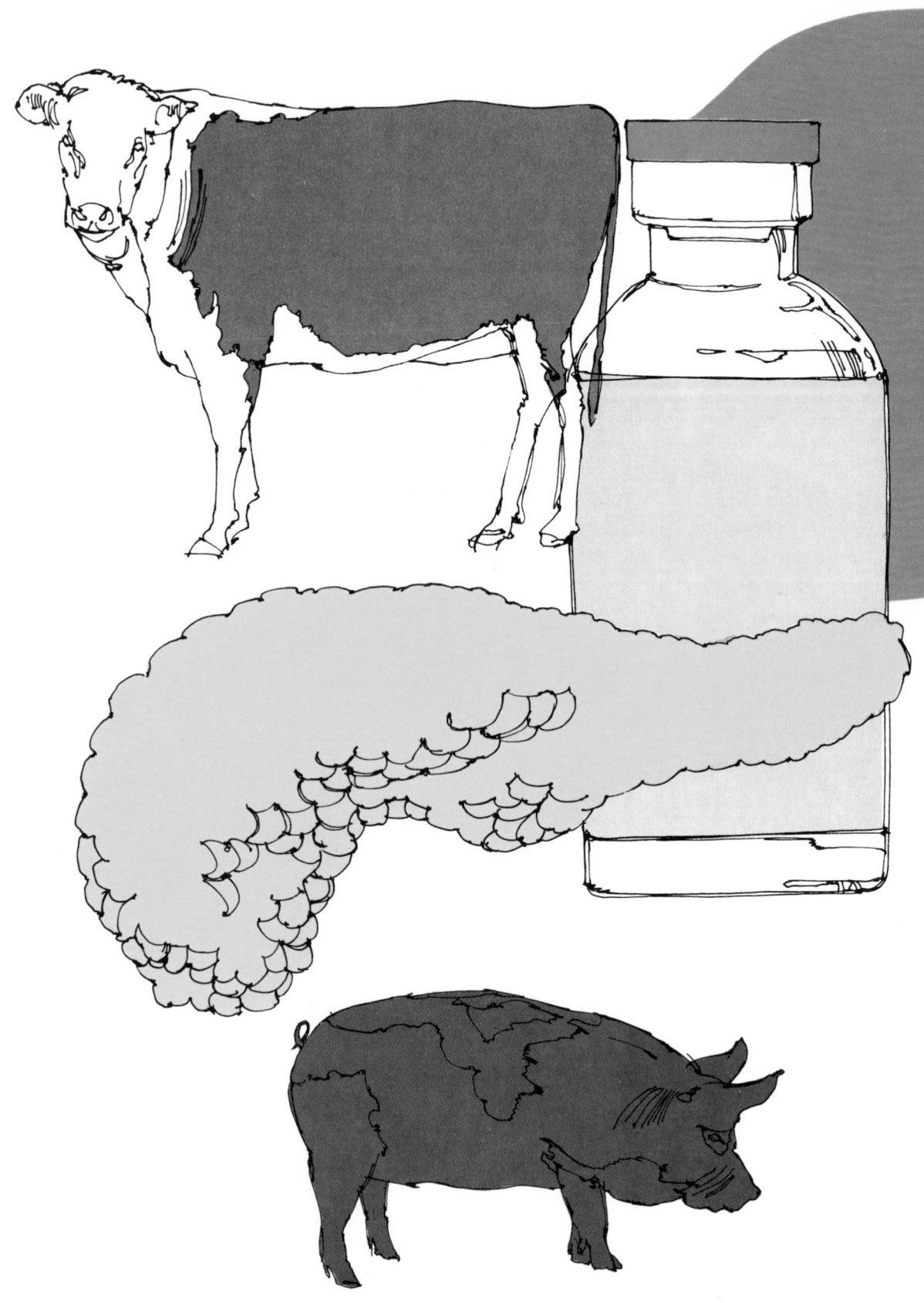

Insulin

4

THE SOURCE OF INSULIN

The islands of Langerhans of the pancreas are now known to consist of at least two types of cells, although there seems to be some species variation (Figure 8).

In 1926, Ukai developed a procedure which enabled him to stain some cells red (called "A cells") and others blue (called "B cells") and thus to differentiate two distinct types in the rabbit islet. In 1931, using special fixatives, Bloom observed a third type of cell in the human pancreas and termed it the "D cell."

The typical B (or beta) cell is many-sided and irregular in outline. The A (or alpha) cell is also irregular but is somewhat elongated and larger in size. Each type of cell contains granules but of a size and number peculiar to it. In order to bring out the distinguishing features of granules and other structures in islet cells, it is necessary to apply certain fixing and staining procedures to the tissue.

Cells of the islands

A successful method, devised by Gomori, makes use of chrome alum hematoxylin phloxine. With this procedure, the granules of the beta cell stain a deep blue from the chrome hematoxylin. They are rather coarse, and their number per cell varies greatly. Some cells in a given islet are literally filled with granules; others are almost empty. Furthermore, the granules are not distributed evenly throughout a cell; they are often densely packed in that portion of the cell which borders on a capillary.

Figure 8. A three-dimensional reconstruction of a normal human island of Langerhans emphasizing alpha (A) and beta (B) cells and the extensive vasculature.

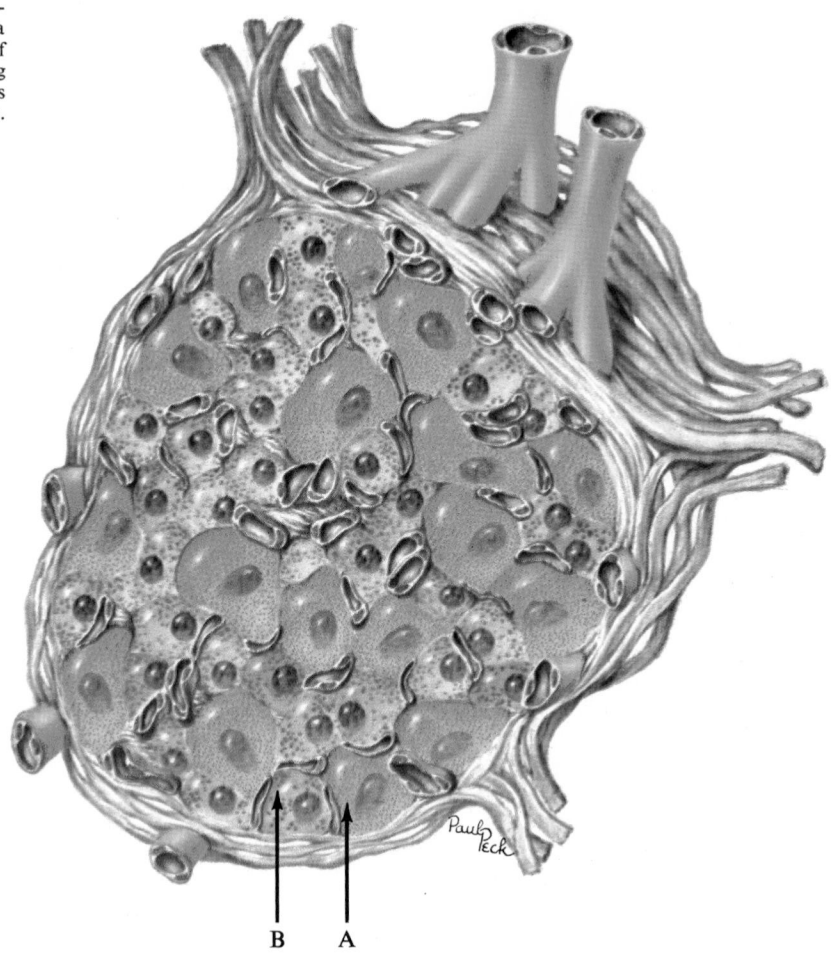

B   A

In contrast, the alpha-cell granules stain red with phloxine (used in the Gomori technic) and are finer than the granules of beta cells. They are also more numerous, more evenly distributed within a cell, and subject to less variation in number from one cell to another (Figure 9).

Beta cells outnumber all other kinds of islet cells. They are generally scattered throughout the islet but may be concentrated at its edge. Many beta cells lie next to capillaries; no intervening membrane appears to separate these two structures.

The discovery that discrete cells in the islands of Langerhans, the D (delta) cells, produce somatostatin, a substance which inhibits the secretion of insulin and glucagon (see Chapter 5), highlights the possibility that the anatomic proximity of the alpha, beta, and delta cells has great functional significance.[1]

ULTRASTRUCTURE OF ISLET CELLS

In electron micrographs taken at relatively low magnification (2,300×), islet cells stand out from the surrounding acinar tissue because of the abundance of endoplasmic reticulum, or ergastoplasm, which in section and under low magnification resembles approximately parallel rows of strings studded with irregularly spaced knots of various sizes. The knot-like enlargements are believed to be ribosomes. No other cell in the pancreas is so richly endowed with endoplasmic reticulum. The acinar cell contains structures generally present in all cells, such as a nucleus and mitochondria.

Islet cells lie close together, with only an occasional space between them. Each cell is apparently surrounded by its own plasma membrane, although at times it is difficult to determine the limits of individual membranes, especially along those portions of a cell which adhere to adjacent cells.

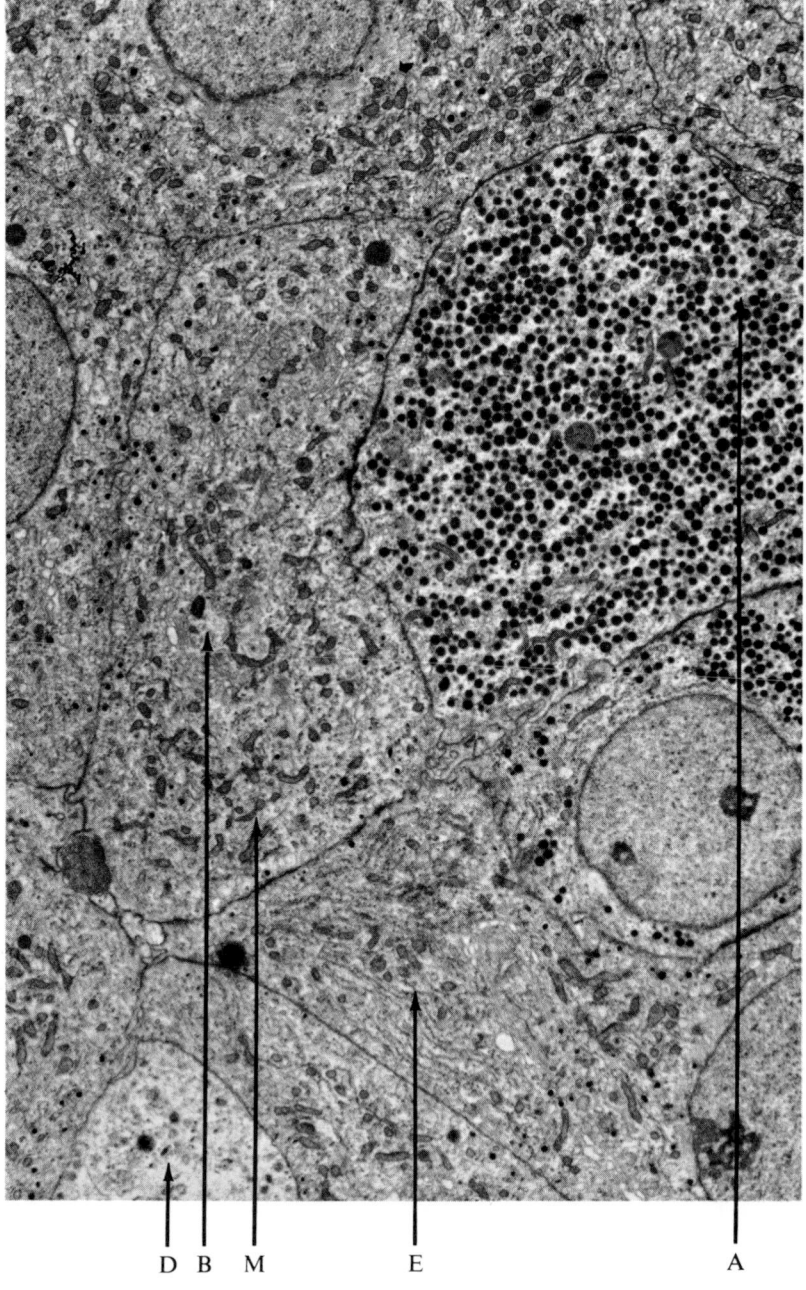

Figure 9. Electron micrograph of normal rabbit islet showing alpha cells (A) with numerous dark granules. In the beta cells (B) are insulin-bearing granules within capsule-like structures. Mitochondria (M) are numerous, and some endoplasmic reticulum is evident (E). The pale cells are delta cells (D).

D B M   E   A

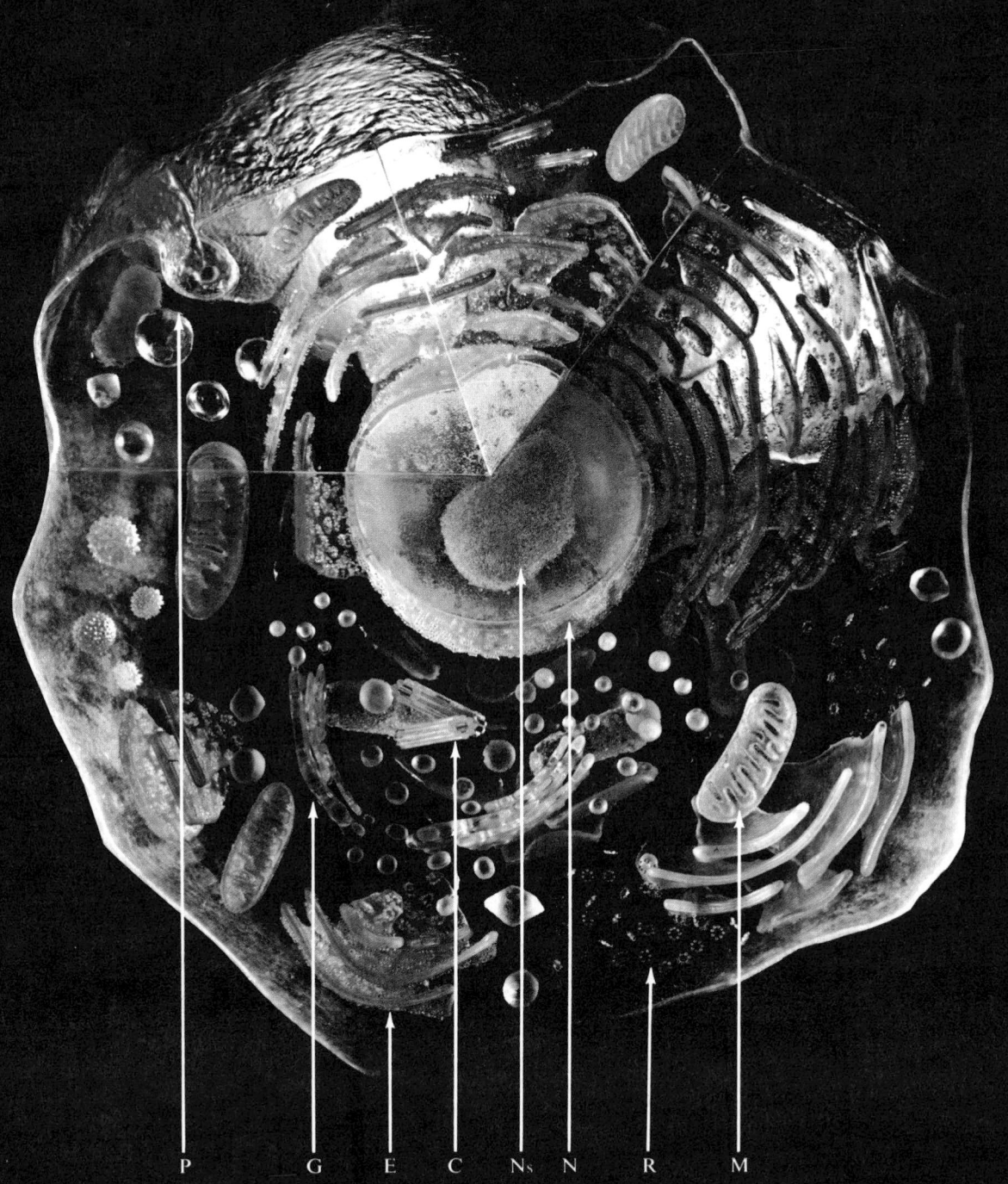

P   G E C Nₛ N   R   M

Figure 10. Three-dimensional model of a cell idealized to illustrate various cell structures as seen in electron micrographs. These include mitochondria (M); ribosomes, both free (R) and those part of the endoplasmic reticulum (E); double-walled nucleus (N); nucleolus (Ns); centriole (C); Golgi body (G); and an invagination of the cell surface which may depict entrance of either solid or fluid material into the cell's interior (P).

ULTRASTRUCTURE AND FUNCTION OF BETA CELLS

Electron micrographs obtained at considerably higher magnification (i.e., 24,000× to 40,000×) than those useful for purposes of orientation have revealed the ultrafine structure of the various types of cells encountered in the pancreas.

At this high magnification, the endoplasmic reticulum resembles canals liberally dotted along their outer surface with electron-dense granules, which are ribosomes (Figure 10). A number of these canals are often arranged in approximately parallel rows. Singly or in groups, they appear to span a considerable distance through the cytoplasm without interruption. Here, as with mitochondria, only a thin section of a large entity can be observed. The canals are actually slices of sandwich-like structures, the outer sides of which are sprinkled with beadlike ribosomes. The "sandwiches" vary in dimension, and all are not necessarily oriented in parallel rows.

In any cell in which it is present, the endoplasmic reticulum is considered to be the site of protein synthesis. Its function in the beta cell is probably no different. Various cell proteins are formed within its confines, including insulin, which is uniquely a product of beta-cell endoplasmic reticulum.

Possibly because insulin is a highly specialized protein with powerful hormonal action, it is associated with special structures while in the beta cell. These structures and the activities which they engender appear to be necessary for the synthesis, storage, and ultimate release of insulin into the bloodstream.

INSULIN SYNTHESIS: THE ENDOPLASMIC RETICULUM

The earliest morphological evidence of insulin synthesis is observed in characteristic alterations of the endoplasmic reticulum. These changes begin as slight swellings which distend the wall of the canal-like reticulum (Figure 11). As the irregularly spaced areas gradually increase in size, connecting segments become less conspicuous; they finally disappear altogether and leave only oval or globular structures. These bear little resemblance to the typical slender canal-like endoplasmic reticulum, but they carry marks of their origin; that is, each globule has adhering to it a number of ribosomes.

The globules look pale in the electron micrograph and may even appear to be empty since the material within does not greatly hinder the passage of the electron beam. The chemical nature of this material is not known, but it is generally considered to be the precursor of insulin.

INSULIN STORAGE: THE BETA GRANULES

The substance within the globule soon changes in appearance (and probably also in chemical composition) by becoming increasingly electron-dense. The process is described as a condensation because, when it is complete, well-defined granules containing insulin have been formed. These are virtually opaque to the electron beam and seem to take up less volume than did the precursor material. Granules and clear space are in turn en-

Figure 11. Rat islet tissue at beginning of beta granule synthesis. The endoplasmic reticulum E_2 is slightly distended in comparison with E_1, which is normal. Other structures are nucleus (N) and Golgi bodies (G).

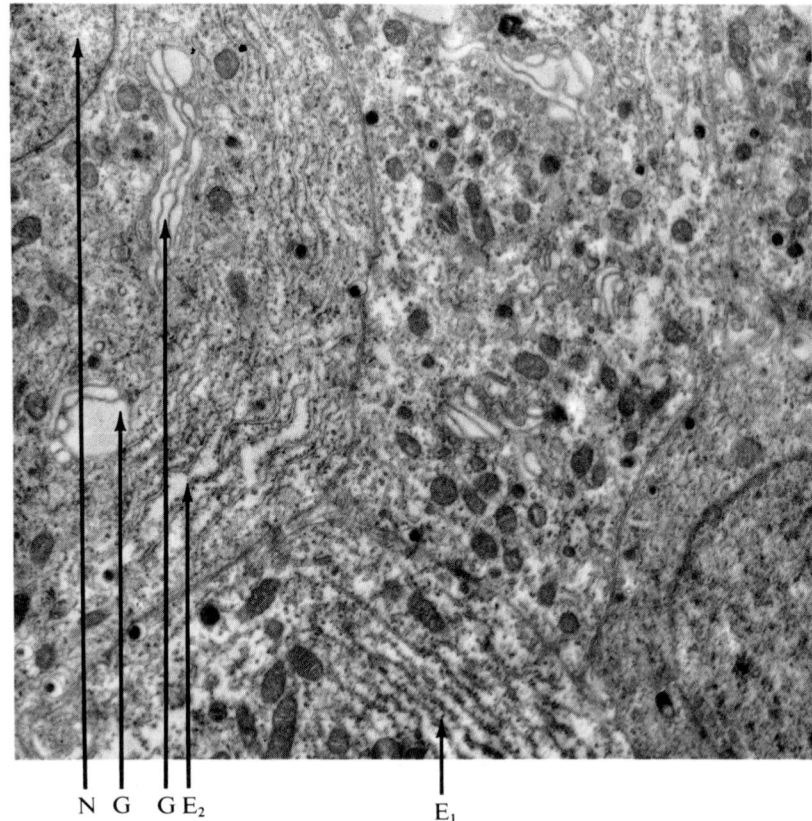

N G G E_2 E_1

closed by a membrane which, in the early stages of granule development (i.e., during condensation), is dotted with ribosomes, as were the globules. Ultimately the ribosomes disappear, perhaps coincident with the maturation of the beta granules, and a smooth outer membrane remains.

Insulin-bearing capsules, or sacs, have been observed in various animals, including man. They have a smooth external membrane in all instances, but the actual form taken by the granules within is often characteristic of the species. In man, the granule may be rectangular in outline and crystalline in appearance.

Variation in granule shape may reflect differences in insulin structure or in the type of materials with which insulin is associated in the granules. Granules are too large to represent single molecules of insulin. Thus, the actual amino acid sequence in the insulin might influence the way the molecules can be arranged in the granule. Similarly, the structure of the protein which binds insulin may impart certain characteristics of form to the granule.

INSULIN RELEASE: EMIOCYTOSIS

Insulin seems to function as a hormone only when it is in certain tissues. To reach these sites of action, it must first break out of its capsule and leave the beta cell. Then it must negotiate a route through several kinds of barriers which stand between it and a capillary. Only after it reaches the lumen of the capillary is it transported via the bloodstream to appropriate tissue, such as muscle and fat.

The events which ultimately bring insulin to its "target tissue" begin with migration of fully formed insulin sacs from their formation sites to the surface of the beta cells. The mechanism of this movement is not known, nor is it clear how the insulin-containing granules are released from the capsule when it reaches the cell surface. However, it has been proposed that the cell's plasma membrane and the capsule membrane fuse upon contact and that these membranes then rupture at the point of fusion. As a result, a passageway is thereby provided for the granule across two membranes and thus out of the beta cell. The rupture at the point of fusion of the plasma and capsule membranes may be expected to leave fragments of these structures at the sides of each space formerly occupied by the granule. The finding of these fragments (or "microvilli," as they are called) in association with spaces resembling empty capsules is the basis for the idea that insulin-containing granules are released, or ejected, from the beta cell in the manner described. The process of ejection is called "emiocytosis."

Although it is presumed that granules of insulin shed their enveloping capsules when they leave the beta cell, as described, free granules have not been observed. Therefore, it is likely that each insulin granule (which may consist of many molecules of insulin held within a protein matrix) undergoes a drastic transformation at the moment of emiocytosis. Consequently, the insulin that continues to the lumen of the nearest capillary is probably in a nongranular form, or it may even be in the soluble state, although perhaps bound to protein.

Insulin granules

On the basis of the foregoing discussion, it is now possible to summarize the events that result in the production and release of insulin from the beta cell.[1A,1B] Insulin synthesis is initiated by a signal (or signals), the chief one being glucose. As a result, in the region of the rough endoplasmic reticulum (RER), m-RNA from the insulin gene (or genes) directs the synthesis of a "pre-region" of a precursor of insulin called "preproinsulin." This material has a molecular weight of about 13,000 and serves to bind ribosomes to the membrane of the RER and thus guide the formation of preproinsulin chains. The pre-region is quickly depleted and leaves proinsulin, which consists of insulin and a connecting peptide (C-peptide) (see page 45 and Figure 16, page 46). The purpose of the connecting peptide in proinsulin is to promote the correct folding of the parts of the molecule with proper positioning of the disulfide bonds.

Proinsulin is then transferred to the Golgi apparatus, where the process of granule formation and the conversion to insulin begins. When cleavage of the connecting peptide from proinsulin and the formation of insulin occur, the beta granules are released into the cytoplasm, where they attach to a microtubular-microfilament system. Glucose, acting by increasing Ca^{++} binding in the beta cell, stimulates conformational changes in the microvilli that result in the ascent of insulin-containing granules to the cell surface, where they are released by emiocytosis to the intercellular and thence to the extracellular space.

THE CHEMISTRY OF INSULIN

Insulin, the antidiabetic hormone produced in the pancreas by the beta cells of the islands of Langerhans, is a protein consisting of fifty-one amino

Figure 12. A Portrayal of the Polypeptide Backbone of Pork Insulin[1C,1D]

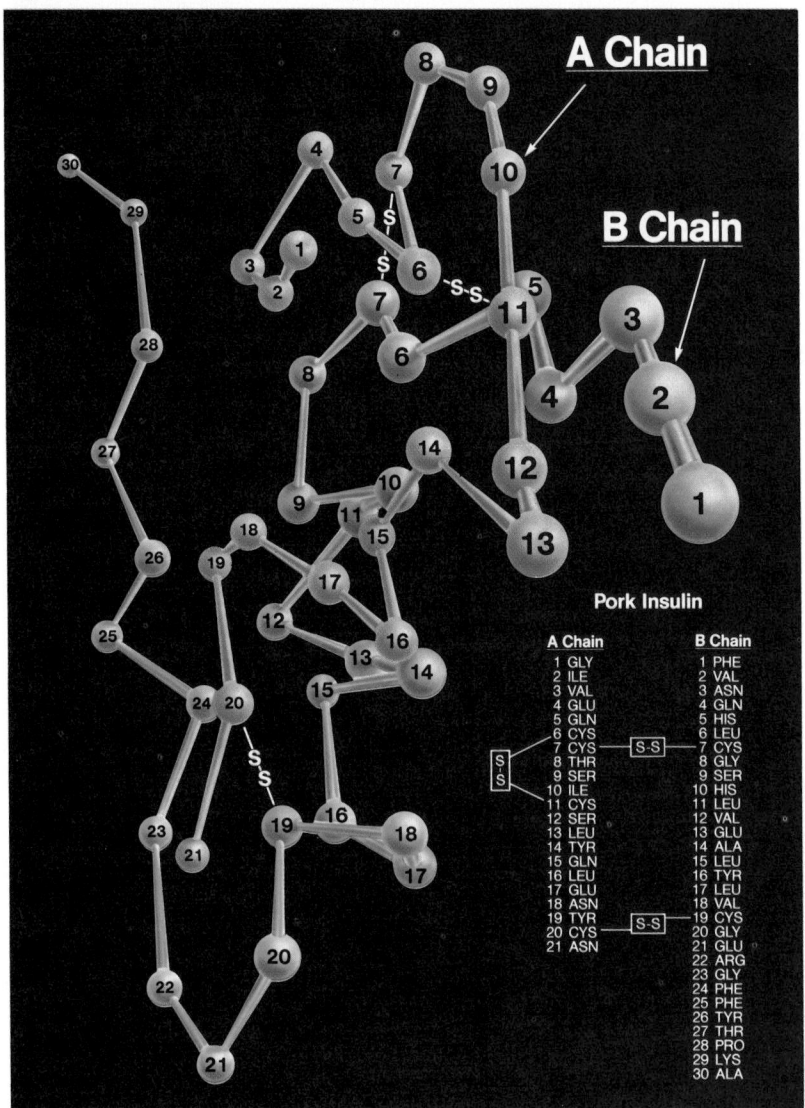

Pork Insulin

A Chain		B Chain
1 GLY		1 PHE
2 ILE		2 VAL
3 VAL		3 ASN
4 GLU		4 GLN
5 GLN		5 HIS
6 CYS		6 LEU
7 CYS	S-S	7 CYS
8 THR		8 GLY
9 SER		9 SER
10 ILE		10 HIS
11 CYS		11 LEU
12 SER		12 VAL
13 LEU		13 GLU
14 TYR		14 ALA
15 GLN		15 LEU
16 LEU		16 TYR
17 GLU		17 LEU
18 ASN		18 VAL
19 TYR	S-S	19 CYS
20 CYS		20 GLY
21 ASN		21 GLU
		22 ARG
		23 GLY
		24 PHE
		25 PHE
		26 TYR
		27 THR
		28 PRO
		29 LYS
		30 ALA

acids and having a minimum molecular weight of 6,000. It is quite stable in dilute acid solutions at a pH of 2.5 to 3.5.

The insulin molecule is composed of two polypeptide chains, designated "A" and "B," which are connected by two interchain disulfide bridges of cystine. These are depicted schematically in Figure 12.

The "A" chain of insulin contains an intrachain disulfide bridge within which a species difference in amino acid composition occurs, primarily at positions 8, 9, and 10. Pork, dog, and human insulin have a similar amino acid composition at these positions and differ only in the carboxyl terminal end of the "B" chain. Pork insulin, like that of beef, has alanine at this position; human insulin has threonine (Table 8).

Most commercial Insulin* preparations in this country are made from a combination of beef and pork zinc-Insulin crystals. Regular, NPH, Protamine Zinc, and Lente® Insulins are available also as beef and pork Insulins. The species source of all Lilly Insulins is indicated on the labels.

---

*In this book, "Insulin" with a capital letter refers to the commercial product to distinguish it from "insulin," the natural hormone.

Table 8. Species Differences in Amino Acid Sequence of Mammalian Insulins

| | "A" CHAIN | | | "B" CHAIN |
	8	9	10	30
Beef	Alanine	Serine	Valine	Alanine
Pork	Threonine	Serine	Isoleucine	Alanine
Human	Threonine	Serine	Isoleucine	Threonine
Other Species				
Dog	Threonine	Serine	Isoleucine	Alanine
Sperm whale	Threonine	Serine	Isoleucine	Alanine
Rabbit	Threonine	Serine	Isoleucine	Serine
Horse	Threonine	Glycine	Isoleucine	Alanine
Sheep	Alanine	Glycine	Valine	Alanine
Sei whale	Alanine	Serine	Threonine	Alanine

HISTORY

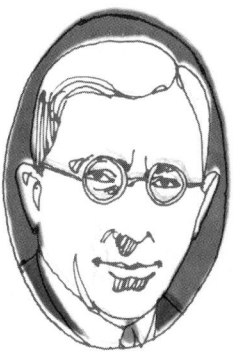

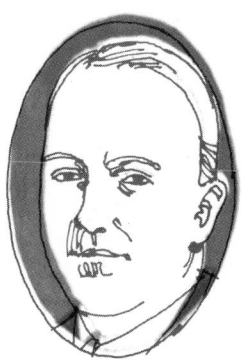

The discovery of Insulin in 1921 by Frederick G. Banting and Charles H. Best, working in the laboratory of J. J. R. Macleod in Toronto, revolutionized the outlook for the diabetic patient. In December, 1921, following the first report of the action of Insulin in dogs, Eli Lilly and Company offered its facilities and co-operation to Banting and Best, through the University of Toronto, for the development and production of Insulin. Soon afterward, clinical studies confirmed the value of Insulin in the treatment of human diabetes, and by April, 1922, the two groups were actively collaborating in an effort to make a purified Insulin in a sufficient amount to treat all diabetics whose disease could not be controlled by diet alone. In 1923, only two years after the laboratory breakthrough, Eli Lilly and Company produced the first commercially available Insulin. Presented in the order of their commercial availability, the Insulins below have been produced and tested clinically at Eli Lilly and Company.

REGULAR (UNMODIFIED) INSULIN

The first Insulin developed for clinical use was amorphous Insulin; it was the only one available until considerably later, when regular Insulin crystals, a purified form of which is now labeled "Regular Insulin," were produced. Regular Insulin made from zinc-Insulin crystals is a clear solution. However, the antidiabetic effect of Regular Insulin is essentially the same whether the solution is made from crystalline or noncrystalline preparations of the active antidiabetic principle. The rapid onset of hypoglycemic effect of Insulin made from zinc-Insulin crystals is identical with that of Insulin of amorphous origin.

Regular Insulin is ordinarily administered subcutaneously one-half to two hours before a meal so that its physiological effects will parallel the absorption of glucose. Regular Pork Insulin (Concentrated) containing 500 units per ml. is employed in Insulin coma therapy and in cases of Insulin resistance requiring very large doses.

NEUTRAL REGULAR INSULIN

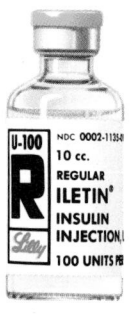

Until 1973, Lilly Regular Insulin was produced at a *p*H of 2.8 to 3.5. This was necessary because particles formed in the vial when the *p*H was increased above the acid range. However, following recent changes in the manufacturing methods which result in Insulin of increased purity, it was found that Regular Insulin could be maintained in solution over a wide *p*H range even when unbuffered (e.g., when the *p*H is adjusted upward with sodium hydroxide). Moreover, neutral Regular Insulin (that is, Insulin with a neutral *p*H, or NRI) was found to have increased stability over acid Regular Insulin (ARI), probably because of a slower rate of deamination at the higher *p*H. Thus, NRI maintains nearly full potency when stored up to eighteen months at 5° and 25°C. (Figure 13). After twelve months of storage at 37°C., NRI still maintains 95 percent of its potency. With ARI, on the other hand, decreases in potency of about 25 percent are seen after six months of storage conditions at 25°C. or warmer.[2] These data support the clinical practice of not refrigerating the vial of Insulin that has been opened and is currently being used.

Figure 13. Effect of *p*H on the Stability of Regular Insulin

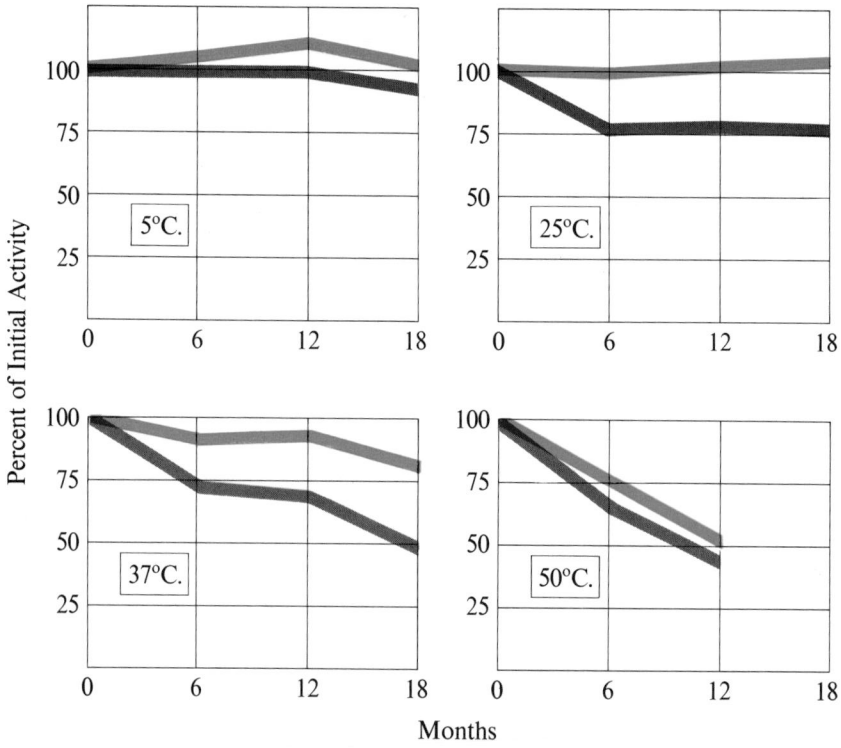

The blue line represents neutral Regular Insulin (*p*H 7.4), and the olive line represents acid Regular Insulin (*p*H 3). Values at 5° and 25°C. (41° and 77°F.) were determined by rabbit assay; at 37° and 50°C. (98.6° and 122°F.), by immunoassay.

Studies in animals have established that NRI may be mixed with NPH and Lente® Insulin in any proportion desired, and the mixture may be prepared two to three months before use.[3] This is in contrast to ARI; because of its low *p*H, it should not be added to the modified Insulins (which have a neutral pH) in a ratio greater than 1:1. Clinical studies in normal fasted subjects have disclosed that, although there are small differences between ARI and NRI in absorption and time action, these are of neither statistical significance nor practical importance[4] (Figure 14).

By early 1973, Lilly Regular Insulin was being produced at a neutral instead of an acid pH.

Figure 14. A Comparison of the Blood Glucose and Serum Insulin Responses Following Administration of Neutral Regular Insulin and Acid Regular Insulin, 0.3 Unit per Kg. Subcutaneously

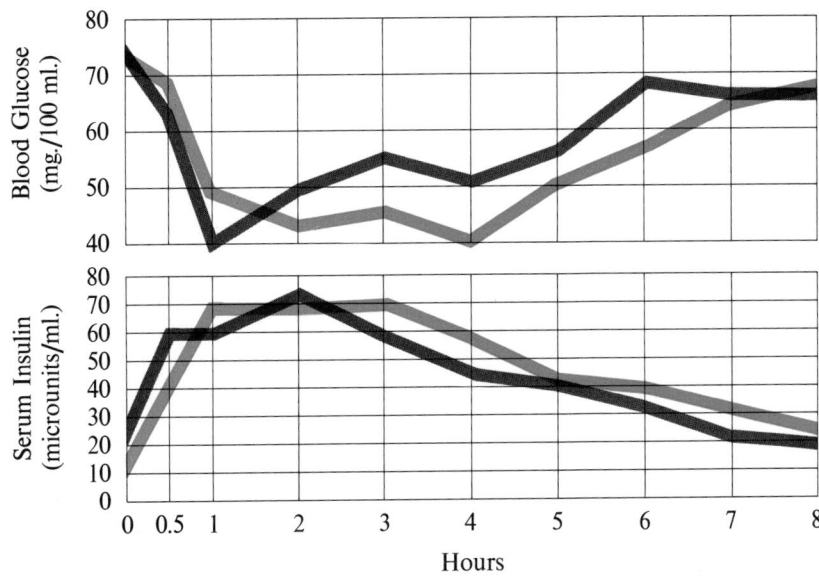

Neutral Regular Insulin

Acid Regular Insulin

The values represent the mean of four normal male subjects after an overnight fast.

PROTAMINE ZINC INSULIN

Beginning as early as 1923, attempts were made to prolong the blood-sugar-lowering effect of Regular Insulin, but none of the methods employed were found to be of practical advantage in the treatment of diabetes. Regular Insulin, which has its minimum solubility at approximately pH 5, is completely soluble at the pH of the body fluids (approximately 7.4). Therefore, following injection, it is almost immediately taken up by these fluids. Hagedorn and his co-workers, of Copenhagen, reasoned that an Insulin preparation which has a very low solubility at the pH of the body fluids might be absorbed with much less rapidity. Consequently, they developed a series of protamine Insulin preparations. It was found that when Insulin is mixed with a properly buffered solution containing protamine, the result is a protamine Insulin precipitate which has poor solubility and is slowly absorbed from body tissue. Therefore, subcutaneous injection of a suspension of the precipitate makes available a depot of supply from which Insulin is slowly dissolved by the body fluids.

Investigators in Toronto, studying the effect of adding small amounts of zinc to protamine Insulin, found that protamine Insulin preparations

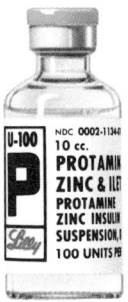

of low ash content were not as effective in the prolongation of hypoglycemic activity as were corresponding preparations to which zinc had been added. Protamine Zinc Insulin is now prepared by mixing Insulin, protamine, and zinc with a buffered solution. When this combination is brought into uniform suspension, each ml. contains 40, 80, or 100 units of Insulin, together with approximately 1.2 mg. of protamine and approximately 0.2 mg. of zinc per 100 units of Insulin.

Estimates of the duration of action of protamine Insulin preparations naturally have varied with the methods employed for its measurement. In a patient receiving food at two-hour intervals, the greatest effect of a large dose of Protamine Zinc Insulin develops from fourteen to twenty hours after its administration, and there is evidence of duration of action well beyond a twenty-four-hour period. In fasting patients, a single injection of Protamine Zinc Insulin has maintained hypoglycemic levels for as long as forty-eight to seventy-two hours. As in the case of unmodified Insulin, the larger the dose given, the more prolonged will be the effect.

GLOBIN INSULIN

Globin, another basic protein, was found to combine with Insulin in a manner similar to that of protamine. Globin Insulin was prepared and placed on clinical trial. However, since it failed to provide adequate effect for twenty-four hours, Lilly abandoned interest in this Insulin. It is available on the market through E. R. Squibb & Sons.

NPH (ISOPHANE) INSULIN

NPH Insulin was developed as a consequence of clinical investigations of a large series of intermediate-acting Insulin modifications and of mixtures of Regular Insulin and Protamine Zinc Insulin given as a single daily dose in the management of diabetes. In the majority of cases, it was found that such mixtures (usually in the ratio of two parts of Regular Insulin to one part of Protamine Zinc Insulin), administered once in the morning, would have the pharmacologic effect of doses of Protamine Zinc Insulin supplemented by separate injections of Regular Insulin.

Because of the possibility of errors in dosage and the relative inconvenience of extemporaneous mixtures, a preparation was sought that would be as stable as Protamine Zinc Insulin yet incorporate the desirable time activity of a mixture. At the Hagedorn laboratories in Copenhagen, it was discovered that careful control of the ratio of protamine and Insulin made it possible to produce a crystalline entity which contained both Insulin and the modifier. "Isophane," the generic name applied to this Insulin, was coined by Hagedorn and was based on the Greek *iso* and *phane* meaning "equal" and "appearance." The isophane point describes those conditions in which the amounts of protamine and Insulin approach stoichiometric proportion so that the crystals being formed leave behind no protamine or Insulin. The resulting product became known as NPH Insulin (NPH was a code designation used during the clinical trial; the

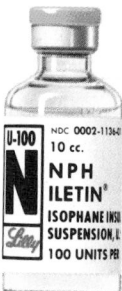

"N" indicated a neutral *p*H, the "P" denoted the presence of protamine, and the "H" referred to Hagedorn, its discoverer).

From studies of a large series of possible modifications, NPH Insulin was found to duplicate very closely the clinical effects and timing which seem most suitable for the greatest number of cases. Because of its more rapid intensity of action after injection plus its moderate overlapping effect, NPH Insulin incorporates some of the advantages of Regular Insulin and eliminates some of the disadvantages of Protamine Zinc Insulin. The duration of effect of NPH Insulin, although not as great as that of Protamine Zinc Insulin, usually is sufficiently long to protect the patient from one day to the next.

LENTE® INSULIN PREPARATIONS

As previously stated, the basic principle involved in the prolongation of action of Insulin has been the production of a material with low solubility at the *p*H of the body fluids. Relative insolubility of different modifications has accounted for the various intermediate timing characteristics observed with NPH Insulin, Globin Insulin with zinc, or mixtures of Protamine Zinc and unmodified Insulin.

However, a new concept in the chemistry of Insulin and zinc was made possible through the formulation of a relatively insoluble Insulin without the need for a modifying protein. Although it had been shown as early as 1935 that zinc had a delaying action on the absorption of Insulin, the precise mechanism was not extensively investigated until 1951, when Hallas-Møller and his associates[5] clarified this relationship.

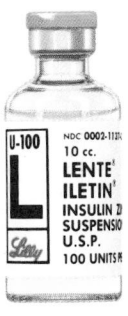

When the concentration of zinc was increased to ten times the amount required for the formation of soluble zinc-Insulin crystals and when the buffer solution was simultaneously changed from phosphate to acetate, the higher concentration of zinc could be made to combine with the Insulin in such a way that the resulting product was insoluble at *p*H 7.4. Two physical forms of the high-zinc Insulin compound can be produced by careful adjustment of the *p*H, one crystalline and one either amorphous or microcrystalline. The crystalline form is much more insoluble and, therefore, is very long acting. The amorphous form presents more surface area to the body fluids and is more quickly absorbed. With the basic term "Lente®" to indicate slow action, the two preparations were designated "Ultralente®" for the very long-acting crystalline form and "Semilente®" for the shorter-acting amorphous form.

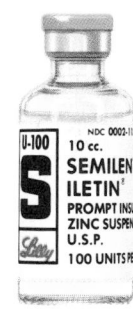

Clinical evaluation disclosed that perhaps the most practical timing could be achieved by utilizing a portion of each physical form in a mixture combining approximately 70 percent of the Ultralente and 30 percent of the Semilente form. This mixture, designated simply as "Lente Insulin," has almost precisely the same characteristics as NPH Insulin or the 2:1 mixture of unmodified Insulin and Protamine Zinc Insulin. These preparations are similar in clinical effectiveness, but Lente Insulin is free of a foreign modifying protein. By the addition of Ultralente or Semilente, mixtures can be "tailor-made" for patients not adequately controlled by Lente alone. Activity curves of these Insulins are shown in Figure 15.

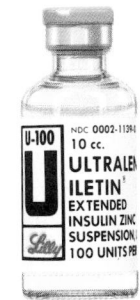

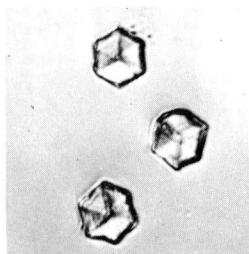

Crystalline Zinc Insulin
(300×)

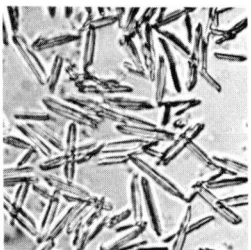

NPH Insulin (300×)

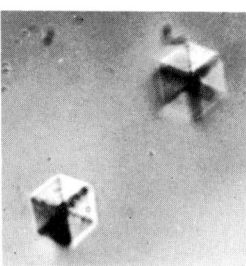

Ultralente Insulin (300×)

Ultralente® Insulin has been found to be satisfactory when given in single doses, but it is most useful when mixed with Lente® Insulin in the treatment of patients who manifest inadequate control of the blood sugar in the fasting phase.

Semilente® Insulin is particularly useful in accelerating the action of Lente Insulin when control of the postprandial blood sugar with Lente Insulin alone is less than satisfactory.

The types and characteristics of the Insulins available in the United States from Lilly are summarized in Table 9. The crystals of zinc Insulin, NPH Insulin, and Ultralente Insulin are shown on the left.

Table 9. Lilly Insulin Preparations Used in the United States

TYPE OF INSULIN	APPEARANCE	ACTION	PEAK ACTIVITY (HOURS)	DURATION (HOURS)	ZINC CONTENT (MG./100 UNITS)	pH BUFFER	PROTEIN TYPE	PROTEIN MG./100 UNITS
Regular Crystalline	Clear	Rapid	2-4	5-7	0.01-0.04	7.2	None	—
NPH	Turbid	Intermediate	6-12	24-28	0.01-0.04	Phosphate 7.2	Protamine	0.4
Protamine Zinc	Turbid	Prolonged	14-24	36+	0.15-0.25	Phosphate 7.2	Protamine	1-1.5
Semilente	Turbid	Rapid	2-4	12-16	0.14-0.25	Acetate	None	—
Lente	Turbid	Intermediate	6-12	24-28	0.14-0.25	Acetate 7.2	None	—
Ultralente	Turbid	Prolonged	18-24	36+	0.14-0.25	Acetate 7.2	None	—

UNIT OF INSULIN

One of the first tasks confronting the early workers in the development of Insulin was that of establishing a reference standard for determining its potency. The first standards were based on the hypoglycemic effect of Insulin on rabbits. However, with improved technics of extraction and manufacture, the potency of the Insulin solutions became greater, and this resulted in increasing variations in the value of the unit in terms of actual hypoglycemic activity. To insure uniformity in all laboratories, a number of Insulin manufacturers and researchers joined efforts in the preparation of a quantity of Insulin in a dry, stable form. With this material, the unit was carefully determined with respect to the standard preparation and redefined in terms of exact weight. As the quantity of standard became exhausted, new standards were prepared and assayed co-operatively; the increasing potency with improvement in manufacturing procedures was taken into account. The first standard of Insulin contained approximately 8 units per mg. By 1935, the unit was defined as 1/22 mg., and the present standard is 24 units per mg.

Originally the unit of Insulin was based on the physiological reaction of rabbits, but now it is based on an absolute weight of Insulin prepared from a recrystallized composite sample. The U.S.P. standard and the International standard are the same.

Figure 15. Comparative Time Activities of the Various Insulins

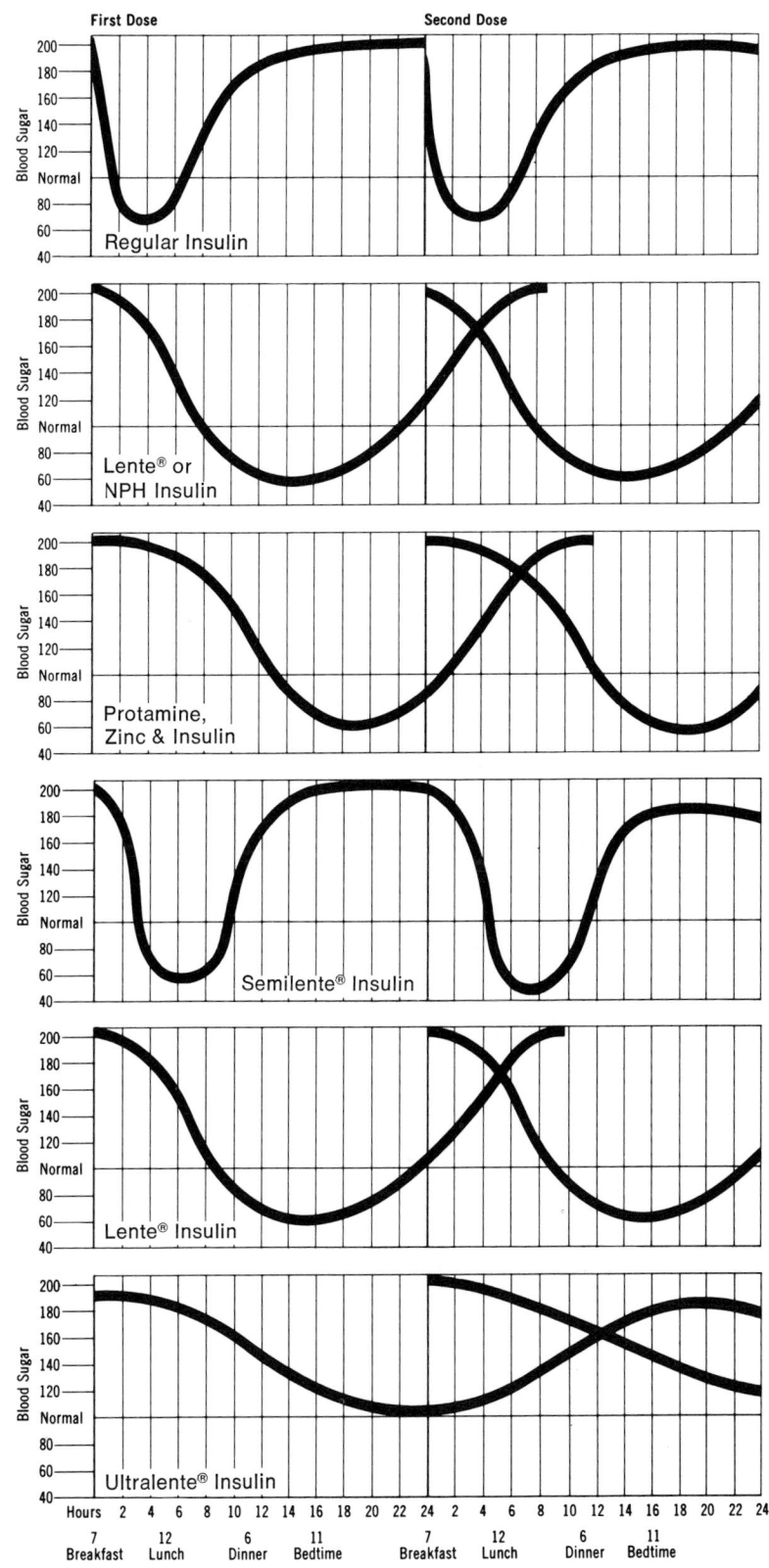

PROINSULIN

Although it had been widely held that insulin was formed in the beta cells by a joining of the "A" and "B" chains, Givol et al.[6] suggested that the biosynthesis of insulin was accomplished by transformation of a single-chain precursor. Two groups of scientists, working independently, made discoveries which unequivocally support this concept.

At the University of Chicago, Steiner and Oyer[7] found that if leucine was labeled with tritium and incubated with tissue from an islet-cell adenoma and the tumor was then extracted and purified, two peaks of radioactivity occurred. One clearly represents insulin. The other, present in smaller quantities, was of a larger molecular size than insulin but reacted with insulin antiserum and, following treatment with trypsin, was converted to an insulin-like material. This larger molecule could be further transformed into "A" and "B" chains of insulin. Their findings led Steiner and Oyer to conclude that the larger-molecular-weight material was, in fact, a precursor of insulin, or "proinsulin." Additional studies with commercial beef Insulin crystals[8,9] confirmed the presence not only of proinsulin but of intermediate forms between proinsulin and insulin as well as aggregates of insulin.

At about the same time, Chance, Ellis, and Bromer,[10] working with porcine Insulin at the Lilly Research Laboratories in an effort to improve the purity of the product, also found a larger-molecular-weight material which appeared as a single band when separated on columns containing diethylaminoethyl (DEAE) cellulose and urea-containing buffers. This

Figure 16. The Primary Structure of Porcine Proinsulin (After Chance[11])

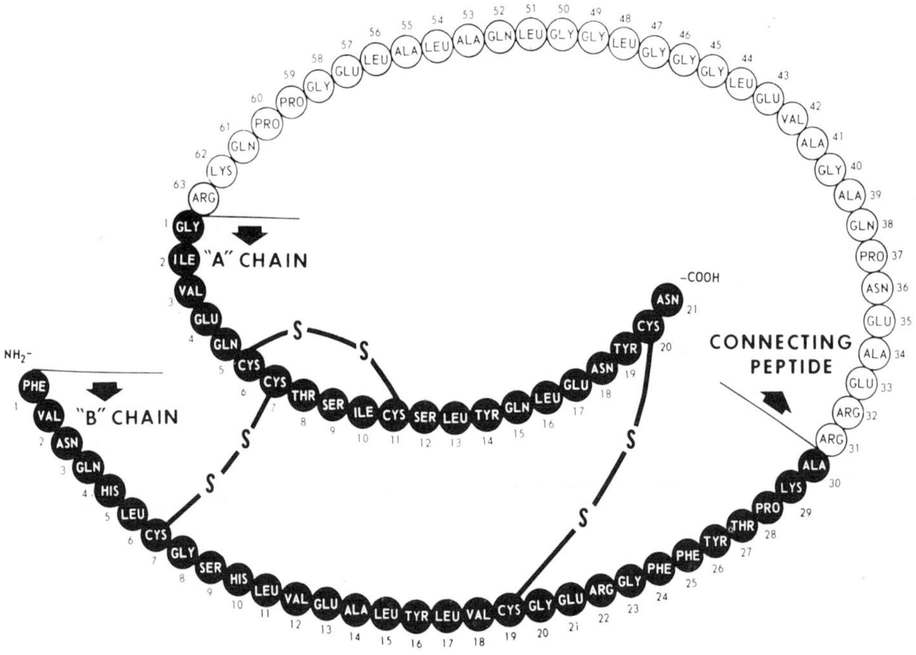

The sequence of porcine proinsulin is represented by the amino acids in the darker circles. The sequence of the connecting peptide reported by Chance, Ellis, and Bromer[10] is depicted by the amino acids in the open circles.

Figure 17a. Purity Profiles of Lilly Beef-Pork Insulins

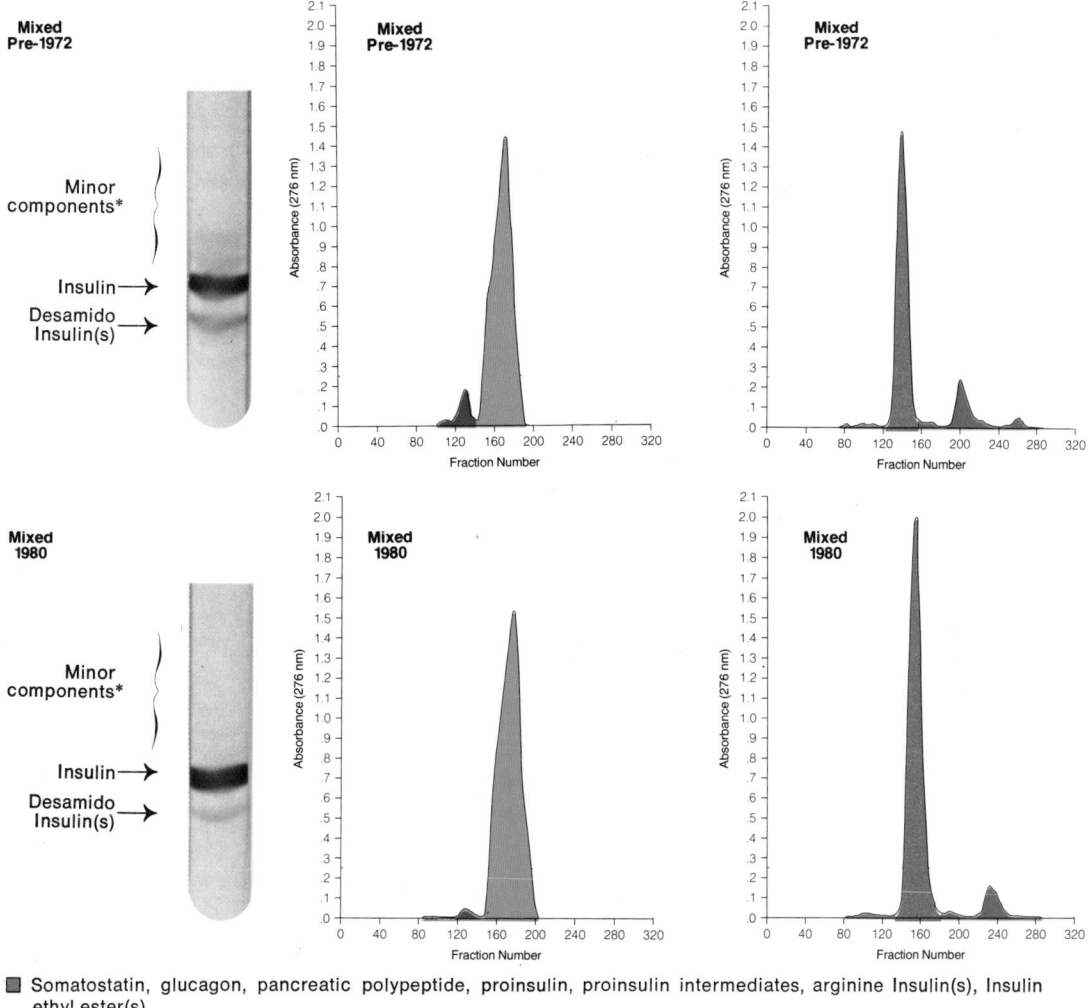

* ■ Somatostatin, glucagon, pancreatic polypeptide, proinsulin, proinsulin intermediates, arginine Insulin(s), Insulin ethyl ester(s)

■ Insulin

■ Desamido Insulin(s)

■ Proinsulin, proinsulin intermediates, Insulin dimer(s), unidentified proteins

■ Insulin, desamido Insulin(s), arginine Insulin(s), Insulin ethyl ester(s), glucagon, pancreatic polypeptide, somatostatin

fraction (proinsulin) consisted of about 1 percent of the Insulin material and had a biological and immunologic activity approximately 10 to 20 percent that of Insulin. Specifically, porcine proinsulin in the mouse convulsion assay has a potency of about 3 units per mg. Further research showed that its molecular structure consisted of the "A" and "B" chains of Insulin plus thirty-three amino acids (Figure 16).

In addition to extensive work on commercial Insulin preparations, studies have been made of endogenous human proinsulin and C-peptide, the fragment released from proinsulin during the formation of insulin (see Chapter 5).

Although many additional technics probably will be developed to simplify the procedures now needed for the synthesis of Insulin, it seems unlikely that Insulin prepared by total chemical synthesis will be available for general use for many years. However, the chemical synthesis of Insulin does afford a valuable new approach to such research problems as the structure-activity relationships of Insulin and the mechanism of its action. Insulins may be specifically modified or changed to test a hypothesis as to the role of certain specific parts or functional groups of the molecule or to facilitate tracing the fate of the molecule in the living organism and thus aid in the unraveling of the mysteries of diabetes itself.

PURITY OF INSULIN

The chromatographic technics used in the identification of proinsulin[7-10] have been employed to assess the composition of commercial Insulins. These recently developed analytical methods include:

1. *Polyacrylamide gel electrophoresis* (PAGE)—separates proteins in an electrical field on the basis of both net electrical charge and molecular size.

2. *Gel-filtration chromatography* (e.g., Sephadex™ G-50)—separates substances on the basis of molecular size.

3. *Ion-exchange chromatography* (e.g., DEAE-cellulose)—separates molecules on the basis of net electrical charge.

These procedures, supplemented by even newer analytical tools, such as high-pressure liquid chromatography (HPLC) and specific radioimmunoassays for proinsulin, proinsulin-like materials, glucagon, pancreatic polypeptide (PP), and somatostatin, provide an impressive battery of assay technics to evaluate and monitor Insulin purity. More than twenty different proteins and polypeptides have been identified in the conventional U.S.P. Insulin made by Lilly prior to 1972; the primary purification procedures used then were isoelectric precipitation and crystallization.

In 1972, Lilly incorporated gel-filtration chromatography into its manufacturing processes to produce Insulin with greatly reduced levels

---

Table 10. Proinsulin Content of Insulins Commercially Available in the United States in 1980

TYPE OF INSULIN	PROINSULIN CONTENT (P.P.M.)
Conventional U.S.P.	10,000-20,000
"Single peak"*	300-3,000
"Improved single peak"†	<50
Purified pork and/or purified beef‡	<10

*All Lilly Insulins manufactured from 1972-1979.
†All Lilly mixed beef-pork Insulins marketed beginning in 1980.
‡Lilly purified pork (formerly termed "single component" or "special pork") and purified beef Insulins manufactured after late 1979.

Figure 17b. Purity Profiles of Lilly Pork Insulins

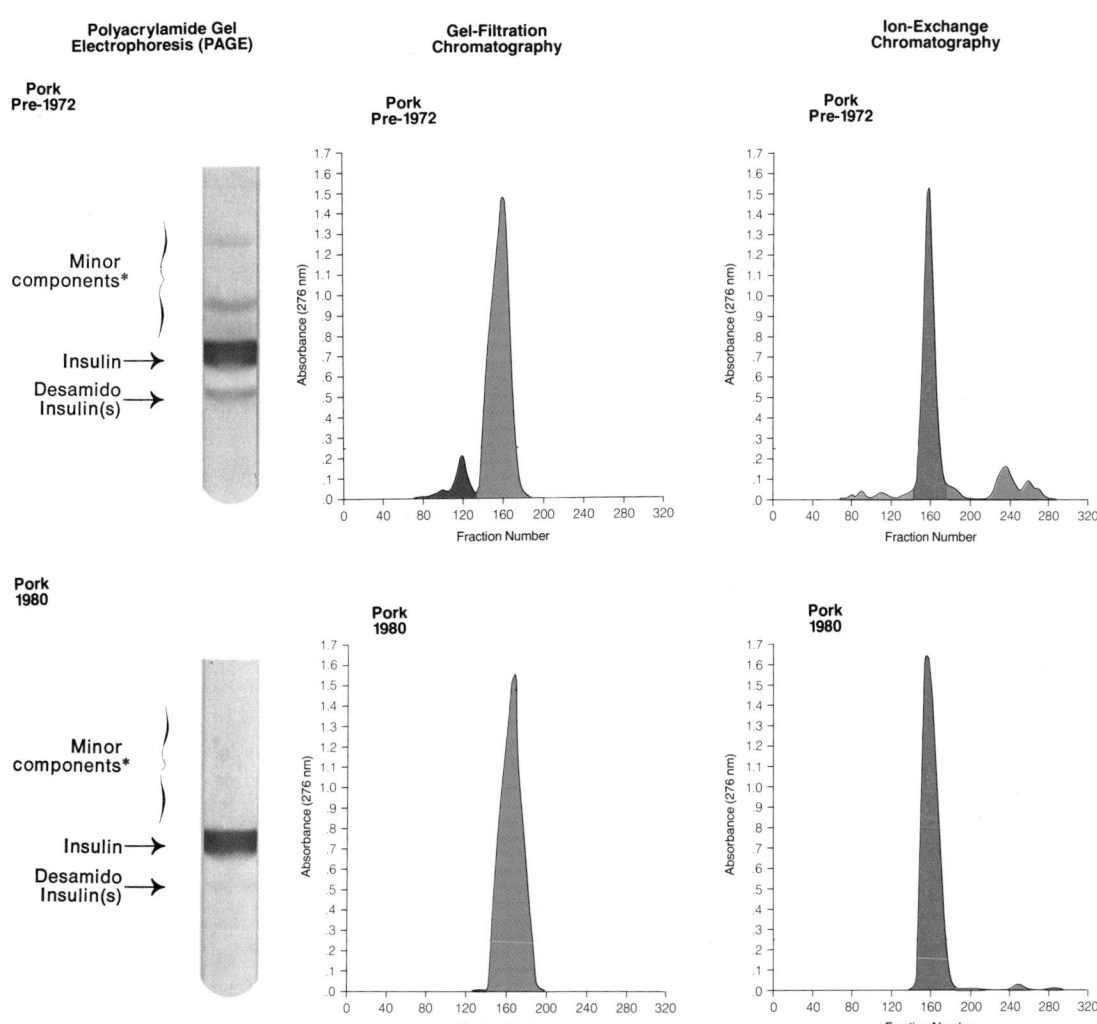

| Polyacrylamide Gel Electrophoresis (PAGE) | Gel-Filtration Chromatography | Ion-Exchange Chromatography |

Pork Pre-1972

Pork 1980

Minor components*

Insulin→

Desamido Insulin(s)→

Pork Pre-1972

Pork 1980

Pork Pre-1972

Pork 1980

Absorbance (276 nm)

Fraction Number

* ▨ Somatostatin, glucagon, pancreatic polypeptide, proinsulin, proinsulin intermediates, arginine Insulin(s), Insulin ethyl ester(s)

◻ Insulin

▨ Desamido Insulin(s)

■ Proinsulin, proinsulin intermediates, Insulin dimer(s), unidentified proteins

▨ Insulin, desamido Insulin(s), arginine Insulin(s), Insulin ethyl ester(s), glucagon, pancreatic polypeptide, somatóstatin

of large-molecular-weight materials, some of which may be immunogenic[12] and/or may play a role in the development of Insulin lipodystrophy (see pages 106 to 108) and Insulin allergy (see pages 98 to 102).[13] Insulin marketed between 1972 and 1979 yields a chromatographic profile consisting chiefly of a single peak and has been designated unofficially as "single peak."

In 1980, all Lilly Insulins began to be manufactured with the additional purification procedure of ion-exchange chromatography. Unofficially termed "improved single peak," this material contains less than 0.005

percent proinsulin, or less than 50 p.p.m. This represents approximately a 60-fold improvement over "single peak" Insulin (less than 3,000 p.p.m.) and up to a 400-fold improvement over conventional U.S.P. Insulin, which contains proinsulin in the range of 10,000 to 20,000 p.p.m. (see Table 10). Figure 17a illustrates the PAGE patterns, gel-filtration chromatography elution profiles, and ion-exchange chromatography elution profiles of Lilly mixed beef-pork Insulins produced prior to 1972 and after 1980.

Eli Lilly and Company also makes further purified pork and beef Insulins (Regular, Protamine Zinc, NPH, and Lente® only) for the small percentage of diabetic patients who demonstrate a true clinical need for such products (see Chapter 7, pages 98 to 108). These Insulins have a slightly higher degree of purity than that of "improved single peak" (see Figure 17b). Specifically, the proinsulin content of purified Insulins is in the range of 4 to 8 p.p.m. (see Table 10).

CONCENTRATION OF INSULIN

The first Insulin sold by Eli Lilly and Company in 1923 contained about 3 units per ml. With increases in purity and the desirability of reducing the volumes of fluid injected with Insulin, the concentrations available progressively increased to 10, 20, 40, 80, 100, and 500 units per ml. During the past thirty years, the chief concentrations used have been U-40 and U-80. However, in numerous instances, patients have confused the amount, concentration, or correct syringe to be used and have injected more or less than their proper doses, with ensuing hypoglycemia or hyperglycemia. As a result, the American Diabetes Association, the FDA, and Insulin suppliers agreed in 1971 that one concentration of Insulin be made available.

U-100 INSULIN

This concentration of Insulin was introduced in the United States early in 1973. Since U-80 Insulin is no longer certifiable by the FDA, it is likely that, by the end of 1980, more than 90 percent of the units used in the United States will be U-100. Now that the potential for patient dosage errors that result from having Insulin available in two different high concentrations has been reduced, the true clinical need for a low-strength Insulin (U-40) is being evaluated.

THE CHEMICAL SYNTHESIS OF INSULIN

Probably the most significant achievement in the chemistry of Insulin since the determination of its primary structure by Sanger and his colleagues[14] is the total synthesis of material having insulin activity. Accomplishment of this enormous undertaking was achieved by three groups[15-17] working independently in West Germany, China, and Pittsburgh. The approach used was to synthesize the "A" and "B" chains of the molecule (see Figure 12) separately and then to join the two groups through formation of disulfide bonds between the chains. Later, using over 170 complex chemical reactions, another group[18] constructed the insulin molecule by starting with the three disulfide bonds. Although some regard chemically synthesized Insulin as eventually being a viable source of supply,[1B] the complexity of the procedure reduces the likelihood of its being feasible in the foreseeable future for the production of the tens of billions of Insulin units required to meet world needs.

HUMAN INSULIN PRODUCTION BY BACTERIA

One of the more exciting recent developments in medical research has been the production of Insulin by bacteria that have been genetically altered. Recent research by scientists at the City of Hope National Medical Institute and at the Genentech Company has led to the chemical synthesis and cloning of the "A" and "B" chains of human insulin. *Escherichia coli* bacteria transformed with these recombinant plasmids have produced small amounts of the "A" and "B" peptide chains. These chains are then chemically recombined to form immunologically active insulin. Just what clinical advantages this procedure will have and how economically practical it may prove to be remain to be seen. Nevertheless, such a scientific accomplishment has exciting potential.

BIBLIOGRAPHY

1. Orci, L.: The Microanatomy of the Islets of Langerhans, Metabolism, *25:*1303, 1976.

1A. Lacy, P. E.: Beta Cell Secretion—from the Standpoint of a Pathobiologist, Diabetes, *19:*895, 1970.

1B. Steiner, D. F.: Insulin Today, Diabetes, *26:*322, 1977.

1C. Hodgkin, D. C.: Diabetes, *21:*1131, 1972.

1D. Blundell, T. L., Dodson, G., Hodgkin, D., and Mercola, D.: Adv. Protein Chem., *26:*279, 1972.

2. Jackson, R. L., Størvick, W. D., Hollindeu, C. S., Stroeh, L., and Stilz, J. G.: Neutral Regular Insulin, Diabetes, *21:*235, 1972.

3. Jackson, R. L.: Personal communication.

4. Galloway, J. A., and Root, M. A.: New Forms of Insulin, Diabetes, *21*(Supplement 2):637, 1972.

5. Hallas-Moller, K., Jersild, M., Petersen, K., and Schlichtkrull, J.: Clinical Investigations on New Insulin Preparations with Protracted Action; Insulin-Zinc Preparations Used in One Daily Injection, Ugesk. læger, *113:*1767, 1951.

6. Givol, D., De Lorenzo, F., Goldberger, R. F., and Anfinsen, C. B.: Disulfide Interchange and the Three-Dimensional Structure of Proteins, Proc. Nat. Acad. Sc., *53:*676, 1965.

7. Steiner, D. F., and Oyer, P. E.: The Biosynthesis of Insulin and a Probable Precursor of Insulin by a Human Islet Cell Adenoma, Proc. Nat. Acad. Sc., *57:*473, 1967.

8. Steiner, D. F., Clark, J. L., Nolan, C., Rubenstein, A. H., Margoliash, E., Aten, B., and Oyer, P. E.: Proinsulin and the Biosynthesis of Insulin, Recent Progr. Hormone Res., *25:*207, 1969.

9. Steiner, D. F., Hallund, O., Rubenstein, A. H., Cho, S., and Bayliss, C.: Isolation and Properties of Proinsulin, Intermediate Forms, and Other Minor Components from Crystalline Bovine Insulin, Diabetes, *17:*725, 1968.

10. Chance, R. E., Ellis, R. M., and Bromer, W. W.: Porcine Proinsulin: Characterization and Amino Acid Sequence, Science, *161:*165, 1968.

11. Chance, R. E.: Amino Acid Sequences of Proinsulins and Intermediates, Diabetes, *21* (Supplement 2): 461, 1972.

12. Root, M. A., Chance, R. E., and Galloway, J. A.: Immunogenicity of Insulin, Diabetes, *21* (Supplement 2):657, 1972.

13. Galloway, J. A., Root, M. A., Chance, R. E., Jackson, R. L., Wentworth, S. M., and Davidson, J. A.: New Forms of Insulin, in Endocrinology and Diabetes (edited by L. J. Kryston and R. A. Shaw), p. 329. New York: Grune & Stratton, Inc., 1975.

14. Ryle, A. P., Sanger, F., Smith, L. F., and Kitai, R.: The Disulphide Bonds of Insulin, Biochem. J., *60:*541, 1955.

15. Meienhofer, J., Schnabel, E., Bremer, H., Brinkhoff, O., Zabel, R., Sroka, W., Klostermeyer, H., Brandenburg, D., Okuda, T., and Zahn, H.: Synthese der Insulinketten und ihre Kombination zu insulinaktinen Präparaten, Ztschr. Naturforsch., *18b:*1120, 1963.

16. Katsoyannis, P. G., Fukuda, K., Tometsko, A., Suzuki, K., and Tilak, M.: Insulin Peptides. X. The Synthesis of the B-Chain of Insulin and Its Combination with Natural or Synthetic A-Chain to Generate Insulin Activity, J. Am. Chem. Soc., *86:*930, 1964.

17. Wang, Y., Hsu, J. Z., Chang, W. C., Cheng, L. L., Hsing, C. Y., Chi, A. H., Loh, T. P., Li, C. H., Shi, P. T., and Yieh, Y. H.: A Preliminary Report on the Synthesis of the A-Chain of Bovine Insulin, Sc. sinica, *8:*2030, 1965.

18. Brandenburg, D., and Wollmer, A.: The Effect of Nonpeptide Interchain Cross-Link on the Reoxidation of Reduced Insulin, Hoppe Seylers Z. Physiol. Chem., *354:*613, 1973.

Glucose-Regulating Substances in Blood

5

The measurement of insulin and other hormones that occur only in minute concentrations in body fluids, chiefly plasma or serum,* has posed a major stumbling block to the understanding of the pathophysiology of diabetes and other endocrine disorders. Among the technics employed were in-vivo assays using adrenalectomized, hypophysectomized diabetic rats and in-vitro bioassays using rat diaphragm or epididymal fat pad together with human serum or plasma.[1-5]

However, about twenty years ago, Berson, Yalow, and associates[6,6A,7] pursued their observation that, in Insulin-treated diabetics, the disappearance of intravenously administered radio-labeled Insulin was delayed (a phenomenon that they attributed to the formation of antibodies to therapeutic Insulin). They immunized guinea pigs with Insulin and utilized the immune serums in their procedure. Their assay was based on two phenomena: First, when Insulin is added to insulin antibody, insulin is bound by the antibody in a reversible reaction which follows the Law of Mass Action. In other words, after equilibrium has been obtained, the amount of insulin bound (B) to antibody depends on the quantities of free insulin (F) and antibody in the system.

Second, whereas free insulin (F) moves only slightly in an electrical field (hydrodynamic electrophoresis) when applied to a strip of filter paper, antibody-bound insulin (B) migrates down the strip away from the point of application. By use of tracer amounts of radioactive Insulin, the amount of the hormone in the two zones representing the bound and free forms can be measured. The binding ability of the antibody produced in a guinea pig by administration of Insulin is tested against a known amount

---

*When the insulin content of the blood is determined, the term "serum" or "plasma" is used, depending on the preference of the investigator. There is no evidence that red blood cells contain insulin.

of the hormone by calculating the ratio of bound to free (B:F) insulin. Plasma samples can be substituted for the known insulin standard. The B:F ratio will indicate the amount of insulin present.

Modifications in the Berson-Yalow insulin immunoassay have been made by Morgan and Lazarow[8] and others[9-13] and have resulted in simplified but accurate methods which are now widely used.

INSULIN SECRETION IN HEALTH AND DISEASE

The availability of accurate methods to measure insulin in the blood has been a major breakthrough in the understanding of insulin secretion in health and disease. In particular, it has been possible to identify a number of stimuli which affect the insulin secretory response to glucose and other substances and to assess the importance of insulin and contra-insulin factors in various stages and degrees of severity of diabetes. Finally, the immunoassay for insulin has been the prototype for the accurate measurement of other polypeptide hormones which are important in carbohydrate homeostasis.[14]

Measurement of plasma insulin has brought about a major revision of the former view that the chief, if not sole, stimulus for insulin secretion is the concentration of glucose in the blood supplying the beta cell. In experiments[15] comparing the plasma insulin and blood glucose levels after intravenous and intragastric administration of glucose (by nasogastric tube), plasma insulin levels are higher and more sustained following the latter method of glucose administration.

Perley and Kipnis[16] confirmed and added to these findings by infusing glucose intravenously at a rate calculated to simulate blood glucose levels achieved by the oral route. They found that, in normal-weight and obese diabetic and nondiabetic subjects, the response to intravenous glucose was only 30 to 40 percent of that to oral glucose. The fact that this phenomenon occurred also in patients whose portal circulation is diverted to (i.e., connected with) the systemic circulation made it possible to localize the factor(s) which augment insulin secretion in the intestinal tract after oral glucose. These have been reviewed by Dupré and Chisholm.[17] For instance, secretin, pancreozymin-cholecystokinin, gastrin, "gut glucagon,"* and neutral factors have been shown to have an effect on insulin secretion. Although, to date, the effect of none of these factors alone has been demonstrated to be sufficient to account for the increased insulin response to oral over intravenous glucose, available data suggest that several of these factors may work in concert, perhaps with other substances associated with the gastro-intestinal tract, to augment the release of insulin and disposal of glucose administered orally.

Stimuli that release insulin

---

*Unger et al.[18,19] identified material from the gastro-intestinal tissues of several species, including man, which cross-reacted with antibodies against pancreatic glucagon. Because this material did not react consistently with pancreatic glucagon antiserums, these workers surmised that the material was "glucagon-like" and not glucagon. Although increased concentrations of this material occur in the plasma after administration of glucose, a number of absorbable monosaccharides have a similar effect. However, the potential importance of glucagon-like substance is minimized somewhat by the fact that it fails to stimulate insulin secretion in the absence of glucose and is a weak stimulus in concentrations found under physiological conditions.

In addition to glucose and intestinal factors, certain amino acids have also been shown to be capable of stimulating release of pancreatic insulin.[20] For instance, plasma insulin is increased following intravenous or oral administration of leucine. Subsequent studies[20] have disclosed that the most potent of the essential amino acids is arginine and the least potent is histidine. These effects can be demonstrated in the absence of glucose. However, no amino acid is more potent as an insulin secretagogue than a mixture of all ten essential acids. These findings indicate that the various amino acids exert their effects synergistically. Synergism has also been reported between glucose and the amino acids. Thus, under physiological conditions, glucose and amino acids work together to effect insulin release from the beta cell, and this in turn enhances the metabolic disposition of such nutrients.

Whatever the complete mechanisms are for initiating the secretion of insulin following ingestion of carbohydrates by normal subjects, they function nearly instantaneously and shut off when the need has subsided[21] (Figure 18).

In normal individuals on standard diets during the glucose tolerance test (Figure 19), plasma insulin levels rise quickly, reach a peak after thirty to sixty minutes, and then fall to normal levels.[23] In adult-onset diabetics,[7] the secretion of insulin is delayed, and at the end of two hours the level is considerably higher than normal. These findings have been interpreted as indicating not an excessive secretory response of plasma insulin but "a reflection of impaired insulin sensitivity, which results in persistence of hyperglycemia and a continuing stimulus to insulin secretion."[24]

The remarkable synchronization of insulin release with metabolic need has been studied both in vitro[25,26] and in vivo.[27-29]

Grodsky *et al.*[26] have perfused isolated rat pancreas preparations with glucose solutions (containing 300 mg. per 100 ml.) and other substances for periods up to fifty minutes and observed a multiphasic response. During the first five to six minutes, a brisk outpouring of insulin occurred. This was followed by a reduction in insulin output, after which the insulin slowly increased to its initial peak level.

On the basis of studies, these workers proposed that the insulin release system is composed of a small and a larger compartment.[25] The small one contains about 2 percent of the insulin that can be extracted from the pancreas and responds promptly to pulse delivery of such stimulants as glucose and tolbutamide. The larger compartment, storing about 98 percent of the insulin in the pancreas system studied, replenishes insulin for the small compartment in response to a protracted period of exposure to increased concentration of glucose in the perfusate.

In-vivo studies have been carried out in normal and diabetic subjects immediately after the intravenous administration of glucose and/or glucagon[27] and other substances.[28,29] Normals respond to glucose and to glucagon in three to five minutes with a brisk increase in plasma insulin.

Potential diabetics (offspring of two diabetic parents) have a subnormal response in the early phase of insulin release, and nonobese, non-Insulin-dependent diabetics have no response to glucose. Thus, ex-

Figure 18. Serum Insulin Responses to Oral Glucose in Obese Normals, Obese Diabetics, Thin Normals, and Thin Diabetics (After Bagdade *et al.*[22])

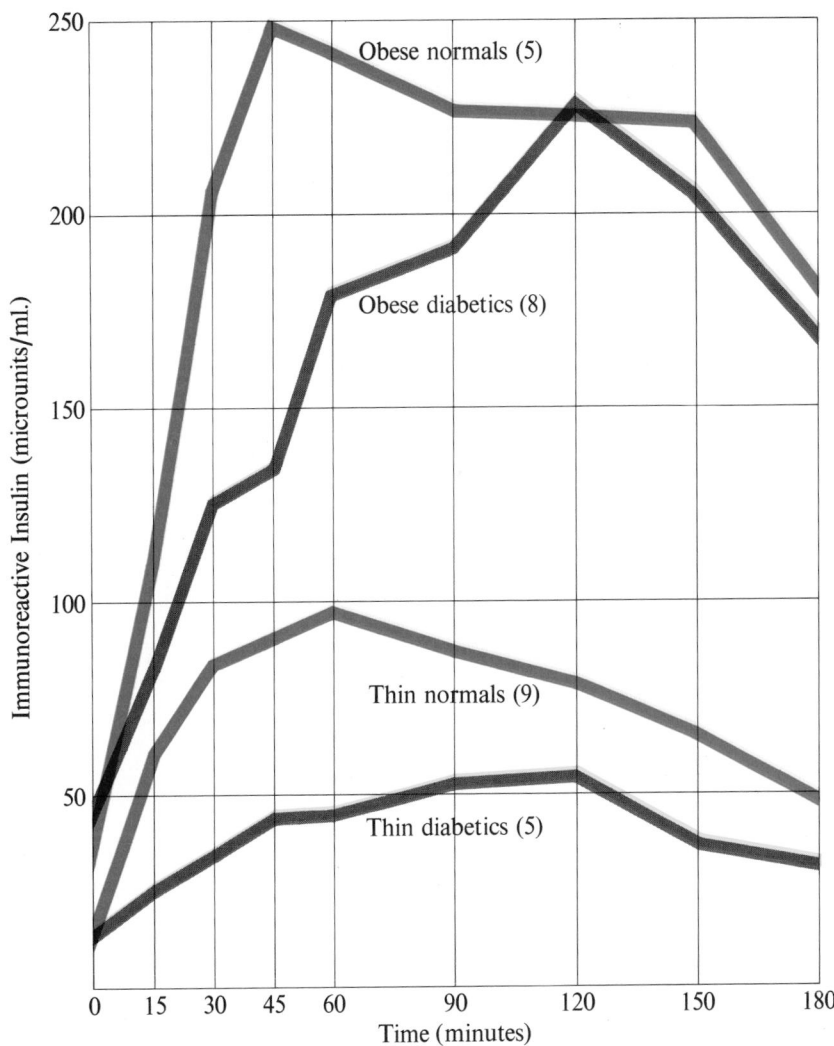

These data show that (1) the insulin response of normal-weight diabetics is less than that of normal subjects, (2) the insulin response of obese diabetics is less than that of obese normals, and (3) obesity is associated with increased insulin levels. Note also that both thin and obese diabetics have a slow rise and delayed peak in serum concentration of insulin in relation to their normal counterparts.

perimental models have been designed which can both detect and, in part, explain early abnormalities in beta-cell function.

Because plasma insulin levels are elevated also in obesity,[30] it has been speculated that the reported hyperinsulinism is due to obesity. In order to examine this point, investigators categorized nondiabetic subjects and untreated nonketotic diabetic patients according to body weight and plasma insulin response during glucose tolerance testing.[31] This study confirmed that obesity combined with abnormal glucose tolerance resulted in the highest insulin levels. However, when the insulin responses were examined on the basis of glucose tolerance (severely impaired glucose tolerance

Insulin levels in obesity

is defined as a blood sugar higher than 300 mg. per 100 ml. at two hours), it was found that the patients with the greatest impairment of glucose tolerance had the lowest plasma insulin levels in both the nonobese and obese groups. Higher plasma insulin levels were found in the obese and nonobese patients who had a better ability to metabolize carbohydrate.

Seltzer *et al.*[32] confirm that, during the latter portion of the glucose tolerance tests, plasma insulin levels in adult-onset diabetics may be higher than those found in normal individuals. However, they point out that, in relation to the blood sugar value, the amount of insulin secreted is less than normal.

Figure 19. Blood Glucose and Serum Insulin Response of Normal Subjects to Feeding and Fasting

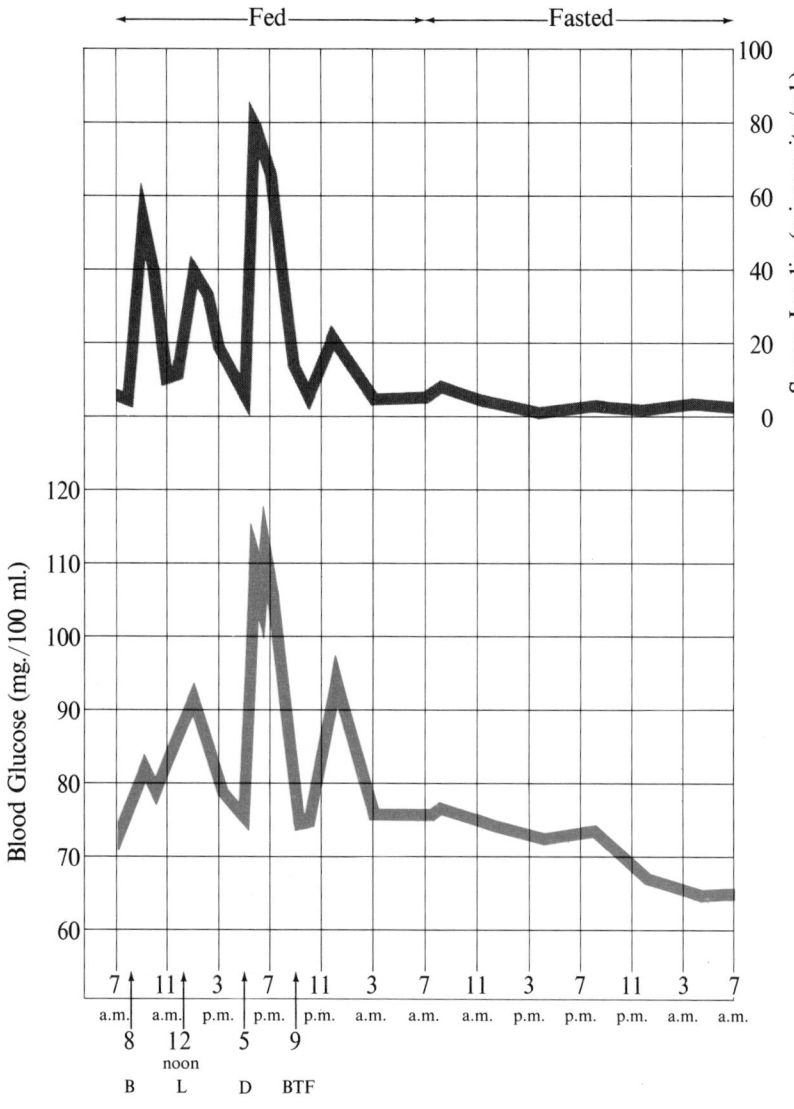

Six normal men received a balanced daily diet consisting of 30 calories per Kg. of body weight: 2/7 with breakfast (B), 2/7 with lunch (L), 2/7 with dinner (D), and 1/7 as a bedtime feeding (BTF). This figure demonstrates the insulin response to fasting as well as to feeding.[23]

Measurement of insulin by the fat pad method has produced a number of interesting and curious findings. Insulin measured by this method is called "insulin-like activity," because the values often exceed those reached by the diaphragm and immunologic methods and suggest the presence of other factors or substances in addition to insulin. In prediabetics as compared with controls, elevated levels of ILA were observed both in the fasting state and after an intravenous glucose load.[33] In another study, abnormally elevated ILA and delayed response to glucose loading were found in adult-onset patients but not in dogs following pancreatectomy.[34] Diabetes subsequently developed in two of seven "normal" subjects (from a group of twenty-seven) who had elevated ILA.

Insulin-like activity

The finding of hyperinsulinism by both methods after glucose loading provides an explanation for the report[35] that postprandial hypoglycemia is a manifestation of early adult-onset diabetes.

The fasting and postprandial blood glucose and ILA were measured in untreated diabetics and in patients treated with Insulin. Reaven and Salans[36] noted that hyperglycemia frequently persisted in both groups in the presence of elevated ILA values. These findings suggest that interference with the hypoglycemic effect of insulin may represent an important characteristic of diabetes.

Very low plasma insulin levels are seen in patients with growth-onset diabetes and in chronic pancreatitis.[37] When the immunologic method is used, low plasma insulin levels are also observed in diabetic ketosis.[37-39] However, when the rat diaphragm method is used, insulin has been detected in the serum and protein fractions in most patients with diabetic ketosis. By means of an immunologic method, infants of diabetic mothers were found to have elevated insulin levels at birth; in two of five instances, this high level persisted for more than twenty hours.[40]

HYPOGLYCEMIA

POSTPRANDIAL HYPOGLYCEMIA IN THE POSTGASTRECTOMY SYNDROME

Several investigators[41,42] have reported high insulin levels as a result of the hyperglycemia seen with the absorption of glucose in patients after gastrectomy. Hypoglycemia occurs because of an "overshoot" of the insulin response;[41] i.e., after the initial stimulus, there is an insufficiency of glucose to offset the insulin which has been elaborated.

FASTING HYPOGLYCEMIA

It had been thought that insulin determinations would obviate the need for repeated and extended glucose tolerance tests in those patients with hypoglycemia due to islet-cell tumor. However, fasting plasma insulin levels have been elevated in only about 50 percent of the cases. The variability of these fasting insulin levels has been explained by the fact that the plasma concentration is subject to rapid, spontaneous fluctuations.

Fortunately, it is now fairly well established[43] that the secretion of insulin in patients with islet-cell tumor can be stimulated by tolbutamide. The plasma insulins, in most instances, can then be demonstrated to be elevated to diagnostic levels by all three methods of in-vitro assay discussed here.

Non-islet-cell tumors which are associated with hypoglycemia usually do not contain insulin as determined by immunologic methods.[44] However, in a recent review, Ginsberg[45] recorded several instances of high insulin activity as determined by the rat fat pad and diaphragm assays. Nonetheless, the mechanism of hypoglycemia is not known in many cases.

One of the enigmas of insulin-like activity is that hypophysectomy in dogs[46] results in 50 percent reduction in serum ILA and that subsequent pancreatectomy fails to reduce ILA further. Hypophysectomized dogs have no insulin measurable by immunoassay. Another paradox about ILA is that its activity is not suppressed by insulin antibodies.[47,48]

HUMAN PROINSULIN—"BIG" AND "LITTLE" INSULIN

If samples of human serum or urine are extracted with acid-ethanol and filtered on G-50 Sephadex, two peaks of immunologic activity can be detected, one corresponding to insulin and the other to proinsulin.[49] When Roth et al.[50] also found two peaks, they called one "big" insulin and the other "little" insulin. The conclusion that "big" insulin is proinsulin and "little" insulin is insulin is supported by the finding that tryptic digestion of the proinsulin peak converted proinsulin to insulin-like components.[51]

Experience with G-50 Sephadex separation and immunoassay for insulin calls attention to several assay problems in the evaluation of circulating levels of proinsulin and insulin. First, because human proinsulin is extremely difficult to obtain, the amount available has been insufficient to permit preparation of human antiproinsulin serum for use in an immunoassay. Secondly, even if human proinsulin serum were available, the cross-reactivity between insulin and proinsulin makes it necessary for the two substances to be separated before assay.

Another difficulty with the present methods for measuring human proinsulin is that proinsulin and some of the intermediate forms between proinsulin and insulin which may be present in the serum have an almost identical reaction to antiproinsulin serum.[52] These intermediate forms cannot be removed by gel filtration.

In the fasting state, normal subjects have proinsulin values in the range of 0.05 to 0.4 ng. per ml., and these account for 5 to 48 percent of the fasting insulin concentration.[51] During the performance of glucose tolerance tests, proinsulin levels normally rise along with the insulin level. In obese subjects with hyperinsulinemia, the insulin-proinsulin ratio is comparable to that found in normal individuals. Furthermore, in their oral glucose tolerance tests, the percentage of proinsulin tends to diminish during the first hour of the test but increases by the second hour to the fasting level. These findings are consistent with those of Gorden and Roth,[53] who speculate that the insulin released within the first hour of the oral glucose tolerance test represents already synthesized material but that the levels of proinsulin found at two hours represent newly synthesized insulin.

The data on proinsulin and "big" insulin have raised many questions about the significance of past results of the immunoassay. Goldsmith et al.[54] did Sephadex separation followed by immunoassay on samples from a number of patients, including healthy normal and diabetic subjects (lean and obese) and a patient with islet-cell adenoma. Although the "big" insulin fraction constituted 24 to 55 percent of the insulin immunoreactivity in blood samples from the patient with the islet-cell adenoma, in none of the other subjects tested did the amount of proinsulin exceed 20 percent.

Because it was recognized that proinsulin is substantially less potent than insulin on a weight basis (3 units per mg. versus 25 units per mg.), Yalow and Berson[55] investigated the possibility that the lack of sensitivity to Insulin observed in some diabetic patients could be due to disproportionate increases in proinsulin levels. However, in none of twenty-five obese patients with hyperinsulinism was the "big" insulin more than 10 to 12 percent of the total Insulin concentration as measured in the routine immunoassay of Insulin with crystalline Insulin used as a standard. When corrections were made for differences in potency of the Insulin antiserum for binding proinsulin, the total amount of proinsulin measured on a molar basis was less than 15 to 18 percent of the Insulin present. Although such studies have yielded much interesting data, they have disclosed no consistent abnormality in proinsulin in diabetes.[56]

C-PEPTIDE IN HEALTH AND DISEASE

As indicated previously, the conversion of proinsulin to insulin in the beta cell results in the production of equimolar quantities of insulin and C-peptide (connecting peptide). Because insulin and C-peptide concentrations correlate over a wide range and commercial Insulin is essentially free of C-peptide, the evaluation of C-peptide in Insulin-dependent diabetics provides a useful index to the amount of residual endogenous insulin produced. Human C-peptide is measured by radioimmunoassay according to procedures similar to those outlined earlier. Because this material reacts with antibodies to proinsulin and other substances present in the serum of Insulin-treated patients, these substances are separated by chromatographic means from the C-peptide before the immunoassay is performed. The source of C-peptide for the assay is either material extracted from human pancreas or synthesized peptide.

Clinical studies have disclosed that, during acute hyperglycemia with ketosis, serum concentrations of C-peptide are negligible. However, when the blood glucose is returned to normal levels, C-peptide concentrations rise. In adult-onset diabetics, the serum C-peptide may be at normal or near-normal levels, and this is associated with mild diabetes. In juvenile diabetics at the time of the initial acute hyperglycemic phase, the C-peptide concentrations are exceedingly low but may then increase even to near-normal levels during remission. However, in the remission phase, C-peptide rises in response to protein but not to carbohydrate stimuli.[57] Following remission, the usual pattern in juvenile diabetes is for the C-peptide to decrease during the first few years of the disease. Unmeasurable C-peptide concentrations are the rule in labile, or brittle, juvenile diabetes.

Serum C-peptide measurement is a useful procedure in distinguishing patients with hypoglycemia secondary to endogenous hyperinsulinism (e.g., islet-cell tumors) from those with factitious hyperinsulinism resulting from exogenous Insulin. Normally, hypoglycemia shuts off insulin secretion, but islet-cell tumors behave autonomously. In this condition, the blood glucose will be reduced, but serum insulin and C-peptide will be elevated. In factitious hyperinsulinism, blood glucose and serum C-peptide will be reduced, but serum insulin will be elevated.

C-peptide measurements have provided new insights into the natural history of insulin secretion in both normal subjects and patients with diabetes of varying degrees of severity. It is hoped that an extension of such studies will lead to ways of preserving endogenous insulin secretion and thereby reduce the severity of the metabolic disorder in patients with diabetes mellitus.

GLUCAGON AND OTHER HORMONES

Shortly after the development of the immunoassay for insulin, Unger[58] devised a similar assay for glucagon, which has been used to elucidate the role of this hormone in normal and diabetic subjects. The current concept (at least for Type I diabetes) is that glucagon exerts many actions that oppose those of insulin. As a result, diabetes is viewed not only as a disease of insulin deficiency but also of glucagon excess, i.e., a bihormonal disorder. Insulin deficiency is the prime cause of hyperglycemia and other abnormalities seen in diabetes, but these aberrations are amplified by the glucagon excess. Consequently, uncontrolled diabetes is associated not only with insulinopenia but also with hyperglucagonemia; however, the extent to which hyperglucagonemia contributes to hyperglycemia is controversial. (It is of interest that strict diabetic control does not significantly change the elevated plasma glucagon concentration in diabetics.)

The contribution of hormonal abnormalities in the metabolic derangements of severe diabetes, as elaborated by Raskin and Unger (Med. Clin. North Am., *62:*713, 1978), is listed below.

DERANGEMENT	INSULIN DEFICIENCY	GLUCAGON EXCESS
Underutilization of glucose	+ + + +	0
Overproduction of glucose	+ +	+ + + +
Increased lipolysis	+ + + +	+ + (?)
Increased ketogenesis	+ + (?)	+ + + +

Two other gluco-regulatory hormones in the blood that have been measured by immunoassay are growth hormone and placental lactogen.[59] Growth hormone is elevated in diabetics but can be normalized by exercise and improved control.[60] Placental lactogen has a number of contra-insulin actions, the sum effect of which is to assure an adequate flow of glucose to the fetus.[61] Its concentration in the maternal circulation is a function of placental size.

SOMATOSTATIN

A recently discovered and intensely studied gluco-regulatory substance is somatostatin.[62] It was first isolated by Guillemin and co-workers, who were investigating the growth-hormone-releasing activity of various hypothalamic extracts. One such substance had an opposite effect—inhibiting release of growth hormone from anterior pituitary cells. Subsequent studies disclosed that it was a single-chain tetradecapeptide that contained a disulfide bridge. Because initial studies suggested that this material was a specific hypothalamic hormone, it was called "growth-hormone (somatotropin)-release-inhibiting factor (S.R.I.F.)," or "somatostatin."

Studies have disclosed that somatostatin is found in a variety of human tissues, including the pancreas, and has a great many effects, e.g., suppression of endogenous glucagon, growth hormone, and insulin. Although no clear-cut clinical indication for somatostatin has yet been demonstrated, it is hoped that a related substance which specifically suppresses glucagon will eventually be developed and perhaps be found useful in the treatment of human diabetes.

BIBLIOGRAPHY

1. Yalow, R. S., and Berson, S. A.: Plasma Insulin in Man, Am. J. Med., 29:1, 1960.

2. Vallance-Owen, J.: Assays of Insulin in the Plasma, in Diabetes (edited by R. H. Williams), p. 423. New York: Paul B. Hoeber, Inc., 1960.

3. Bornstein, J.: Discussion on Plasma Insulin, in Aetiology of Diabetes Mellitus and Its Complications, Ciba Foundation Colloquia on Endocrinology, 15:148, 1964.

4. Vallance-Owen, J., and Hurlock, B.: Estimation of Plasma-Insulin by the Rat Diaphragm Method, Lancet, 1:68, 1954.

5. Martin, D. B., Renold, A. E., and Dagenais, Y. M.: An Assay for Insulin-Like Activity Using Rat Adipose Tissue, Lancet, 2:76, 1958.

6. Yalow, R. S., Bauman, A., Rothschild, M. A., and Newerly, K.: Insulin I131 Metabolism in Human Subjects: Demonstration of Insulin Binding Globulin in the Circulation of Insulin Treated Subjects, J. Clin. Invest., 35:170, 1956.

6A. Yalow, R. S., and Berson, S. A.: Immunoassay of Endogenous Plasma Insulin in Man, J. Clin. Invest., 39:1157, 1960.

7. Yalow, R. S., and Berson, S. A.: Plasma Insulin Concentrations in Nondiabetic and Early Diabetic Subjects. Determinations by a New Sensitive Immuno-Assay Technic, Diabetes, 9:254, 1960.

8. Morgan, C. R., and Lazarow, A.: Immunoassay of Insulin Using a Two-Antibody System, Proc. Soc. Exper. Biol. & Med., 110:29, 1962.

9. Grodsky, G. M., and Forsham, P. H.: An Immunochemical Assay of Total Extractable Insulin in Man, J. Clin. Invest., 39:1070, 1960.

10. Genuth, S., Frohman, L. A., and Lebovitz, H. E.: A Radioimmunological Assay Method for Insulin Using Insulin-125I and Gel Filtration, J. Clin. Endocrinol., 25:1043, 1965.

11. Hales, C. N., and Randle, P. J.: Immunoassay of Insulin with Insulin-Antibody Precipitate, Biochem. J., 88:137, 1963.

12. Goetz, F. C., Greenberg, B. Z., Ells, J., and Meinert, C.: A Simple Immunoassay for Insulin. Application to Human and Dog Plasma, J. Clin. Endocrinol., 23:1237, 1963.

13. Meade, R. C., and Klitgaard, H. M.: A Simplified Method for Immunoassay of Human Serum Insulin, J. Nucl. Med., 3:407, 1960.

14. Potts, J. T., Jr., Sherwood, L. M., O'Riordan, J. L. H., and Aurback, G. D.: Radioimmunoassay of Polypeptide Hormones, Advances Int. Med., 13:183, 1967.

15. Elrick, H., Stimmler, L., Hlad, C. J., Jr., and Arai, Y.: Plasma Insulin Response to Oral and Intravenous Glucose Administration, J. Clin. Endocrinol., 24:1076, 1964.

16. Perley, M. J., and Kipnis, D. M.: Plasma Insulin Responses to Oral and Intravenous Glucose: Studies in Normal and Diabetic Subjects, J. Clin. Invest., 46:1954, 1967.

17. Dupré, J., and Chisholm, D. J.: Gastrointestinal Factors and Insulin Release, in Diabetes Mellitus: Diagnosis and Treatment (edited by S. S. Fajans and K. E. Sussman), III:47. New York: American Diabetes Association, Inc., 1971.

18. Unger, R. H., Ketterer, H., and Eisentraut, A. M.: Distribution of Immunoassayable Glucagon in Gastrointestinal Tissues, Metabolism, 15:865, 1966.

19. Unger, R. H.: Pancreatic Glucagon in Health and Disease, Advances Int. Med., 17:265, 1971.

20. Floyd, J. C., Jr.: Dietary Stimulants to Insulin Secretion, in Diabetes Mellitus: Diagnosis and Treatment (edited by S. S. Fajans and K. E. Sussman), III:25. New York: American Diabetes Association, Inc., 1971.

21. Lerner, R. L., and Porte, D., Jr.: Insulin Secretion in Diabetes and Other Pathological States, in Diabetes Mellitus: Diagnosis and Treatment (edited by S. S. Fajans and K. E. Sussman), III:31. New York: American Diabetes Association, Inc., 1971.

22. Bagdade, J. D., Bierman, E. L., and Porte, D., Jr.: The Significance of Basal Insulin Levels in the Evaluation of the Insulin Response to Glucose in Diabetic and Nondiabetic Subjects, J. Clin. Invest., 46:1549, 1967.

23. Matsuda, A., Galloway, J. A., Diller, E. R., Rodda, B. E., and Young, E. C.: The Effect of Weight Change and Sulfonylurea Treatment on Circadian Blood Glucose and Serum Insulin in Maturity-Onset Diabetes, Diabetes, 20 (Supplement 1):366, 1971.

24. Berson, S. A., and Yalow, R. S.: Some Current Controversies in Diabetes Research, Diabetes, 14:549, 1965.

25. Grodsky, G., Landahl, H., Curry, D., and Bennett, L.: A Two-Compartmental Model for Insulin Secretion, in Early Diabetes (edited by R. A. Camerini-Dávalos and H. S. Cole), p. 45. New York: Academic Press Inc., 1970.

26. Grodsky, G. M., Bennett, L. L., Smith, D. F., and Schmid, F. G.: Effect of *Pulse* Administration of Glucose or Glucagon on Insulin Secretion in Vitro, Metabolism, 16:222, 1967.

27. Simpson, R. G., Benedetti, A., Grodsky, G. M., Karam, J. H., and Forsham, P. H.: Early Phase of Insulin Release, Diabetes, 17:684, 1968.

28. Porte, D., Jr.: Beta Adrenergic Stimulation of Insulin Release in Man, Diabetes, 16:150, 1967.

29. Siegal, A. M., Kreisberg, R. A., Owen, W. C., and Fox, O. J.: Some Aspects of "Acute Phase" Insulin Release in Healthy Subjects, Diabetes, 21:157, 1972.

30. Karam, J. H., Grodsky, G. M., and Forsham, P. H.: Excessive Insulin Response to Glucose in Obese Subjects as Measured by Immunochemical Assay, Diabetes, 12:197, 1963.

31. Yalow, R. S., Glick, S. M., Roth, J., and Berson, S. A.: Plasma Insulin and Growth Hormone Levels in Obesity and Diabetes, Ann. New York Acad. Sc., 131:357, 1965.

32. Seltzer, H. S., Allen, E. W., Herron, A. L., Jr., and Brennan, M. T.: Insulin Secretion in Response to Glycemic Stimulus: Relation of Delayed Initial Release to Carbohydrate Intolerance in Mild Diabetes Mellitus, J. Clin. Invest., 46:323, 1967.

33. Steinke, J., Soeldner, J. S., Camerini-Dávalos, R. A., and Renold, A. E.: Studies on Serum Insulin-Like Activity (ILA) in Prediabetes and Early Overt Diabetes, Diabetes, 12:502, 1963.

34. Power, L., Reyes-Leal, B., and Conn, J. W.: Serum Insulin-Like Activity in Genetic and Experimental Diabetes Mellitus, Metabolism, 13:1297, 1964.

35. Seltzer, H. S., Fajans, S. S., and Conn, J. W.: Spontaneous Hypoglycemia as an Early Manifestation of Diabetes Mellitus, Diabetes, 5:437, 1956.

36. Reaven, G., and Salans, L.: Insulin-Like Activity in Insulin-Treated Patients with Diabetes Mellitus, Ann. Int. Med., 61:680, 1964.

37. Berson, S. A., and Yalow, R. S.: Immunoassay of Plasma Insulin, in Immunoassay of Hormones, Ciba Foundation Colloquia on Endocrinology, 14:182, 1964.

38. Randle, P. J., Garland, P. B., Hales, C. N., and Newsholme, E. A.: The Glucose Fatty-Acid Cycle. Its Role in Insulin Sensitivity and the Metabolic Disturbances of Diabetes Mellitus, Lancet, 1:785, 1963.

39. Ehrlich, R. M., and Bambers, G.: Immunologic Assay of Insulin in Plasma of Children, Diabetes, 13:177, 1964.

40. Stimmler, L., Brazie, J. V., and O'Brien, D.: Plasma-Insulin Levels in the Newborn Infants of Normal and Diabetic Mothers, Lancet, 1:137, 1964.

41. Yalow, R. S., and Berson, S. A.: Dynamics of Insulin Secretion in Hypoglycemia, Diabetes, 14:341, 1965.

42. Roth, D. A., and Meade, R. C.: Hyperinsulinism-Hypoglycemia in the Postgastrectomy Patient, Diabetes, 14:526, 1965.

43. Samols, E., and Marks, V.: Insulin Assay in Insulinomas, Brit. M. J., 1:507, 1963.

44. Samols, E.: Hypoglycaemia in Neoplasia, Postgrad. M. J., 39:634, 1963.

45. Ginsberg, D. M.: Hypoglycemia Associated with Extrapancreatic Neoplasms. With a Note on Other Unusual Forms of Hypoglycemia, Advances Int. Med., 12:33, 1964.

46. Schoeffling, K., Ditschuneit, H., Petzoldt, R., Beyer, J., Pfeiffer, E. F., Sirek, A., Geerling, H., and Sirek, O. V.: Serum Insulin-Like Activity in Hypophysectomized and Depancreatized (Houssay) Dogs, Diabetes, 14:658, 1965.

47. Froesch, E. R., Bürgi, H., Ramseier, E. B., Bally, P., and Labhart, A.: Antibody-Suppressible and Non-suppressible Insulin-Like Activities in Human Serum and Their Physiologic Significance. An Insulin Assay with Adipose Tissue of Increased Precision and Specificity, J. Clin. Invest., 42:1816, 1963.

48. Samaan, N., and Fraser, R.: "Typical" and "Atypical" Serum Insulin-Like Activity in Untreated Diabetes Mellitus, Lancet, 2:311, 1963.

49. Rubenstein, A. H., Cho, S., and Steiner, D. F.: Evidence for Proinsulin in Human Urine and Serum, Lancet, 1:1353, 1968.

50. Roth, J., Gorden, P., and Pastan, I.: "Big Insulin": A New Component of Plasma Insulin Detected by Immunoassay, Proc. Nat. Acad. Sc., 61:138, 1968.

51. Melani, F., Rubenstein, A. H., and Steiner, D. F.: Human Serum Proinsulin, J. Clin. Invest., 49:497, 1970.

52. Bromer, W. W.: Proinsulin, BioScience, 20:701, 1970.

53. Gorden, P., and Roth, J.: Circulating Insulins; "Big" and "Little," Arch. Int. Med., 123:237, 1969.

54. Goldsmith, S. G., Yalow, R. S., and Berson, S. A.: Significance of Human Plasma Insulin Sephadex Fractions, Diabetes, 18:834, 1969.

55. Yalow, R. S., and Berson, S. A.: Dynamics of Insulin Secretion in Early Diabetes in Humans, in Early Diabetes (edited by R. A. Camerini-Dávalos and H. S. Cole), p. 95. New York: Academic Press Inc., 1970.

56. Horwitz, D. L., Rubenstein, A. H., and Steiner, D. F.: Proinsulin and C-Peptide in Diabetes, Med. Clin. North Am., 62:723, 1978.

57. Heinze, E., Beischer, W., Keller, L., Winkler, G., Teller, W. M., and Pfeiffer, E. F.: C-Peptide Secretion during the Remission Phase of Juvenile Diabetes, Diabetes, 27:670, 1978.

58. Unger, R. H.: Pancreatic Glucagon in Health and Disease, Adv. Intern. Med., 17:265, 1971.

59. Potts, J. T., Jr., Sherwood, L. M., O'Riordan, J. L. H., and Aurbach, G. D.: Radioimmunoassay of Polypeptide Hormones, Adv. Intern. Med., 13:183, 1967.

60. Cahill, G. F., Jr., and Soeldner, J.: Editorial: Diabetes, Glucagon, and Growth Hormone, N. Engl. J. Med., 291:577, 1974.

61. Mintz, D. H., Skyler, J. S., and Chez, R. A.: Diabetes and Pregnancy, Diabetes Care, 1:49, 1978.

62. Gerich, J. E.: Somatostatin: Diabetes and Acromegaly, Adv. Intern. Med., 22:251, 1977.

Dietary Treatment

6

Although the current availability of several Insulins with various durations of action and the oral hypoglycemic compounds constitutes a significant contribution to the welfare of the diabetic patient, proper dietary management still remains the most important factor in the practical treatment of diabetes. No hypoglycemic agent yet developed can restore to the diabetic patient a normal metabolic response to the usual nondiabetic diet. In addition, for reasons that are largely unexplained, carbohydrate tolerance in the diabetic patient is reduced by the presence of obesity and frequently improves when normal body weight is achieved. Thus, dietary therapy for the diabetic patient has two goals: (1) to provide in proper quantities and at regular intervals that food, especially carbohydrate, which meets the metabolic needs of the patient with the least strain on impaired homeostatic mechanisms; and (2) to maintain the patient at a body weight that is compatible with the greatest longevity, i.e., the so-called ideal body weight, or IBW.

There are many valid methods for arriving at the proper dietary prescription for a given diabetic patient. Although these methods differ in the way in which the final prescription is determined, all strive:

1. To supply the total caloric requirement (carbohydrate, protein, and fat) of the patient for maintenance of his ideal body weight.

2. To satisfy special considerations—i.e., modifications in the amounts and types of food allowed as dictated by the presence of complications of diabetes or other diseases.

3. To provide adequate intake of vitamins and minerals.*

THE TOTAL DAILY CALORIC ALLOTMENT

The total daily allotment of calories is based upon the requirements of the patient and depends upon his nutritional status when the diet is instituted and upon an estimate of his daily activity. Patients who are sedentary and overweight seldom need more than 20 calories per Kg. of *ideal* body weight per day. On the other hand, individuals whose weights are normal and who are engaged in moderate activity require approximately 35 calories per Kg. of ideal body weight daily. Table 11 provides a guide to the

---

*In the dietary management of the diabetic, it is particularly important for the physician to insure a sufficient vitamin intake. Although a well-planned diet provides an adequate supply of the essential vitamins, supplementation with a well-balanced formula is convenient and reassuring.

number of calories that should be prescribed. This table is an amplification of the amounts advised in the folder of the *Lilly Diabetes Diet Packet and Patient Instruction Guide*.

For example, an obese sedentary patient whose ideal body weight is 70 Kg. needs only from 1,400 to a maximum of 1,700 calories daily. An underweight individual engaged in heavy activity, such as construction work or furniture moving, with an ideal body weight of about 80 Kg. (ca. 200 pounds) may require up to 4,000 calories a day.

During their peak growth period, active adolescent boys need from 3,100 to 3,600 calories a day and adolescent girls from 2,400 to 2,700. In general, children require 1,000 calories a day plus an additional 100 for every year of age. Accordingly, a ten-year-old should receive approximately 2,000 calories daily. *One of the most common errors in the dietary management of juvenile diabetics is the failure to allow an adequate caloric intake.*

Table 11. Diabetic Diet Calculation (Calories/Kg./Day)

	SEDENTARY	MODERATE ACTIVITY	MARKED ACTIVITY
Overweight	20-25*	30	35
Normal	30	35	40
Underweight	35	40	45-50

*The value ordinarily used for elderly sedentary patients is 20 calories per Kg.

CARBOHYDRATE REQUIREMENTS

Formerly, carbohydrates in the standard diabetic diets comprised 38 to 45 percent of the total calories. The revised Lilly diets now reflect the new thinking[1,1A,1B] of the American Diabetes and American Dietetic Associations in that they include 47 to 51 percent of the total calories as carbohydrate (see Table 12, page 65). The routine use of less than 80 Gm. is not advisable, since such a low level frequently leads to ketosis. Whereas diets high in carbohydrate formerly were thought to be unsuitable for diabetics, current medical thinking[1] holds that high-carbohydrate diets are acceptable for most patients (except those with carbohydrate-induced hyperlipidemia—see below) if the total calorie intake is not increased and concentrated sugars are not used.

PROTEIN REQUIREMENTS

The amount of protein that should be prescribed also depends upon the nutritional state of the patient. Factors determining the amount of protein in the dietary prescription include the total caloric requirements of the patient as well as the presence of pregnancy, protein-losing or debilitating disease, or disorders in which protein may have adverse effects (e.g., uremia and hepatic coma). The American Diabetes Association recently recommended that the amount of protein in the diabetic diet should reflect approximately 20 percent of the total calories for children and pregnant women and a minimum of 0.5 Gm. per pound of ideal body weight for adults. The protein level of the revised Lilly diets meets these criteria (see Table 12).

FAT IN THE DIET

Authorities generally agree on the type of protein and carbohydrate to be included in the diabetic diet, but there is considerable variation of opinion as to the kind and amount of fat that should be prescribed. Concern about fat intake is based upon results of studies in nondiabetic animals and humans which indicate that pathological changes may be found in the vessels when blood lipids are elevated. This elevation appears to be associated with diets high in total fat and/or saturated fats.

Since nondiabetics with elevated serum lipids (serum cholesterol or triglyceride or both) and diabetics face a high death and disability risk because of large-vessel involvement from atherosclerosis (see Chapter 14), reduction of elevated serum lipids in diabetics is a logical therapeutic goal. Former attempts to decrease blood fats were based almost exclusively upon restriction of fat and total calories in the diet. More recently, new biochemical knowledge and technics have delineated mechanisms that elevate lipid fractions in the blood and have disclosed ways of not only identifying but also correcting specific abnormalities by dietary and other measures. (The details of the biochemical advances in this area are reviewed elsewhere.[2,3]) One of these technics is electrophoresis. With this method, hyperlipidemic states can be categorized from the electrophoretic pattern produced by the migration of lipoproteins. One of the most common lipid abnormalities observed in diabetes has been termed the "type IV," or "carbohydrate-induced," variety, so named because excessive intake of carbohydrate results in elevations of triglycerides and, to a lesser extent, cholesterol. Special diets based on recommendations of the American Heart Association[4] are lower in carbohydrate and saturated (animal) fat and higher in unsaturated fat than their standard counterparts. It should be emphasized, however, that (1) the serum lipid abnormalities in overweight patients with a type IV abnormality may respond to weight reduction alone without these special diets, and (2), although these diets may lead to a reduction in serum triglyceride concentration and cholesterol, there are as yet no firm data to prove that this will lower the incidence of complications of large-vessel disease, e.g., myocardial infarction or cerebrovascular thrombosis.

Types of lipid abnormalities

Another lipid abnormality frequently encountered in diabetics and identified by lipoprotein electrophoresis is "type II," which is primarily associated with elevated blood cholesterol concentrations. Dietary treatment[2] consists in reducing the fat intake to about 30 percent of total calories and, ideally, using only about one-third of the fat in the saturated form, i.e., as animal fat in meat exchanges. The remainder of the dietary fat is made up of polyunsaturated fats of vegetable origin, such as soft margarine, corn oil, and safflower oil. Very important is the omission or sparing use of foods high in cholesterol, such as eggs, shellfish, and organ meats (liver, sweetbreads, kidney). In addition to lean meat, fish and poultry are recommended.

HOW TO CALCULATE A DIABETIC DIET

The following scheme is recommended for calculating the diet for the diabetic patient. There are many methods for arriving at the proper dietary prescription; the one outlined below is merely an attempt to simplify the task and to incorporate the important aspects of the commonly accepted methods:

STEP 1   Calculate the ideal body weight in pounds. This is usually done by reference to standard height-weight tables (Tables 13-15). When such tables are not readily available, a rough approximation may be obtained by means of the following formula. For women, allow 100 pounds for the first 5 feet and 5 pounds for each additional inch. For men, allow 106 pounds for the first 5 feet and 6 pounds for each additional inch. For patients with small frames, 10 percent is subtracted; with large frames, 10 percent is added to the calculation.

STEP 2   Convert ideal body weight from pounds to Kg. (divide pounds by 2.2).

STEP 3   Using Table 11, calculate the total amount of calories the patient needs per day for each Kg. of ideal body weight.

At this point, one of the revised (1979) Lilly diets (1,000, 1,200, 1,500, 1,800, 2,000, 2,500, or 3,000-calorie allowance) may be selected. These diets are listed in Table 12 and are presented in full on pages 73 through 79.

If a prepared diet is not available for the caloric value or amount of protein, carbohydrate, or fat desired, follow steps 4 through 6.

STEP 4   Divide the total calories into carbohydrate, protein, and fat approximately as follows—carbohydrate, 50 percent; protein, 20 percent; and fat, 30 percent. Thus, if X = total calories in the diet:

$$\text{Grams of carbohydrate} = \frac{50\% \ X}{4 \ (\text{cal./Gm.})} = \text{Number of calories in Gm.}$$

$$\text{Protein} = \frac{20\% \ X}{4 \ (\text{cal./Gm.})} = \text{Number of calories in Gm.}$$

$$\text{Fat} = \text{remainder, or } \frac{30\% \ X}{9 \ (\text{cal./Gm.})} = \text{Number of calories in Gm.}$$

STEP 5   Using the exchange lists adapted from those of the American Diabetes Association and The American Dietetic Association (Table 16), translate the diet into food servings and distribute these as desired among the three regular meals and extra feedings, according to the eating habits of the patient and the time activity of the hypoglycemic agent he is taking. Patients receiving Insulin may require a bedtime feeding to protect against late-evening or early-morning hypoglycemia. In the revised Lilly diets, 2/7 of the total daily calories are distributed at each of the three main meals and 1/7 at bedtime. The general recommendation of the American Diabetes Association diets allows 2/10 to 4/10 of total daily calories and carbohydrates at each main meal and 1/10 for between-meal snacks and at bedtime. For the 3,000-calorie diet, a distribution of approximately 2/9 is used for each main meal and 1/9 each for the two between-meal snacks and a bedtime feeding. Other diet patterns, such as 1/5, 2/5, 2/5, can be devised by consulting the exchange lists in Table 16 and reapportioning the foods until the desired distribution is achieved.

Divide the diet into the desired number of feedings and food exchanges by listing across the top of a sheet of paper the total amount of carbohydrate, protein, and fat desired. Then, in a vertical column on the left-hand side of the page, indicate the meals and feedings over which the total is to be distributed. Exchanges may then be selected one meal at a time and the amounts deducted with the completion of each meal.

STEP 6

Add special instructions regarding foods to be avoided or favored on the basis of other conditions (see page 81 for low-sodium diet).

EXAMPLE OF DIET CALCULATION

Elderly female housewife who does light housekeeping in a small apartment. Height, 5′6″ (66″); presenting weight, 150 pounds; slight frame.

Step 1—Ideal body weight for 5′6″ is about 132 pounds.

Step 2—132 pounds (divided by 2.2) equals 60 Kg.

Step 3—Patient is overweight and sedentary.
$60 \times 20\text{-}25$ cal./Kg. (from Table 11) = approximately 1,200 calories.

Step 4—Distribution of calories into carbohydrate, protein, and fat:
Carbohydrate: $50\% \times 1{,}200 = 600 \div 4$ (cal./Gm.) = 150 Gm.
Protein: $20\% \times 1{,}200 = 240 \div 4$ (cal./Gm.) = 60 Gm.
Fat: $30\% \times 1{,}200 = 360 \div 9$ (cal./Gm.) = 40 Gm.
(Usual practice is to round amount off to nearest 5 Gm.)

Step 5—List across the top of a scratch sheet the total quantities of protein, fat, and carbohydrate to be allowed; then, using the exchange lists, prepare the exchange pattern for each meal.

Table 12. Revised Diabetic Diets (1979)

DIET (CALORIES)	CARBO-HYDRATE (GM.)	PROTEIN (GM.)	FAT (GM.)	ACTUAL CALORIES	PERCENT OF CALORIES AS		
					CARBO-HYDRATE	PROTEIN	FAT
1,000	132	55	30	1,018	52	22	27
1,200	144	65	40	1,196	48	22	30
1,500	194	77	50	1,534	51	20	29
1,800	224	89	60	1,792	50	20	30
2,000	246	111	65	2,013	49	22	29
2,500	314	122	85	2,500	50	20	31
3,000	376	150	100	3,004	51	20	30

Table 13. Normal Height-Weight, 1/2 to 21 Years

Age	Male		Female	
	HEIGHT	WEIGHT	HEIGHT	WEIGHT
YEARS	INCHES	POUNDS	INCHES	POUNDS
1/2	26	17	26	16
1	29	21	29	20
2	33	26	33	25
3	36	31	36	30
4	39	35	39	34
5	42	38	41	37
6	45	43	44	43
7	47	50	47	47
8	49	55	49	54
9	51	61	51	60
10	53	67	53	67
11	55	75	55	74
12	57	81	57	82
13	59	90	60	94
14	62	103	62	105
15	64	112	63	112
16	66	126	64	117
17	67	133	64	122
18	68	138	65	124
19	69	138	65	126
20	69	139	65	126

Table 14. Desirable Weights for Men[5] According to Height and Frame, Ages 25 and Over

HEIGHT (IN SHOES, 1-INCH HEELS)		WEIGHT IN POUNDS (IN INDOOR CLOTHING)		
FEET	INCHES	SMALL FRAME	MEDIUM FRAME	LARGE FRAME
5	2	112–120	118–129	126–141
5	3	115–123	121–133	129–144
5	4	118–126	124–136	132–148
5	5	121–129	127–139	135–152
5	6	124–133	130–143	138–156
5	7	128–137	134–147	142–161
5	8	132–141	138–152	147–166
5	9	136–145	142–156	151–170
5	10	140–150	146–160	155–174
5	11	144–154	150–165	159–179
6	0	148–158	154–170	164–184
6	1	152–162	158–175	168–189
6	2	156–167	162–180	173–194
6	3	160–171	167–185	178–199
6	4	164–175	172–190	182–204

Table 15. Desirable Weights for Women[5] According to Height and Frame, Ages 25 and Over

| HEIGHT (IN SHOES, 2-INCH HEELS) | | WEIGHT IN POUNDS (IN INDOOR CLOTHING) | | |
FEET	INCHES	SMALL FRAME	MEDIUM FRAME	LARGE FRAME
4	10	92– 98	96–107	104–119
4	11	94–101	98–110	106–122
5	0	96–104	101–113	109–125
5	1	99–107	104–116	112–128
5	2	102–110	107–119	115–131
5	3	105–113	110–122	118–134
5	4	108–116	113–126	121–138
5	5	111–119	116–130	125–142
5	6	114–123	120–135	129–146
5	7	118–127	124–139	133–150
5	8	122–131	128–143	137–154
5	9	126–135	132–147	141–158
5	10	130–140	136–151	145–163
5	11	134–144	140–155	149–168
6	0	138–148	144–159	153–173

ADDITIONAL COMMENTS

1. The physician or nutritionist must be prepared to consult often and freely with the patient and, within the limits of the diet, to make adjustments and changes to fit the patient's needs and preferences.

2. In all diet therapy, there may be a daily variation of as much as 15 percent in the absolute number of calories received by patients on a calculated diet. These differences are due both to inaccuracies in measurement and to variations in the actual protein, fat, and carbohydrate content of the many foodstuffs.

3. After a diet has been properly calculated and successfully instituted, the physician must adjust Insulin and/or oral hypoglycemic treatment.

4. In high-calorie diets, it may be necessary to have supplemental feedings in midmorning and midafternoon. This is recommended not only to prevent reaction to the large doses of Insulin that may be needed but also to reduce to a reasonable amount the quantity of food taken at each of the regular meals.

5. When a diabetic, especially one who is dependent on Insulin, is unable to take his usual solid feedings, the carbohydrate content of the diet must be replaced gram for gram either with 10 percent beverage (orange juice, soft drinks, ginger ale, etc.) or with parenteral glucose in order to prevent Insulin reaction. Table 31 (page 146) shows the quantity of 10 percent beverage required to replace the various carbohydrate-containing exchanges in the Lilly diet sheets.

By examination of the food uneaten, it is possible to calculate the amount of 10 percent beverage required. On the basis of the standard exchange lists (Table 16), the amount of carbohydrate in each item of food can be ascertained. Accordingly, the replacement for three meat exchanges, a potato, and a half cup of carrots would be estimated as follows:

Three meat exchanges—no carbohydrate replacement*
One potato (same as a bread exchange)   15 Gm.
1/2 cup of carrots (same as a List 2 vegetable)   5 Gm.
Total amount of carbohydrate to be replaced   20 Gm.

The 20 Gm. of carbohydrate would be replaced with 200 ml. (about 7 ounces) of 10 percent beverage, such as orange juice.

Replacement should be started immediately and continued until an hour or so before the next meal. A common cause of Insulin reaction is failure to observe this simple principle of diet therapy.

In general, dietary strategy varies for the two major types of clinical diabetes (Table 15A).

Table 15A. Dietary Strategy for Different Types of Diabetes

	TYPE I	TYPE II
Total calories	If underweight, caloric increases frequently needed	Patients commonly overweight; caloric restriction needed
Calorie distribution over several feedings	Essential	Desirable
Consistency in intake of protein, fat, and carbohydrate	Important	Desirable
Consistency in timing of meals	Crucial	Desirable but not absolutely essential
Extra food for increase in exercise	Very important	Indicated if patient well controlled on an oral agent

GENERAL RULES

Patients should be urged to measure foods with standard measuring cups and spoons. For more accuracy, some patients should be advised to use an ounce scale for weighing meat servings.

Food Preparation

Diabetic meals need not be tasteless or unappetizing. Any fresh or dried herbs and spices can be used as seasoning. For additional flavor, vegetables may be cooked in bouillon. Many good diabetic recipe books are available to facilitate meal planning.

Most cooking methods can be used, including slow cookery (Crockpot®) and microwave ovens. The one exception is frying, unless a specially coated (Teflon®) skillet and/or fat allowed in the meal plan is used.

*Some authorities replace the carbohydrate value which they estimate is lost when the patient fails to take the meat exchanges offered in a given meal. This ordinarily is calculated as 50 percent of protein value, i.e., 3 to 4 Gm. for each meat exchange.

Food Selection

Food items should be selected from among the same foods purchased for the rest of the family. Patients should be discouraged from buying or using unnecessary dietetic foods. Before a diabetic food is incorporated into a diet plan, the label should always be checked for protein, carbohydrate, fat, and calorie content.

Foods to Be Avoided Unless Permitted by the Physician

The physician or the diet counselor should discuss with the patient obvious foods to avoid, such as sugar, candy, honey, jellies, jams, marmalade, syrups, condensed milk, and candy-coated gum.

Only the physician can determine whether the patient can have alcoholic beverages. This should be discussed with the patient or the diet counselor as soon as possible.

Patients should be advised *to eat meals at the same time every day and not to skip meals.* They should be told not to save food from one meal to the next. (Patients requiring Insulin should know how to increase their calories when physical activity is substantially increased.)

A professional consultation with the physician or a nutrition counselor is recommended when diet therapy begins and at regular intervals thereafter. Although the Lilly diabetic diet plans are limited in content, they offer basic information and examples, especially for new diabetics. One feature of the revised Lilly diets is the use of skim milk at all calorie levels. Because of limited space, only one meat exchange list is shown.

Lilly recommends writing to the American Diabetes Association, 600 Fifth Avenue, New York, New York 10020, for its more complete diet booklet "Exchange Lists for Meal Planning." The booklet is helpful in selecting a diet high in polyunsaturated fat from the exchange lists and uses three meat groups to indicate high, medium, and low fat content.

Table 16. Foods Allowed in Various Exchanges

MILK VALUES   LIST 1

Each portion supplies approximately 12 Gm. of carbohydrate and 8 Gm. of protein; the fat content and total calories vary with the type of milk. (One fat exchange equals 5 Gm. of fat.)

	MEASUREMENT	FAT EXCHANGES	CALORIES
Milk			
Buttermilk	1 cup	—	80
Evaporated, undiluted			
Skim	1/2 cup	—	80
Whole	1/2 cup	2	170
Nonfat dry milk mixed according to directions on box	1 cup	—	80
Nonfat dry milk powder	1/3 cup	—	80
Skim	1 cup	—	80
1% butterfat	1 cup	1/2	107
2% butterfat	1 cup	1	125
Whole	1 cup	2	170
Yogurt, plain, made with skim milk	1 cup	—	80

If substitution for the milk indicated in the diet plan is desired, either choose a milk product that contains the same number of fat exchanges or allow for the difference in the meal plan. For example, if the diet plan calls for 1 cup of skim milk (no fat exchange), substitute 1 cup of 2% milk by omitting one fat exchange.

LIST 2 VEGETABLE EXCHANGES

Each portion (except for vegetables marked with an *) supplies approximately 5 Gm. of carbohydrate and 2 Gm. of protein, or 25 calories. One serving equals 1/2 cup.

Asparagus
Beans, green or yellow
Bean sprouts
Beets
Broccoli
Brussels sprouts
Cabbage
Carrots
Cauliflower
Celery
*Chicory
*Chinese cabbage

Cucumbers
Eggplant
*Endive
*Escarole
Greens: beet, chard, collard,
    dandelion, kale, mustard,
    spinach, turnip
*Lettuce
Mushrooms
Okra
Onions
*Parsley

Peppers, green or red
*Radishes
Rutabagas
Sauerkraut
Squash, summer
Tomatoes
Tomato juice
Turnips
Vegetable juice cocktail
*Watercress
Zucchini

*May be used as desired.

LIST 3 FRUIT EXCHANGES (fresh, dried, or frozen or canned without sugar or syrup)

Each portion supplies approximately 10 Gm. of carbohydrate, or 40 calories.

	MEASUREMENT		MEASUREMENT
Apple	1 small (2″ diam.)	Honeydew melon	1/8 (7″ diam.)
Apple juice or cider	1/3 cup	Mandarin oranges	3/4 cup
Applesauce	1/2 cup	Mango	1/2 small
Apricots, fresh	2 med.	Nectarine	1 small
Apricots, dried	4 halves	Orange	1 small
Banana	1/2 small	Orange juice	1/2 cup
Berries (boysenberries, blackberries, blueberries, raspberries)	1/2 cup	Papaya	3/4 cup
		Peach	1 med.
Cantaloupe	1/4 (6″ diam.)	Pear	1 small
Cherries	10 large	Persimmon, native	1 med.
Dates	2	Pineapple	1/2 cup
Figs, fresh	1 large	Pineapple juice	1/3 cup
Figs, dried	1 small	Plums	2 med.
Fruit cocktail	1/2 cup	Prunes	2 med.
Grapefruit	1/2 small	Prune juice	1/4 cup
Grapefruit juice	1/2 cup	Raisins	2 tbsp.
Grapes	12	Strawberries	3/4 cup
Grape juice	1/4 cup	Tangerine	1 large
		Watermelon	1 cup

LIST 4 BREAD EXCHANGES

Each portion supplies approximately 15 Gm. of carbohydrate and 2 Gm. of protein, or 70 calories.

	MEASUREMENT		MEASUREMENT
Bread, French, raisin (without icing), rye, white, whole-wheat	1 slice	Flour	2 1/2 tbsp.
Bagel	1/2	Matzoth	1 (6″ diam.)
Biscuit, roll	1 (2″ diam.)	Popcorn, popped, unbuttered, small-kernel	1 1/2 cups
Bread crumbs, dried	3 tbsp.	Pretzels (3-ring)	6
Bun (for hamburger or wiener)	1/2	Rice or grits, cooked	1/2 cup
Cornbread	1″ x 2″ x 2″	Spaghetti, macaroni, noodles, cooked	1/2 cup
English muffin	1/2	Tortilla	1 (6″ diam.)
Muffin	1 (2″ diam.)	Vegetables	
Cake, angel or sponge, without icing	1 1/2″ cube (1/20 of 10″-diam. cake)	Beans, baked, without pork	1/4 cup
Cereal, cooked	1/2 cup	Lima, navy, etc., dry, cooked	1/2 cup
Dry (flakes or puffed)	3/4 cup	Corn	1/3 cup
Cornstarch	2 tbsp.	Corn on the cob	1/2 med. ear
Crackers, graham	2 (2 1/2″ sq.)	Parsnips	2/3 cup
Oyster	20 (1/2 cup)	Peas, dried (split peas, etc.) or green, cooked	1/2 cup
Round	6	Potatoes, sweet, or yams, fresh	1/4 cup
Rye wafer	3 (2″ x 3 1/2″)		
Saltine	6		
Variety	5 small		

White, baked or boiled........1 (2″ diam.)	Squash, winter (acorn or butternut)........1/2 cup
White, mashed.....1/2 cup	
Pumpkin...........3/4 cup	Wheat germ...........1/4 cup

MEAT EXCHANGES   LIST 5

Each portion supplies approximately 7 Gm. of protein and 5 Gm. of fat, or 73 calories.

MEASUREMENT   MEASUREMENT

Cheese, cheddar, American, Swiss....................1-oz. slice (3 1/2″ sq., 1/8″ thick)	Meat and poultry Beef, lamb, pork, veal, ham, liver, chicken, etc. (med. fat)..............1-oz. slice (4″ x 2″ x 1/4″)
Cottage.................1/4 cup	
Egg.......................1	
Fish and seafood Halibut, perch, sole, etc....1-oz. slice (4″ x 2″ x 1/4″)	Cold cuts...............1 1/2-oz. slice (4 1/2″ sq., 1/8″ thick)
Oysters, clams, shrimp, scallops...............5 small	Vienna sausages...........2
Salmon, tuna, crab........1/4 cup	*Weiner.................1 (10 per lb.)
Sardines................3 med.	Peanut butter (omit two additional fat exchanges)..............2 tbsp.

*Limit wieners to one exchange per day.

FAT EXCHANGES   LIST 6

Each portion supplies approximately 5 Gm. of fat, or 45 calories.

MEASUREMENT   MEASUREMENT

Avocado...................1/8 (4″ diam.)	Dressing, French............1 tbsp.
Bacon, crisp...............1 slice	Italian...................1 tbsp.
Butter or margarine........1 tsp.	Mayonnaise..............1 tsp.
Cream, half-and-half.......3 tbsp.	Mayonnaise-type..........2 tsp.
Heavy, 40%.............1 tbsp.	Roquefort...............2 tsp.
Light, 20%.............2 tbsp.	Nuts.....................6 small
Sour....................2 tbsp.	Oil or cooking fat...........1 tsp.
Cream cheese.............1 tbsp.	Olives....................5 small

MISCELLANEOUS FOODS

The following foods may be used if you wish, but they must be figured into the daily diet plan, with the food exchanges allowed as indicated.

	MEASUREMENT	EXCHANGES
Fish sticks, frozen................................3 sticks		1 bread, 2 meat
Fruit-flavored gelatin..............................1/4 cup		1 bread
Ginger ale......................................7 oz.		1 bread
Ice cream, vanilla, chocolate, strawberry................1/2 cup		1 bread, 2 fat
Low-calorie dressing, French or Italian.................1 tbsp.		†
Potato or corn chips...............................10 large or 15 small		1 bread, 2 fat
Sherbet..1/2 cup		2 bread
Vanilla wafers....................................6		1 bread
Waffle, frozen....................................1 (5 1/2″)		1 bread, 1 fat

†The fat and calorie content do not have to be counted if the amount is limited to 1 tablespoonful.

FOODS ALLOWED IN REASONABLE AMOUNTS

Seasonings

Celery salt	Lemon	Pepper
Cinnamon	Mint	Noncaloric sweeteners
Garlic	Mustard	Spices
Garlic or onion salt	Nutmeg	Vanilla
Horseradish	Parsley	Vinegar

Other Foods

Coffee or tea (no sugar or cream)	Artificially sweetened fruit-flavored gelatin
Diet beverage without sugar	Sour or dill pickles
Fat-free broth or bouillon	Cranberries (without sugar)
Unflavored gelatin	Rhubarb (without sugar)

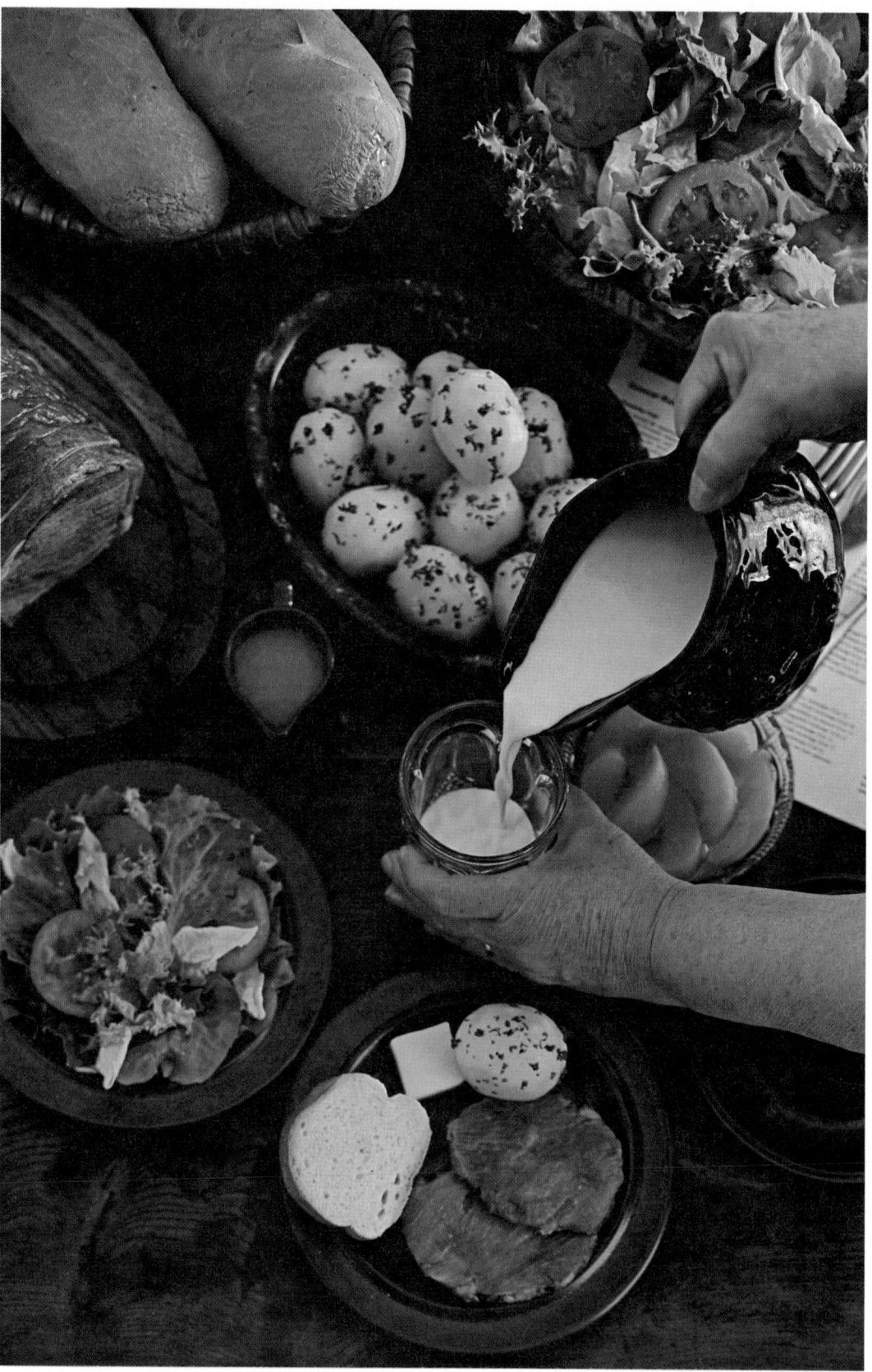

1,000 CALORIES (approximately)

Carbohydrate, 130 Gm. / Protein, 55 Gm. / Fat, 30 Gm.

DAILY MENU GUIDE

These sample menus show some of the ways that the exchange lists may be used to add variety to meals. **The exchange lists in Table 16 may be used to plan different menus.**

Breakfast

1 ½ fruit exchanges (List 3)
2 bread exchanges (List 4)

1 fat exchange (List 6)
½ cup skim milk (List 1)

Lunch

2 meat exchanges (List 5)
1 bread exchange (List 4)
Vegetable(s) as desired (List 2*)
1 fruit exchange (List 3)
½ cup skim milk (List 1)

Dinner

2 meat exchanges (List 5)
1 bread exchange (List 4)
1 vegetable exchange (List 2)
Vegetable(s) as desired (List 2*)
1 ½ fruit exchanges (List 3)
1 fat exchange (List 6)
½ cup skim milk (List 1)

Bedtime Feeding

½ bread exchange (List 4)
½ cup skim milk (List 1)

Breakfast

Orange juice . . . . ¾ cup
Toast . . . . 1 slice
Cereal, dry . . . . ¾ cup
Margarine . . . . 1 tsp.
Skim milk . . . . ½ cup

Lunch

Cheese . . . . 2 1-oz. slices
Bread . . . . 1 slice
Dill pickles, radishes . . . . as desired
Apple . . . . 1 small
Skim milk . . . . ½ cup
Mustard . . . . as desired

Dinner

Chicken, baked . . . . 2 oz.
Peas . . . . ½ cup
Tomatoes . . . . ½ cup
Lettuce, etc. . . . . as desired
Fruit cocktail . . . . ¾ cup
Margarine . . . . 1 tsp.
Skim milk . . . . ½ cup

Bedtime Feeding

Graham cracker . . . . 1 square
Skim milk . . . . ½ cup

73

1,200 CALORIES (approximately)

Carbohydrate, 145 Gm. / Protein, 65 Gm. / Fat, 40 Gm.

DAILY MENU GUIDE

These sample menus show some of the ways that the exchange lists may be used to add variety to meals. **The exchange lists in Table 16 may be used to plan different menus.**

Breakfast

1 ½ fruit exchanges (List 3)
1 bread exchange (List 4)
1 meat exchange (List 5)
1 fat exchange (List 6)
1 cup skim milk (List 1)

Lunch

2 meat exchanges (List 5)

2 bread exchanges (List 4)

1 vegetable exchange (List 2)

1 fruit exchange (List 3)
1 fat exchange (List 6)
½ cup skim milk (List 1)

Dinner

2 meat exchanges (List 5)
1 bread exchange (List 4)
1 vegetable exchange (List 2)
Vegetable(s) as desired (List 2*)
1 fruit exchange (List 3)
1 fat exchange (List 6)

Bedtime Feeding

1 bread exchange (List 4)
½ cup skim milk (List 1)

Breakfast

Orange juice..............¾ cup
Toast....................1 slice
Egg......................1
Margarine...............1 tsp.
Skim milk...............1 cup

Lunch

Cheese..................2 1-oz. slices
Beef bouillon.............as desired
Bread...................1 slice
Saltine crackers...........6
Carrot and celery
  sticks................½ cup
Apple..................1 small
Margarine...............1 tsp.
Skim milk...............½ cup
Mustard.................as desired

Dinner

Chicken, baked...........2 oz.
Potatoes, mashed.......½ cup
Tomatoes...............½ cup
Lettuce, etc.............as desired
Fruit cocktail.............½ cup
Margarine...............1 tsp.

Bedtime Feeding

Graham crackers........2 squares
Skim milk...............½ cup

74

1,500 CALORIES (approximately)

Carbohydrate, 195 Gm. / Protein, 75 Gm. / Fat, 50 Gm.

DAILY MENU GUIDE

These sample menus show some of the ways that the exchange lists may be used to add variety to meals. **The exchange lists in Table 16 may be used to plan different menus.**

Breakfast

2 fruit exchanges (List 3)
2 bread exchanges (List 4)

1 meat exchange (List 5)
1 fat exchange (List 6)
1 cup skim milk (List 1)

Breakfast

Orange juice . . . . 1 cup
Cereal, dry . . . . ¾ cup
Toast . . . . 1 slice
Egg 1
Margarine . . . . 1 tsp.
Skim milk . . . . 1 cup

Lunch

3 meat exchanges (List 5)
2 bread exchanges (List 4)
1 vegetable exchange (List 2)

2 fruit exchanges (List 3)
1 fat exchange (List 6)

Lunch

Cheese . . . . 3 1-oz. slices
Bread . . . . 2 slices
Carrot and celery
   sticks . . . . ½ cup
Apples . . . . 2 small
Mayonnaise-type dressing . . . 2 tsp.

Dinner

3 meat exchanges (List 5)
2 bread exchanges (List 4)

2 vegetable exchanges (List 2)
Vegetable(s) as desired (List 2*)
1 fruit exchange (List 3)
1 fat exchange (List 6)
½ cup skim milk (List 1)

Dinner

Chicken, baked . . . . 3 oz.
Peas . . . . ½ cup
Potatoes, mashed . . . . ½ cup
Tomatoes . . . . 1 cup
Lettuce, etc. . . . . as desired
Fruit cocktail . . . . ½ cup
Margarine . . . . 1 tsp.
Skim milk . . . . ½ cup
French dressing,
   low-calorie . . . . 1 tbsp.

Bedtime Feeding

1 bread exchange (List 4)
½ cup skim milk (List 1)

Bedtime Feeding

Graham crackers . . . . 2 squares
Skim milk . . . . ½ cup

1,800 CALORIES (approximately)

Carbohydrate, 225 Gm. / Protein, 90 Gm. / Fat, 60 Gm.

DAILY MENU GUIDE

These sample menus show some of the ways that the exchange lists may be used to add variety to meals. **The exchange lists in Table 16 may be used to plan different menus.**

Breakfast

2 fruit exchanges (List 3)
2 bread exchanges (List 4)
1 meat exchange (List 5)
1 fat exchange (List 6)
1 cup skim milk (List 1)

Lunch

2 meat exchanges (List 5)

2 bread exchanges (List 4)
1 vegetable exchange (List 2)

2 fruit exchanges (List 3)
2 fat exchanges (List 6)

Dinner

3 meat exchanges (List 5)
3 bread exchanges (List 4)

2 vegetable exchanges (List 2)
Vegetable(s) as desired (List 2*)
1 fruit exchange (List 3)
2 fat exchanges (List 6)
½ cup skim milk (List 1)

Bedtime Feeding

2 bread exchanges (List 4)
1 meat exchange (List 5)
½ cup skim milk (List 1)

Breakfast

Orange juice . . . . 1 cup
Toast . . . . 2 slices
Egg 1
Margarine . . . . 1 tsp.
Skim milk . . . . 1 cup

Lunch

Cold cuts . . . . 1½-oz. slice
Cheese . . . . 1 oz.
Bread . . . . 2 slices
Carrot and celery
  sticks . . . . ½ cup
Banana . . . . 1 small
Mayonnaise-type
  dressing . . . . 4 tsp.

Dinner

Chicken, baked . . . . 3 oz.
Peas . . . . ½ cup
Potatoes, mashed . . . . . ½ cup
Bread . . . . 1 slice
Tomatoes . . . . 1 cup
Lettuce, etc. . . . . as desired
Fruit cocktail . . . . ½ cup
Margarine . . . . 2 tsp.
Skim milk . . . . ½ cup
French dressing,
  low-calorie . . . . 1 tbsp.

Bedtime Feeding

Bread . . . . 2 slices
Roast beef, lean . . . . 1 oz.
Skim milk . . . . ½ cup
Mustard . . . . as desired

2,000 CALORIES (approximately)

Carbohydrate, 245 Gm. / Protein, 110 Gm. / Fat, 65 Gm.

DAILY MENU GUIDE

These sample menus show some of the ways that the exchange lists may be used to add variety to meals. **The exchange lists in Table 16 may be used to plan different menus.**

Breakfast

2 fruit exchanges (List 3)
2 bread exchanges (List 4)

1 meat exchange (List 5)
2 fat exchanges (List 6)

1 cup skim milk (List 1)

Breakfast

Orange juice . . . . 1 cup
Cereal, dry . . . . ¾ cup
Toast . . . . 1 slice
Egg 1
Bacon, crisp . . . . 1 slice
Margarine . . . . 1 tsp.
Skim milk . . . . 1 cup

Lunch

3 meat exchanges (List 5)

2 bread exchanges (List 4)
Vegetable(s) as desired (List 2*)

1 vegetable exchange (List 2)

2 fruit exchanges (List 3)
1 fat exchange (List 6)

1 cup skim milk (List 1)

Lunch

Cold cuts . . . . 2 1½-oz. slices
Cheese . . . . 1 oz.
Bread . . . . 2 slices
Dill pickles,
    radishes . . . . as desired
Carrot and celery
    sticks . . . . ½ cup
Apples . . . . 2 small
Mayonnaise-type
    dressing . . . . 2 tsp.
Skim milk . . . . 1 cup

Dinner

3 meat exchanges (List 5)
3 bread exchanges (List 4)

2 vegetable exchanges (List 2)
Vegetable(s) as desired (List 2*)
1 fruit exchange (List 3)
1 fat exchange (List 6)
1 cup skim milk (List 1)

Dinner

Chicken, baked . . . . 3 oz.
Peas . . . . ½ cup
Potatoes, mashed . . . . . . ½ cup
Bread . . . . 1 slice
Tomatoes . . . . 1 cup
Lettuce, etc. . . . . as desired
Fruit cocktail . . . . ½ cup
Margarine . . . . 1 tsp.
Skim milk . . . . 1 cup
French dressing,
    low-calorie . . . . 1 tbsp.

Bedtime Feeding

2 bread exchanges (List 4)
2 meat exchanges (List 5)
1 fruit exchange (List 3)

Bedtime Feeding

Bread . . . . 2 slices
Roast beef, lean . . . . 2 oz.
Grapes 12
Mustard . . . . as desired

2,500 CALORIES (approximately)

Carbohydrate, 315 Gm. / Protein, 120 Gm. / Fat, 85 Gm.

DAILY MENU GUIDE

These sample menus show some of the ways that the exchange lists may be used to add variety to meals. **The exchange lists in Table 16 may be used to plan different menus.**

Breakfast

2 fruit exchanges (List 3)
3 bread exchanges (List 4)

1 meat exchange (List 5)
2 fat exchanges (List 6)
1 cup skim milk (List 1)

Midmorning Feeding

1 bread exchange (List 4)
½ cup skim milk

Lunch

2 meat exchanges (List 5)
3 bread exchanges (List 4)
3 fat exchanges (List 6)

2 vegetable exchanges

1 fruit exchange (List 3)
1 cup skim milk (List 1)

Midafternoon Feeding

1 bread exchange (List 4)
1 fruit exchange (List 3)

Dinner

3 meat exchanges (List 5)
3 bread exchanges (List 4)

2 vegetable exchanges (List 2)
Vegetable(s) as desired (List 2*)
1 fruit exchange
3 fat exchanges (List 6)
1 cup skim milk (List 1)

Bedtime Feeding

2 bread exchanges (List 4)
2 meat exchanges (List 5)
1 fat exchange (List 6)

½ cup skim milk (List 1)

Breakfast

Orange juice.................1 cup
Cereal, dry...............¾ cup
Toast.....................2 slices
Egg.......................1
Margarine..................2 tsp.
Skim milk..................1 cup

Midmorning Feeding

Graham crackers...........2 squares
Skim milk..................½ cup

Lunch

Cold cuts....1½-oz. slice ⎫
Cheese.......1 oz.   ⎪
Bread.......3 slices   ⎬ triple-
Mayonnaise-   ⎪ decker
  type   ⎪ sandwich
  dressing....2 tsp.   ⎪
Margarine....2 tsp.   ⎭
Carrot and celery
  sticks..................1 cup
Apple.....................1 small
Skim milk..................1 cup

Midafternoon Feeding

Saltine crackers..............6
Pineapple juice..............⅓ cup

Dinner

Chicken, baked..............3 oz.
Peas.......................½ cup
Potatoes, mashed...........½ cup
Bread......................1 slice
Tomatoes...................1 cup
Lettuce, etc...............as desired
Fruit cocktail.............½ cup
Margarine..................3 tsp.
Skim milk..................1 cup

Bedtime Feeding

Hamburger bun..............1
Roast beef, lean...........2 oz.
Mayonnaise-type
  dressing.................2 tsp.
Skim milk..................½ cup

3,000 CALORIES (approximately)

Carbohydrate, 375 Gm. / Protein, 150 Gm. / Fat, 100 Gm.

DAILY MENU GUIDE

These sample menus show some of the ways that the exchange lists may be used to add variety to meals. **The exchange lists in Table 16 may be used to plan different menus.**

Breakfast

2 fruit exchanges (List 3)
3 bread exchanges (List 4)

1 meat exchange (List 5)
2 fat exchanges (List 6)
1 cup skim milk (List 1)

Midmorning Feeding

1½ bread exchanges (List 4)
½ cup skim milk (List 1)

Lunch

3 meat exchanges (List 5)
4 bread exchanges (List 4)
3 fat exchanges (List 6)

2 vegetable exchanges (List 2)

2 fruit exchanges (List 3)
1 cup skim milk (List 1)

Midafternoon Feeding

1 meat exchange (List 5)
2 bread exchanges (List 4)
1 fruit exchange (List 3)

Dinner

4 meat exchanges (List 5)
4 bread exchanges (List 4)

2 vegetable exchanges (List 2)
Vegetable(s) as desired (List 2*)
1 fruit exchange (List 3)
3 fat exchanges (List 6)
1 cup skim milk (List 1)

Bedtime Feeding

2 meat exchanges (List 5)
2 bread exchanges (List 4)
1 fat exchange (List 6)

½ cup skim milk (List 1)

Breakfast

Orange juice . . . . .1 cup
Cereal, dry . . . . .¾ cup
Toast .2 slices
Egg 1
Margarine . . . . .2 tsp.
Skim milk . . . . .1 cup

Midmorning Feeding

Graham crackers . . . . .3 squares
Skim milk . . . . .½ cup

Lunch

Cheese . . . . . . .1 oz.
Bread . . . . .2 slices
Mayonnaise-
    type
    dressing . . . .2 tsp.   } sandwich
Cold cuts . . . . .2 1½-oz. slices
Bread . . . . .2 slices   } sandwich
Margarine . . . .2 tsp.
Carrot and celery
    sticks . . . . .1 cup
Apples . . . . .2 small
Skim milk . . . . .1 cup

Midafternoon Feeding

Wiener .1
Wiener bun 1
Grapefruit juice . . . . .½ cup
Mustard . . . . .as desired

Dinner

Chicken, baked . . . . .4 oz.
Peas . . . . .½ cup
Potatoes, mashed . . . . .½ cup
Bread . . . . .2 slices
Tomatoes . . . . .1 cup
Lettuce, etc. . . . . .as desired
Fruit cocktail . . . . .½ cup
Margarine . . . . .3 tsp.
Skim milk . . . . .1 cup

Bedtime Feeding

Roast beef, lean . . . . .2 oz.
Hamburger bun 1
Mayonnaise-type
    dressing . . . . .2 tsp.
Skim milk . . . . .½ cup

MODIFICATIONS OF THE DIET TO CONFORM WITH THE TREATMENT OF CONCURRENT DISEASES

The ubiquity of diabetes results in the common association of this disease with other medical disorders, many of which require special dietary treatment or restrictions. The most frequently modified diabetic diets are (1) those in which sodium is restricted, as in heart and kidney disease; (2) those in which the consistency of the diet is important, as in gastro-intestinal disorders (peptic ulcer, diverticulitis, gall-bladder disease, and ulcerative colitis); (3) those in which the fat content must be reduced, as in gall-bladder disease; and (4) those disorders in which protein must be restricted, such as uremia and hepatic insufficiency associated with central-nervous-system dysfunction. General comments about each type of special diet are given below. Modified exchange lists for specific diets are found on pages 81 to 83.

When the diabetic diet must be altered in consistency (bland or low-fiber diet) or in seasoning (low sodium content), the following modifications of the exchange lists may be used in conjunction with the desired standard Lilly diet in addition to the prescription of carbohydrate, protein, and fat. It must be clearly understood, however, that the modified exchange lists *replace* the regular exchange lists and that the daily meal pattern as planned should be followed in order to obtain the required prescription of calories, carbohydrate, protein, and fat.

1. SODIUM RESTRICTION

The sodium restriction may range from 500 to 1,000 mg. daily. Although diets containing less than 1 Gm. of sodium are used infrequently as a result of the advent of the thiazide diuretics, the principles of designing diets with lower sodium content should be understood. For all sodium-restricted diets, consult the special food exchange lists on page 81.

500-mg. Sodium Diet

A 500-mg. sodium diet may be constructed by means of the low-sodium diet exchanges without the need for low-sodium or dialyzed milk except when a diet containing more than 70 Gm. of protein has been prescribed.

1-Gm. Sodium Diet

The low-sodium diet exchange list may be used in this diet. In addition, the patient may be permitted to add one-fourth teaspoonful of table salt to his daily intake. This can be done by instructing the patient to use a clean empty saltshaker. Each morning, he must measure out a level quarter teaspoonful of salt—his supplementary salt supply for the day. Each day he should start with an empty saltshaker; otherwise, the total intake of salt for a twenty-four-hour period will exceed the specified limit.

Low-Sodium Diet

Any patient on a sodium-restricted diet should modify the standard exchange lists as suggested below.

Because all the foods in an exchange list contain approximately the same number of milligrams of sodium and have the same caloric value, the patient may substitute freely within the exchange list if he eats only the listed amount of each food.

LOW-SODIUM DIET

FOOD EXCHANGE LIST	ALLOWED	TO BE AVOIDED	
MILK VALUES			LIST 1
120 mg. sodium per 8 oz.	All forms except buttermilk	Buttermilk	
VEGETABLE EXCHANGES			LIST 2
9 mg. sodium per 1/2 cup	All except those listed to be avoided	Celery Hominy Greens Kale Frozen peas Frozen Lima beans Sauerkraut Pickles of any kind Tomato juice, regular	
FRUIT EXCHANGES			LIST 3
2 mg. sodium per serving	All allowed	None	
BREAD EXCHANGES			LIST 4
1 to 5 mg. sodium per serving	Low-sodium bread crumbs and breads Puffed wheat and rice Shredded wheat Unsalted crackers	Regular bread and crackers All other cereals Snack foods Waffles Instant mashed potatoes	
MEAT EXCHANGES			LIST 5
25 mg. sodium per oz. lean meat 65 mg. sodium per egg (limit to 1 per day)	All allowed, including low-sodium cheese, unsalted cottage cheese, and unsalted peanut butter, except those listed to be avoided	Any fish, meat, or poultry that has been smoked, brine-cured, canned, salted and dried, or salted and soaked (kosher), such as cold cuts, frankfurters, bacon, ham, and sausage Brains Heart Clams Kidney Crab Lobster Frozen fish Shrimp	
FAT EXCHANGES			LIST 6
50 mg. sodium per 1 tsp. margarine	Unsalted margarine, butter, oil, mayonnaise, light cream	Salted butter or margarine Sour cream Bacon or ham drippings Commercial mayonnaise French or Italian dressing	

ALLOWED AS DESIRED (need not be measured)

Seasonings—All dried or fresh herbs and spices except onion, garlic, or celery salt, poultry seasoning, and other seasoned salts.

Also: Gelatin, artificially sweetened, low-sodium; coffee or tea (without cream or sugar), as desired; dietetic low-sodium bouillon; dietetic catsup; and salt substitute if recommended by the physician.

Water: The physician should be aware of the sodium content of the water supply where his patient lives to determine whether he may drink as much as he likes. Water that has been treated with water softeners should not be used for cooking or drinking.

2. SPECIAL DIETS FOR DIABETIC PATIENTS WITH GASTRO-INTESTINAL DISORDERS

In these diets, the principal restriction is on coarse or highly seasoned foods, such as bread, crackers containing whole-grain flour or bran, uncooked cereals, fried foods, condiments, herbs, nuts, olives, spices, alcohol, pickles, popcorn, vinegar, clams, and oysters. In addition, patients being treated for ulcer should avoid broth and soups except those which are made with milk and pureed vegetables. On the other hand, those with ulcerative colitis must exclude milk and milk drinks. The bland or low-fiber diet is outlined in detail below. If a peptic ulcer patient must receive milk more than six times a day, skim milk may be used at each feeding and an equal portion of skim milk given at six other times during the twenty-four-hour period. Although such a procedure will keep the diet isocaloric, it will increase the carbohydrate and protein of the diet by 36 and 24 Gm. respectively. An alternative to this use of milk is the utilization of an antacid in place of the interval feedings.

BLAND OR LOW-FIBER DIET

ALLOWED AS DESIRED

Salt, artificially sweetened fruit-flavored gelatin, saccharin, vanilla, and weak tea or decaffeinated coffee.

LIST 1

MILK VALUES

Allowed in the amounts prescribed in the diet. There is no change in this food group.

LIST 2

VEGETABLE EXCHANGES

Only vegetables in the following list should be recommended. Young, tender vegetables should be selected and served cooked. In certain cases, it may be advisable that these vegetables be strained or pureed. **All Raw Vegetables Should Be Omitted.**

Asparagus tips	Green beans, young	Squash, summer (without seeds)
Beets	Peas	Tomato juice
Carrots	Spinach	Tomato puree, unseasoned
Chard		

LIST 3

FRUIT EXCHANGES

Fruits should be cooked or canned without sugar or be artificially sweetened. Only ripe bananas may be served as raw or fresh fruit. All skins and seeds should be avoided. In special situations, fruits may be strained.

Only the fruits listed below should be selected, and they should be served in the amounts indicated.

	MEASUREMENT		MEASUREMENT
Apple, baked	1 small, no skin (2″ diam.)	Grapefruit juice	1/2 cup
Apple juice	1/3 cup	Orange juice	1/2 cup
Applesauce	1/2 cup	Peach, canned	2 halves
Apricots, peeled	2 med.	Pear, canned	2 halves
Banana, ripe	1/2 small	Pineapple juice	1/3 cup
Cherries, canned	10 large	Plums, canned	2 med.

LIST 4

BREAD EXCHANGES

Only enriched white bread, refined cereals, and crackers should be used. Potatoes, sponge cake without frosting, and ice cream in measured amounts are allowed.

The Following Should Not Be Eaten: dried beans, dried peas, Lima beans, baked beans, corn, hominy, parsnips, fried potatoes, potato chips, graham crackers, whole-grain or bran cereals, and whole-grain rice.

MEAT EXCHANGES LIST 5

Only listed amounts of tender cuts (whole, ground, or chopped) of beef, veal, lamb, pork, chicken, or liver are to be used.

The following fish may be eaten in the listed amounts: cod, haddock, halibut, salmon, tuna, and shellfish.

Eggs, cheddar and cottage cheese, and creamy peanut butter are also permitted in the portions indicated.

The Following Should Not Be Eaten: cold cuts, corned beef, frankfurters, fried meats, sardines, and sausages.

FAT EXCHANGES LIST 6

The patient should omit French or Italian dressing, mayonnaise, nuts, olives, and avocados. Other fats may be used in the amounts listed.

3. REDUCED FAT CONTENT

The objectives of dietary treatment in gall-bladder disease are to provide adequate nutrition and to reduce discomfort by limiting those foods which stimulate gall-bladder function, i.e., gas-forming and/or strong-flavored foods (such as those in the cabbage and onion family) and coarse and fatty foods. Since many patients with gall-bladder disease are overweight, low-calorie diets are frequently used.

The details of fat reduction are covered in the discussion under "Fat in the Diet" earlier in the chapter. An absolute reduction in fat ordinarily can be accomplished with a 1,200 to 1,500-calorie diet, the omission of whole milk, fried foods, butter, and margarine, and the use of lean meat. Other foods to be avoided are raw apples, cheeses, melons, sausages, and desserts high in fat, such as ice cream. (Pastries and puddings are not customarily included in diabetic diets.)

4. PROTEIN RESTRICTION

The amount of protein prescribed for patients with renal failure depends upon the amount lost in the urine and for those with hepatic failure, upon the sensorium of the patient; the latter is related to the degree of ammonia retention.

Uremic patients are usually allowed a basal quantity of 40 Gm. of protein, to which may be added the amount that is lost in the urine. Thus, a patient who loses 5 Gm. of protein in the urine might receive 40 plus 5, or 45, Gm. of protein daily. Since it is important to provide adequate caloric intake when the protein allowance is restricted to minimal levels, the carbohydrate and fat allowances must be increased. It should also be remembered that when protein is restricted, all sources become significant, and the quantity supplied by cereals and vegetables must, of necessity, limit the amount of meat exchanges. In cases in which serum phosphorus levels are elevated, it may be necessary to eliminate all milk products.

5. FIBER IN THE DIABETIC DIET

Increased fiber in the diet has been purported to have a number of salutary effects.[6] Specifically, epidemiologic studies suggest that populations which consume diets high in fiber have a lower than expected frequency of cancer of the bowel and diverticular disease.[7] Since such diets increase intestinal bulk and promote the movement of intestinal contents, high-fiber diets are particularly advantageous for diabetic patients with constipation secondary to autonomic neuropathy. An additional benefit of high-fiber diets for diabetic patients is that they reduce the rate of absorption of sugar and starch and therefore reduce the postprandial glucose rise that usually follows the ingestion of carbohydrate substances.[8] The plant fiber content of various foods is listed in Table 17.[9] Energy values and plant fiber content are given for the portion size. A high-fiber diet is one in which the plant fiber content exceeds 40 Gm. per day.

Table 17. Plant Fiber and Energy Content of Selected Foodstuffs

FOOD	PORTION SIZE*	KCALORIES	PLANT FIBER (GM.)
VEGETABLE EXCHANGES			
Asparagus	1/2 cup	15	1.2
Bean sprouts	1/2 cup	17	0.9
Beans, string	1/2 cup	12	1.7
Beets	1/2 cup	22	1.5
Broccoli	1/2 cup	15	2.6
Brussels sprouts	1/2 cup	24	1.8
Cabbage	1/2 cup	11	1.6
Carrots	1/2 cup	19	2.2
Cauliflower	1/2 cup	12	0.9
Celery	1/2 cup	5	1.7
Cucumbers	1/2 cup	7	0.8
Lettuce	1/2 cup	3	0.5
Onions	1/2 cup	25	1.6
Radishes	1/2 cup	9	1.2
Tomatoes	1/2 cup	27	2.0
Turnips	1/2 cup	13	1.3
Zucchini	1/2 cup	9	2.5
FRUIT EXCHANGES			
Apples	1 small	55	3.9
Banana	1/2 small	60	1.3
Cherries	10	44	0.9
Grapefruit	1/2	41	1.3
Grapes	10	34	0.4
Orange	1 small	45	2.1
Peach	1 medium	33	1.0
Pear	1 small	70	2.5
Pineapple	1/2 cup	41	1.3
Strawberries	3/4 cup	36	2.4
BREAD EXCHANGES			
Beans, Lima	1/2 cup	126	1.4
Bran (100%), cereal	1/2 cup	66	10.0
Bread, rye	1 slice	54	2.7
Bread, white	1 slice	74	0.8

*Portion sizes are taken from the ADA exchange lists.

FOOD	PORTION SIZE*	KCALORIES	PLANT FIBER (GM.)
Bread, whole-grain wheat	1 slice	63	2.7
Cornflakes	3/4 cup	64	2.1
Pancakes	1	61	0.4
Peas	1/2 cup	44	5.2
Potatoes, white	1 small	80	3.8
Rice, white	1/2 cup	79	0.5
Spaghetti	1/2 cup	82	0.8
Waffle	1 section	139	0.8
Wheat flour, whole-grain	2 1/2 tbsp.	60	1.8
Wheat flour, white	2 1/2 tbsp.	77	0.7

*Portion sizes are taken from the ADA exchange lists.

BIBLIOGRAPHY

1. Bierman, E. L., Albrink, M. J., Arky, R. A., Connor, W. E., Dayton, S., Spritz, N., and Steinberg, D.: Special Report—Principles of Nutrition and Dietary Recommendations for Patients with Diabetes Mellitus: 1971, Diabetes, 20:633, 1971.

1A. Exchange Lists for Meal Planning, American Diabetes Association, Inc., and The American Dietetic Association, 1976.

1B. A Guide for Professionals: The Effective Application of "Exchange Lists for Meal Planning," American Diabetes Association, Inc., and The American Dietetic Association, 1977.

2. Abel, E. J., and Powell, R. C.: An Approach to the Dietary Management of Hyperlipemia, J. Indiana M. A., 64:827, 1971.

3. Fredrickson, D. S., Levy, R. I., and Lees, R. S.: Fat Transport in Lipoproteins—An Integrated Approach to Mechanisms and Disorders, New England J. Med., 276:34, 94, 148, 215, and 273, 1967.

4. Planning Fat-Controlled Meals for 1200 and 1800 Calories and Planning Fat-Controlled Meals for Approximately 2000-2600 Calories. New York: American Heart Association, 1971.

5. Metropolitan Life Insurance Company: Statistical Bulletin, 40:3 (November-December), 1959.

6. Mendeloff, A. I.: Dietary Fiber and Human Health, N. Engl. J. Med., 297:811, 1977.

7. Wynder, E. L., Reddy, B. S., McCoy, G. D., Weisburger, J. H., and Williams, G. M.: Diet and Cancer of the Gastrointestinal Tract, Adv. Intern. Med., 22:397, 1977.

8. Jenkins, D. J. A., Leeds, A. R., Gassull, M. A., Wolever, T. M. S., Goff, D. V., Alberti, K. G. M. M., and Hockaday, T. D. R.: Unabsorbable Carbohydrates and Diabetes: Decreased Postprandial Hyperglycaemia, Lancet, 2:172, 1976.

9. Anderson, J. W., and Ward, K.: Long-Term Effects of High-Carbohydrate, High-Fiber Diets on Glucose and Lipid Metabolism: A Preliminary Report on Patients with Diabetes, Diabetes Care, 1:77, 1978.

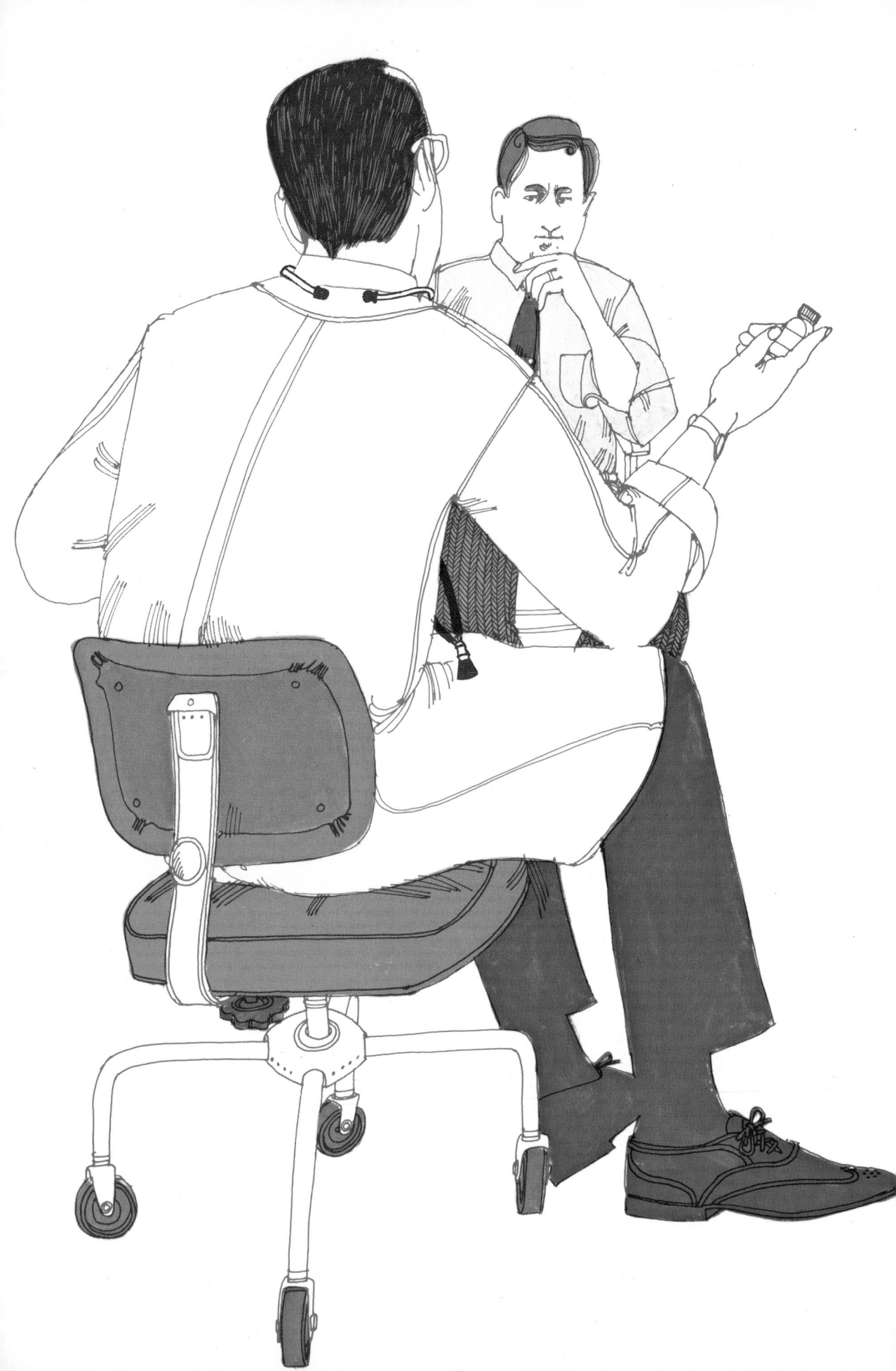

Clinical Use of Insulin

7

The skillful use of Insulin in treating diabetes requires that the physician have a fundamental understanding of the hormone and his patient's response to it as well as of methods of urine testing and their limitations. Useful facts include chemistry and time activity of the various Insulins, how they can be mixed, and how they should be stored and handled when refrigeration is not available. The physician must be constantly on the alert for various factors that may increase or decrease the Insulin requirement of his patient. He must systematically approach the initiation and maintenance of therapy according to the severity of the diabetes and must be aware of complications that may arise as a result of treatment with Insulin.

INFORMATION ABOUT INSULIN

TIME ACTIVITY

The time activities of the various Insulins are compared in Figure 15 (pages 42 and 43). These curves were developed from studies utilizing stable, well-controlled diabetic patients with relatively low daily Insulin requirements. After the patients were stabilized on a metabolic ward, Insulin therapy was interrupted, and the blood sugar was permitted to become elevated. When the blood sugar value rose to more than 200 mg. per 100 ml., a single large dose (usually about 80 units) was given; the blood sugar curve was then followed every four hours, one-sixth of the total diet being given after each blood sample drawn. Such studies were usually pursued for more than thirty-six hours; therefore, the blood sugar levels on which they are based are not strictly analogous to those encountered in clinical practice in patients on long-term Insulin therapy receiving three or four feedings daily. Nevertheless, these curves have provided a useful means of comparing the onset, peak, and duration of action of the various Insulins available for clinical use. It will be noted that the short-acting Insulins (Regular and Semilente®) usually have nearly identical time activities; occasionally with Semilente, however, the onset and peak may be later, and the duration of activity may be longer than with Regular Insulin.

INSULIN COMBINATIONS

When Lilly neutral Regular Insulin became available in 1973, the choice of Insulin combinations was expanded, and the stability of some prepared mixtures was substantially improved. (See pages 38 and 39 for a discussion of acid and neutral Regular Insulin.)

Neutral Regular Insulin (NRI) may be mixed with NPH, Lente®, or Protamine Zinc Insulin (PZI) in any proportion desired. The compatibility of NRI with Lente and NPH has improved the flexibility of using these mixtures in diabetic therapy. As a result, an increasing number of patients are being treated with combinations consisting, for instance, of two parts of NRI and one part NPH or Lente Insulin, a practice which augments diabetic control in selected patients.

Until recently, PZI was an amorphous compound and contained an excess of protamine that bound Regular Insulin. When the two were mixed, the number of units of Regular had to exceed that of PZI in order to achieve an effect from Regular Insulin. Now, however, PZI is in crystalline form, and there is no longer an excess of protamine to combine with added Regular. Consequently, no limitations need to be considered in the ratio of Regular to PZI.

Semilente, Ultralente®, and Lente Insulins may also be combined in any ratio desired.

All mixtures are stable for at least one month if stored at or below room temperature and for three months if refrigerated. Because of this improved stability, it is feasible for the physician to prepare the mixtures during office visits for patients requiring a combination but incapable of preparing it themselves.

The technic for preparing mixtures of Regular and modified Insulins is outlined in Figure 20.

When the two types of Insulin are mixed, it is important to recognize that the hypodermic syringes of different manufacturers may vary in the amount of space between the bottom line in the barrel and the needle.

Figure 20. Technic of Preparing Mixtures of Regular and Modified Insulins for Injection

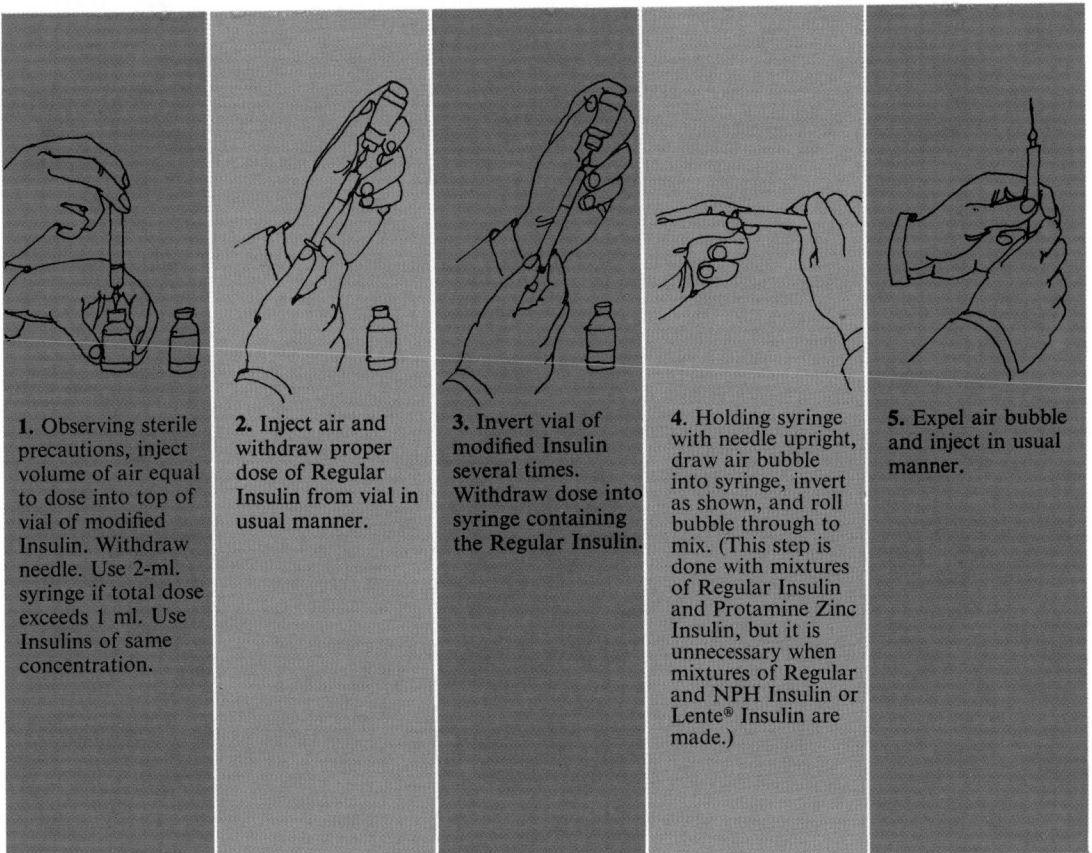

1. Observing sterile precautions, inject volume of air equal to dose into top of vial of modified Insulin. Withdraw needle. Use 2-ml. syringe if total dose exceeds 1 ml. Use Insulins of same concentration.

2. Inject air and withdraw proper dose of Regular Insulin from vial in usual manner.

3. Invert vial of modified Insulin several times. Withdraw dose into syringe containing the Regular Insulin.

4. Holding syringe with needle upright, draw air bubble into syringe, invert as shown, and roll bubble through to mix. (This step is done with mixtures of Regular Insulin and Protamine Zinc Insulin, but it is unnecessary when mixtures of Regular and NPH Insulin or Lente® Insulin are made.)

5. Expel air bubble and inject in usual manner.

This is called "dead space." The problem can be reduced if the patient consistently uses injection equipment of the same manufacturer and does not vary the order in which the Insulins are added to the syringe.

By general agreement of the manufacturers of Insulin, the color of the packaging and the printing on the labels are standardized according to the concentration of the Insulin as indicated: U-40, red; U-80, green; U-100, black; and U-500, brown and white diagonal stripes.

Very rarely (as in the treatment of infants with diabetes mellitus), Insulin with a concentration of less than 40 units per ml. is needed. This can be prepared by use of special materials obtainable from Eli Lilly and Company in Indianapolis, Indiana.

INSULIN IN INTRAVENOUS FLUIDS

In the treatment of diabetic patients undergoing stress, such as surgery, severe illness, or injury, Insulin can be added to intravenous fluids.[1] Insulin is known to be stable in 5 and 10 percent dextrose in water with and without electrolytes, and it does not stratify in these solutions.[2] Data are not available on its stability in other solutions.

Theoretically, the advantage of administering Insulin in intravenous fluids is that both Insulin and glucose are delivered in constant proportions, and smoother diabetes control is thereby achieved. Certain limitations of this procedure, however, can result in unpredictable fluctuations of blood glucose levels. Up to 20 percent of Insulin is bound to the flask and tubing. The greater degree of binding occurs with lower doses of Insulin.[2] If the same set is used for a second infusion, binding sites in the set may have become saturated with Insulin. The resulting increase in the amount of free Insulin can cause a hypoglycemic reaction.

Antibody binding of intravenous Insulin may delay its effect. When antibody-binding sites become saturated, the level of free Insulin rises rapidly and causes hypoglycemia.

STORAGE OF INSULIN

Because Insulin is a heat-labile protein, care must be exercised in storing all preparations so that they may maintain potency and maximum stability.

Although Insulin should be refrigerated, potency is lost so slowly and gradually that it probably will not be affected sufficiently to interfere with the control of diabetes if Insulin preparations are carefully protected from extremes of temperature or direct sunlight. However, the coolest spot available should be used for storage when refrigeration is impossible. The Food and Drug Administration requires that all preparations of Insulin bear the following instructions on the label: "Keep in a cold place. Avoid freezing." Radioimmunoassay has been used to assess the stability of Insulin at various temperatures.[3] These data show that Lente®, Semilente®, and Ultralente® Insulin retain potency when stored at room temperature (75°F.) over a period of twenty-four months. Storage for periods in excess of thirty months is required before there is significant loss of potency. Color changes appear after twenty-four months, and some easily dispersed aggregates form in the layer of the precipitates. Under the same conditions, the potency of Protamine Zinc Insulin and NPH Insulin does not diminish during thirty-six months of storage, but the normally fine precipitate in NPH Insulin forms into aggregates which become increasingly difficult to disperse. In contrast, there is a decline in potency of Regular Insulin.*

At higher temperatures (100° to 122°F.), all Insulin preparations deteriorate. However, the rate of deterioration for Protamine Zinc Insulin and NPH Insulin is so low that brief exposure to 100°F. may not result in notable loss of potency. Exposure to 120°F. should be avoided. Regular Insulin is the least stable at elevated temperatures. At the other extreme, freezing does not seem to cause a significant decrease in activity in any of the Insulins, although it may result in clumping of the suspension and may make it difficult to withdraw a uniform dose.

Storage during travel   Because it is difficult to maintain refrigeration temperatures in all situations, the storage of Insulin products presents a problem during travel. If the traveler's destination will be reached within a few days, the

*All statements here apply to acid Regular Insulin only. See pages 38 and 88 for a discussion of neutral Regular Insulin.

Table 18. Availability of Lilly Insulins in Foreign Countries

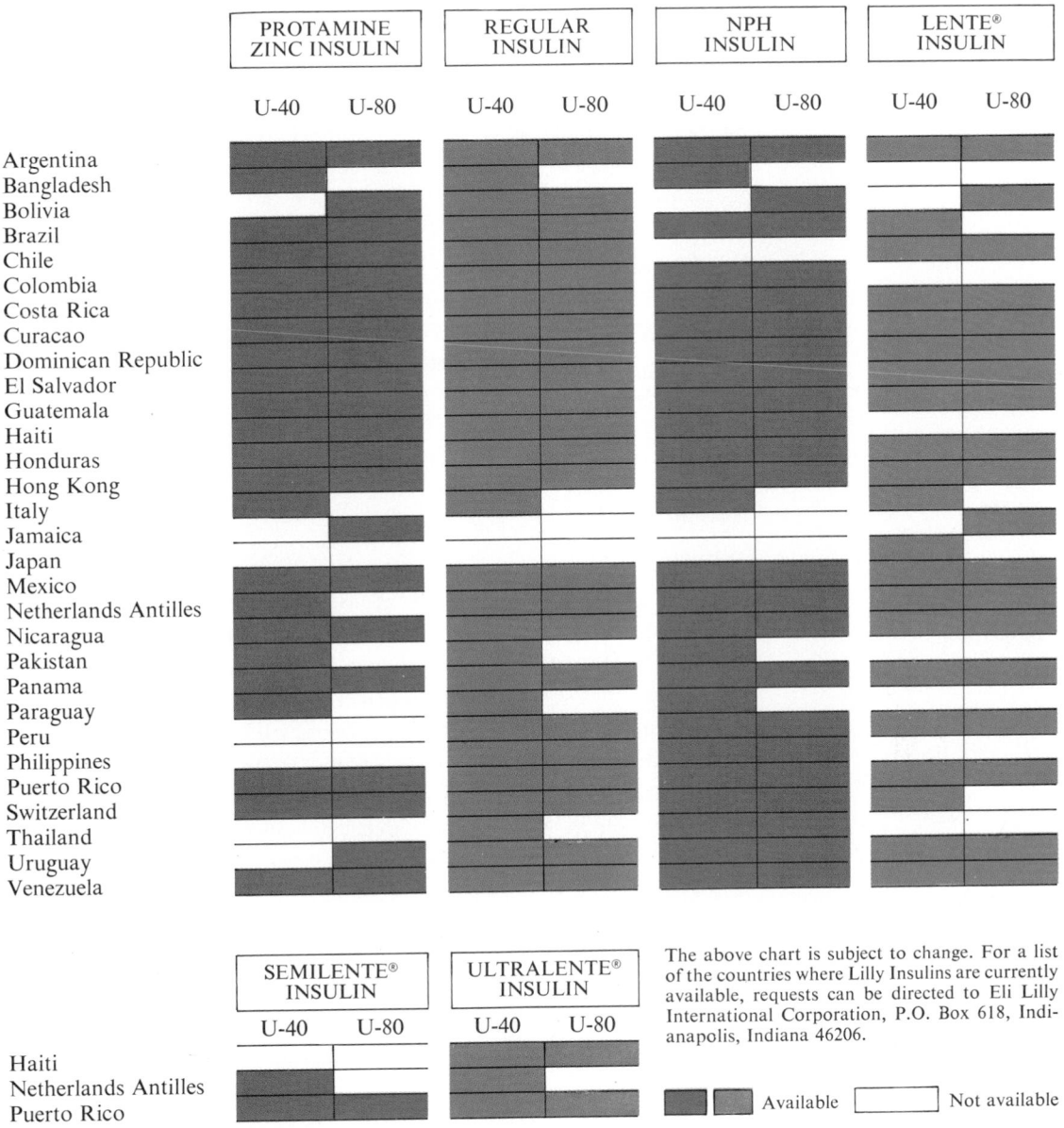

The above chart is subject to change. For a list of the countries where Lilly Insulins are currently available, requests can be directed to Eli Lilly International Corporation, P.O. Box 618, Indianapolis, Indiana 46206.

Available / Not available

Note: U-100 Insulin available in Puerto Rico and U.S. Virgin Islands.

Insulin can be removed from the refrigerator and packed in a suitcase between several layers of clothing. With this insulation, it will keep satisfactorily for several days.

If a diabetic is on an extended trip, it is usually possible to secure refrigeration through the services of personnel on the commercial carrier (e.g., when aboard ship, through the ship's doctor or the purser). When such an arrangement is not possible, a thermos bottle can easily be adapted for this purpose.

When traveling in foreign countries, diabetic patients are advised to take along an extra supply of Insulin and to divide the vials among several pieces of luggage; thus, an adequate supply is assured if anything should happen to any one suitcase. For extended trips, it may be necessary for diabetics to purchase Insulin while abroad. The availability of the various types of Lilly Insulin in foreign countries is indicated in Table 18.

URINE TESTING

Although the blood glucose level is the critical parameter in the continuous assessment of diabetic control, the expense and inconvenience of obtaining this determination, especially on an outpatient basis, justifies the use of urine tests for glucose. The interpretation of results obtained by means of various tests of urinary glucose depends upon the skill with which they are made and reported, the inherent accuracy of the test, and the renal threshold of the patient for glucose. Many clinics carry out a continuing program to instruct patients in the proper technic for urine glucose tests. Patients are told to void approximately one-half hour before urine determinations are performed for glucose; otherwise, glycosuria accumulating prior to the test may give a spurious result.

Tes-Tape   The inherent accuracy of the tests for urinary glucose is indicated in Figure 21, which compares the concentration of glucose or reducing substances per "plus" found with Tes-Tape® (Glucose Enzymatic Test Strip, USP, Lilly) or Benedict's Solution, the prototype of the copper-reduction methods. Tes-Tape, the most sensitive method, is *specific* for glucose, whereas the copper-reduction methods measure all reducing substances. The rapid testing methods for urine glucose are semiquantitative at best, because all indicate a range of concentration, not an absolute value. Thus, Figure 21 illustrates the necessity for the physician to ascertain the test method used when he interprets patient reports based on "pluses" rather than on percent concentrations.

When properly utilized, the renal threshold for glucose can be exceedingly valuable in predicting and confirming the presence of hypoglycemia and hyperglycemia. Although this level is nearly normal when diabetes is first discovered, the threshold for glucose will increase as diabetic nephropathy and other changes in renal function occur. For this reason, urinary glucose determinations are better indexes of blood glucose levels in the lower range in the recently discovered diabetic and of levels in the higher range in the patient who has had diabetes for many years. In patients with

Figure 21. Comparison of Tes-Tape and Tests Based on Benedict's Solution

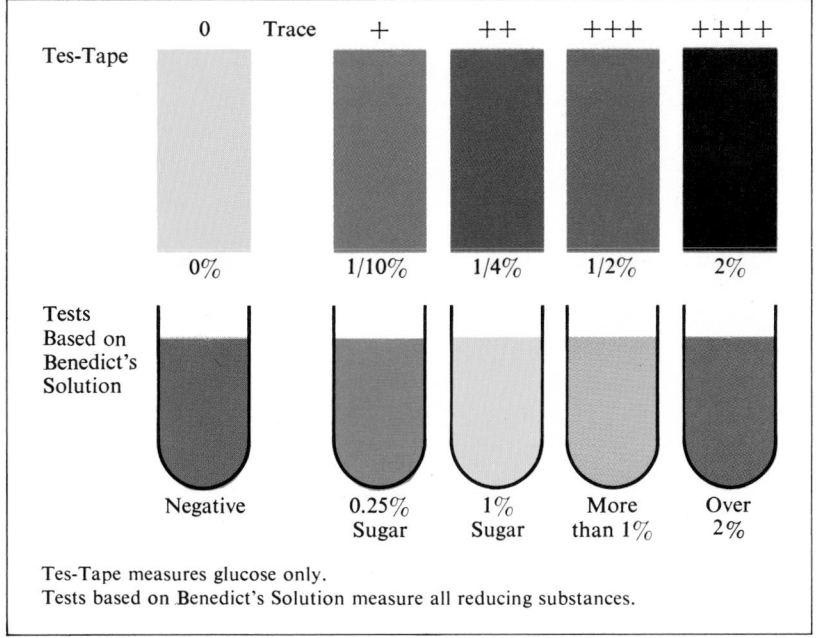

Tes-Tape measures glucose only.
Tests based on Benedict's Solution measure all reducing substances.

mild diabetes, it may be necessary or more useful to obtain this information through a three-hour glucose tolerance test.

GOALS OF TREATMENT

Although there are variations in the acceptable standards of control among different workers in diabetes, the majority strive for normal fasting blood glucose levels and maintenance of the "ideal" body weight, with freedom from acetonuria and hypoglycemia. As far as postprandial blood sugar is concerned, control of the Insulin-dependent diabetic can seldom be expected to approach the status of the normal individual. For instance, among forty-two diabetic males, the average two-hour postprandial blood sugar was 76 mg. per 100 ml. higher than the fasting level, and there was a range from −31 to +206 mg. per 100 ml.[4] No relationship was found between the Insulin requirement and the extent the two-hour postprandial value differed from the fasting value, nor was there any correlation of this difference with the height of the fasting level. In more than half the patients who had good fasting blood glucose values, the two-hour postprandial level averaged 184 mg. per ml., or approximately twice the fasting level. This report is cited not to discourage attempts to achieve optimum control of diabetic patients but to point out that such an objective is difficult to achieve.

PATIENT FACTORS AND METHODS FOR INITIATING AND MAINTAINING THERAPY WITH INSULIN

A patient's response to a dose of Insulin (i.e., his blood glucose level) at any given time is the result of numerous interrelated factors (Table 19).[5]

Table 19. Factors Which May Alter the Need for Insulin

NEED FOR INSULIN INCREASED BY
Increased food intake/weight gain
Reduction or cessation of physical exercise
Pregnancy
Withdrawal of oral hypoglycemic agents
Therapy with thyroid, corticosteroids, etc.
Deep x-ray therapy/ultraviolet-ray burns
Hyperthyroidism
Infections, fever, sepsis
"Idiopathic spontaneous exacerbations"

In general, correction or reversal of these factors decreases the need for Insulin.

In addition to these factors, individual patients show intrinsic variations. They have been categorized by Hallas-Moller,[6] who demonstrated three types of clinical response to a single dose of intermediate-acting (Lente® or NPH) Insulin. These differing patterns are depicted in Figure 22.

The patient with a "B" type of response maintains a normal blood glucose throughout a twenty-four-hour period and develops a tendency toward hyperglycemia only in relation to the ingestion of food. The patient with the "C" response shows a trend toward hyperglycemia during the daytime and toward hypoglycemia during the evening and early morning. The work of Bolinger et al.[7] with Insulin I[131] suggests that the patient with the "C" response is one whose serum protein binds exogenous Insulin, and this results in a delay in the availability of free insulin for metabolic action. The patient with an "A" response tends to be hyperglycemic during the early morning, in the evening, and throughout the night and hypoglycemic during the rest of the day. The selection of appropriate Insulin combinations can be facilitated by the identification of the type of response observed in a given patient.

Figure 22. Types of Response to a Single Daily Dose of NPH Insulin

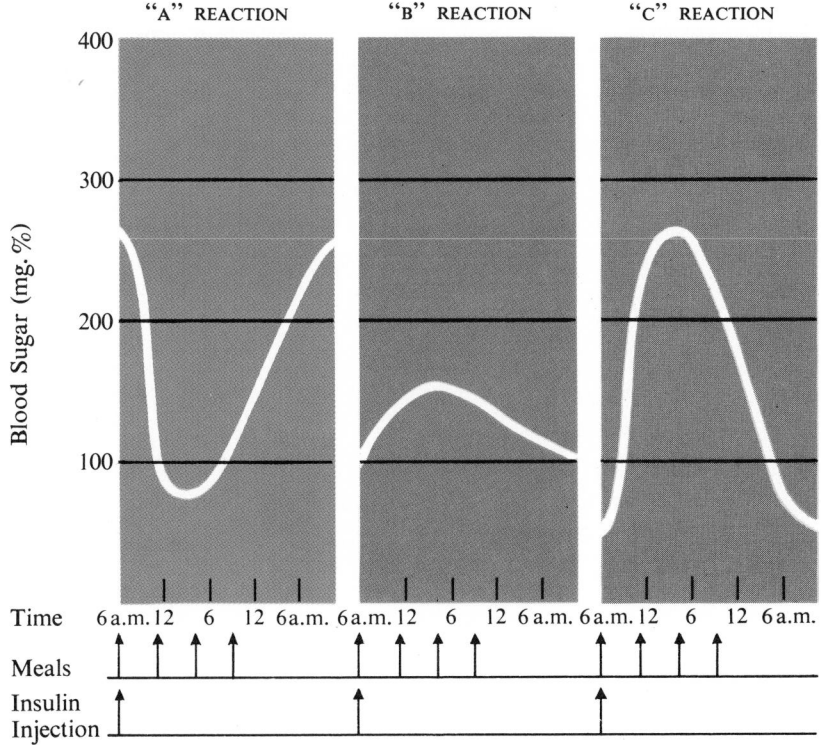

SPECIFIC SCHEMES FOR THE INITIATION AND MAINTENANCE OF INSULIN THERAPY

1. The *uncomplicated, nonketotic diabetic* who ordinarily can be controlled as an outpatient may be given an initial dose of 10 to 20 units of intermediate-acting (NPH or Lente®) Insulin.[8] This should be followed by weekly determinations of the blood sugar level, with fractional urine tests four or five times daily (usually before each meal and at bedtime). If all values obtained with the copper-reduction methods are in a 3 to 4+ range, the patient is instructed to increase the following day's dose of Lente or NPH Insulin by 4 units. If all values are in the range of 0 to 2+, but all are not 0, then the Insulin dose is not changed. On the other hand, if all values show 0 to 1+ by the copper-reduction methods, the patient is instructed to reduce the next day's dose by 4 units.

The uncomplicated case

When he is seen in approximately one week, the record for the urine tests is reviewed. On the basis of this record and the fasting blood sugar taken the morning of the visit, the Insulin dose for the next day is prescribed. Before this dosage is determined, however, the patient should be questioned about the occurrence of signs and symptoms of hypoglycemia (such as intense hunger, nervousness, and sweatiness), especially between 3:00 and 6:00 p.m. Then, on the basis of the fasting blood sugar, the Insulin dose for the next day is adjusted further. This procedure is described below under the alternative method in the section on the management of the ketotic or moderately severe diabetic. Selection of the initial Insulin dose by the physician and subsequent adjustment of that dose by the patient are illustrated in Table 20.

Table 20. The Adjustment of Intermediate-Acting Insulin in the Outpatient Management of an Uncomplicated, Nonketotic Diabetic

DAY	UNITS OF LENTE® INSULIN	FASTING BLOOD SUGAR (MG./ ML.)	URINE TESTS (COPPER-REDUCTION METHODS)				DOSAGE ADJUSTED BY	
			BEFORE BREAK-FAST	BEFORE LUNCH	BEFORE SUPPER	BEFORE BEDTIME	DOCTOR	PATIENT
Monday	20	230	4+	2+	4+	4+	x	
Tuesday	24	—	3+	4+	1+	3+		x
Wednesday	28	—	2+	3+	1+	2+		x
Thursday	28	—	1+	1+	0	0		x
Friday	28	—	1+	2+	0	0		x
Saturday	28	—	1+	0	1+	1+		x
Sunday	24	—	1+	0	2+	2+		x
Monday	24	120	1+	2+	0	0		x
Tuesday	24	—	1+	0	0	0	x	

If, in the attempt to control the diabetes, the dose of Insulin reaches 50 to 60 units daily and the fasting blood sugars still are not adequately controlled (i.e., fasting levels are not under 120 to 130 mg. per 100 ml.), the physician should consider giving two-thirds of the total dose of intermediate-acting Insulin before breakfast and one-third before supper. For the occasional patient whose postprandial morning blood sugar is persistently elevated, Regular or Semilente® Insulin may be added to the program, with beginning doses in the range of 4 to 6 units. For persistent hyperglycemia in the late evening and/or elevated fasting blood sugars, the use of Ultralente® Insulin, or the split dose of intermediate-acting Insulin as described above, may be considered.

It is nearly impossible to eradicate the hyperglycemia and glycosuria that occur after the morning meal by increasing the previous day's dose of Protamine Zinc or Ultralente Insulin without producing marked and dangerous late-evening and early-morning hypoglycemia.

Moderately severe diabetes

2. For the *ketotic or moderately severe diabetic*, standardization is usually carried out in the hospital setting, where frequent blood sugars and urine sugars can be obtained and dietary adherence is assured.[8] For each "plus" of the copper-reduction methods, 4 to 5 units of Regular Insulin are administered before meals and at bedtime. If the diabetic state is severe, a further dose is given at midnight. The Insulin requirement for twenty-four hours is then determined, and two-thirds to three-fourths of this is given in the morning as an intermediate-acting Insulin. Fractional urine tests are continued for twenty-four hours, and Regular Insulin is administered according to the amount of glycosuria found, but in smaller amounts (for instance, 6 units for 2+, 10 units for 3+, 12 units for 4+).

Alternatively, after the first dose of intermediate-acting Insulin, a second dose may be administered before supper on the basis of urine tests or the fasting blood sugar. If the latter is used, 1 unit should be given for each 10-mg. increment over "normal" (100 mg./100 ml.). For instance, if the patient had received 40 units of NPH in the morning on Day 1 and the fasting blood sugar that morning was 260 mg. per 100 ml., the supplementary dose of intermediate-acting Insulin before supper would be 16 units ($260 - 100 = 160$ mg., or 16 units). An amount equal to two-thirds of this dose (approximately 10 units) is then added to the next day's (Day 2) morning dose so that the total would be 50 units. The Insulin doses are subsequently increased until control is achieved. If hypoglycemia occurs in the afternoon or evening during the attempt to correct morning hyperglycemia in the mild, nonketotic diabetic, either a combination of intermediate-acting Insulins or a program of supplementary Insulin doses may be given, usually before the evening meal.

In some patients, the maximum activity of Regular Insulin does not occur until six to eight hours after a dose has been administered. A second dose of Regular Insulin given on the basis of a urine sugar result obtained sooner than six hours would be excessive. This problem can usually be averted by adjusting the dose according to urine sugar tests taken every six to eight hours instead of before meals and at bedtime.

3. The *labile, brittle diabetic* poses one of the greatest of all therapeutic challenges. Brittleness has been defined by Molnar[9] as a syndrome of excessive Insulin sensitivity and ketosis proneness manifested by extreme and unexplainable short-term and long-term fluctuations in the parameters of the disease. In practice, the labile, brittle diabetic is one whose blood glucose fluctuates widely and often rises precipitously in spite of careful quantitation and balance of Insulin dosage with food and exercise. The incidence of labile, brittle diabetes has been estimated to be 2 to 10 percent of the Insulin-dependent diabetic population. Therapy consists primarily in emphasizing precise adherence to the principles of treating the nonbrittle diabetic and using multiple injections of Regular Insulin. The timing of Insulin, exercise, and meals must be accurate. Also, the day-to-day intake of food must be consistent and divided. Instead of three or four meals daily, the labile, brittle diabetic may require four to six feedings, each corresponding with the action of the Insulin administered. Molnar *et al.*[10] suggest that Regular Insulin be administered every six hours day and night or that Regular Insulin be given every five hours during the day and Semilente® used for coverage during the night. Therapy is flexible so that nighttime Insulin reactions may be avoided.

Labile diabetes

Regardless of the method of adjustment used or the total daily Insulin dosage (unless, of course, there is Insulin resistance), when a diabetic has been standardized as an inpatient, it is usually advisable to reduce the Insulin dose by 4 to 6 units upon his leaving the hospital. This reduction will ordinarily offset the effect of increased activity of the patient after his discharge and avert hypoglycemia. Naturally, the zeal for dietary adherence may wane a few days later, and the Insulin dose may have to be increased to the previous level. The Insulin dose of diabetic patients admitted to the hospital for reasons other than control of diabetes should also be

Additional points

reduced, since in most instances the hospital diet program will be much more precise than the one they had been following.

Finally, a problem in diabetes control may be solved more readily by changing the time of a bread or fruit exchange than by changing the Insulin dose. A patient on 40 units of NPH Insulin who complains of nervousness and sweating at three o'clock in the afternoon may do better if a fruit exchange is borrowed from lunch and taken at 2:30 in the afternoon. Late-evening hypoglycemia may be prevented by the addition of a carbohydrate exchange to the bedtime feeding. Similarly, a problem of morning postprandial glycosuria which is not handled by the addition of Regular Insulin to the usual long-acting Insulin dose taken before breakfast may be improved by reducing the carbohydrate content of the breakfast or, possibly, by a supplemental dose of long-acting Insulin before supper.

COMPLICATIONS OF INSULIN THERAPY

The great majority of patients receiving Insulin rarely experience difficulty other than possibly an occasional episode of hypoglycemia which can easily be traced to the omission or delay of a meal, unexpected exercise, or an inappropriate dose of Insulin. Hypoglycemia as a potential hazard of sulfonylurea or Insulin therapy is treated separately in Chapter 10.

The complications of Insulin therapy discussed below are allergy (local and systemic), lipodystrophy (atrophic and hypertrophic), and serum antibody formation resulting in increased Insulin requirements (immunologic resistance). Because these complications apparently do not occur in patients who have received only purified pork Insulins[10A,10B,10C] and are evident with decreasing frequency as Insulin purity is increased,[10D] it is fair to assume that impurities in Insulin preparations contribute significantly to their development. Another etiologic factor in the complications of Insulin therapy is species source. As indicated in Table 8, Chapter 4, the amino acid composition of pork and of human insulin is identical at positions 8, 9, and 10 of the "A" chain. Since this site is an active one immunologically on the insulin molecule, the similarity here of human and pork insulins probably explains why pork Insulin is very well tolerated by diabetic patients. On the other hand, because beef insulin differs from human insulin at this site, it is significantly more immunogenic than pork.[10E] Finally, pharmaceutical form affects Insulin antibody formation; hence Lente®, for instance, is more immunogenic than is Regular Insulin.[10E,10F]

Since purity is a significant factor in the complications of Insulin therapy and purified pork Insulin is recommended for the treatment of such complications, familiarity with the chemical information concerning pork Insulins is desirable (see Chapter 4).

CUTANEOUS REACTIONS TO INSULIN

Cutaneous reactions to Insulin usually are represented by one or the other of two fairly distinct, although not always separate, clinical pictures. In one, there is generally a hivelike or urticarial type of reaction which may be associated with systemic manifestations, including itching, gastrointestinal complaints (gastric distention, nausea, vomiting, and diarrhea), and, rarely, hypotension. The other is a local wheal, or "knot," at the site of injection.

Local cutaneous reactions to Insulin are seen most frequently in diabetics who are receiving Insulin for the first time. Local reactions are also observed after the reinstitution of Insulin in patients whose treatment has been interrupted with the use of diet alone or with diet and oral therapy.

The typical lesion is characterized by the presence of a firm, red, indurated area extending from 1 to 5 cm. around the site of Insulin injection. Such lesions usually begin to form twenty to forty minutes after injection and reach their peak in size and intensity of itching within two to six hours. Occasionally, local reactions begin six to twelve hours after injection and do not develop fully until twenty-four to forty-eight hours afterward. Often they require from seven to ten days to subside, and some may persist for two to three months.

TREATMENT OF LOCAL REACTIONS

For the patient who develops a local reaction to Insulin, the first step is to rule out any errors in injection technic that may result in intradermal rather than subcutaneous injection. For example, since potentially irritating impurities are present in some grades of 70 percent isopropyl alcohol, they may produce redness at the injection site. To avoid this, Isopropyl Alcohol, Lilly, 91%, is recommended.

When problems resulting from faulty injection technic or the type of alcohol used have been ruled out, it may be assumed that the difficulty is related to the Insulin preparation being injected. The condition will subside spontaneously in many instances, probably as a result of desensitization, if the patient continues to use the same vial of Insulin. For relief during this period, an oral antihistaminic preparation may be given one to two hours prior to the Insulin injection; subsequent doses may be administered on a four-hour schedule, depending on the severity of the local reaction. Alternatively, Dolger[11] recommends the parenteral use of the antihistamine Benadryl®, 0.5 to 1 ml. (50 mg. per ml.), before administration of Insulin.

If such measures do not yield satisfactory results, the possibility that the allergy is species-specific must be considered. The standard preparations of Lilly Insulin are made from a combination of beef and pork sources (see Table 21). If local cutaneous reactions fail to subside when the current vial is continued, purified pork Insulin is recommended. If the patient reacts to pork, then purified beef Insulin is used. The species sources of commercial Lilly Insulins available in the United States are indicated in Table 21.

Sheep Insulin is occasionally requested for patients with local reactions to commercial preparations and has been reported to be efficacious in a patient with generalized reaction to Insulin.[12] Because its Insulin-like

Table 21. Species Sources of Lilly Insulins Available in the United States

BEEF:	All Insulins labeled "Beef"
BEEF-PORK:	All commercial Insulins unless otherwise labeled. Up to 90 percent is beef and the remainder pork.
PORK:	All Insulins labeled "Pork" Regular (Concentrated), U-500

proteins may differ from those to which the patient has become sensitive, sheep Insulin is theoretically useful. However, since it differs even more from human Insulin than does beef Insulin (see Table 8), it cannot be expected to prove of lasting value for patients whose reactivity is due to molecular differences that exist between human Insulin and Insulins from other species. Consequently, sheep Insulin is no longer commercially produced.

In the experience of the Lilly Clinic, about 90 percent of patients with persistent local allergy to mixed beef-pork Insulin will improve if treated with purified pork Insulin. About 5 percent of those with local allergy react less to beef than to pork Insulin. A rare patient with persistent local reactions to Insulin will benefit from the addition of a steroid to the Insulin.[10F] Because dexamethasone is compatible with Insulin, it is recommended that it be added to the Insulin in the syringe (total daily dose not to exceed 0.75 mg.). Not infrequently, patients with persistent local reactions develop systemic allergy to Insulin.

GENERALIZED REACTIONS

Generalized reactions are characterized by urticarial, or hivelike, skin eruptions with or without systemic manifestations that may include angioedema, gastrointestinal symptoms (nausea, vomiting, diarrhea), respiratory symptoms (asthma, dyspnea), and, occasionally, hypotension, shock, and death. Generalized reactions have been ascribed to sensitivity to the Insulin molecule proper. Data collected by the Lilly Research Laboratories[13] from studies of a large number of patients showed that those with systemic allergy to Insulin frequently have a history of (1) intermittent treatment with Insulin, (2) allergy to materials other than Insulin (e.g., penicillin), (3) obesity, and (4) increased serum antibody titers to beef Insulin. The last finding suggests that immunologic Insulin resistance would become manifest if such patients were treated with beef Insulin. For this reason, desensitization to pork Insulin is considered first in the management of patients with systemic or persistent local allergy to Insulin.

Although over 80 percent of patients with systemic or persistent local allergy to Insulin will tolerate pork Insulin better than beef Insulin, there is a small but definite group who are markedly sensitive to pork Insulin. Occasionally, these patients can be identified by a history of food allergy to pork. Intradermal testing with 1/1,000 and 1/500 of a unit of Regular Insulin in 0.025 to 0.1-ml. volumes also may identify patients who require beef Insulin. (Fortunately, in the Lilly Clinic experience, patients who clearly cannot tolerate pork Insulin do not demonstrate serum antibody titers in a range that would preclude the use of beef Insulin in the treatment of their disease.)

The methods of desensitization recommended and used by the Lilly Clinic are based on those of Mattson *et al.*,[14] Marble,[15] and Corcoran.[16] Because of the inconvenience of preparing dilutions of Insulin for skin testing and desensitization and the large error that occurs when these solutions are prepared at the bedside or on the ward, Eli Lilly and Company provides Insulin Allergy Desensitization Kits containing purified pork or purified beef Insulin.

Insulin Allergy Desensitization Kits contain 0.1 percent human serum albumin to prevent binding of Insulin to the walls of the glass vial. (Otherwise, as much as 2 units per ml. may be bound.)

When desensitization is to be performed, materials should be available for the treatment of an acute allergic emergency, such as anaphylaxis. Thus, before the procedure is initiated, 5 ml. of epinephrine (1:1,000) in a syringe, oxygen, tourniquets, injectable steroids, and antihistaminic preparations should be ready for emergency use.

Before desensitization is started, the patient should be advised of (1) the possibility of severe allergic reactions during the procedure; (2) the necessity of maintaining the desensitized state once it has been achieved (injection of Insulin is required at least once—and in many cases, twice—a day); and (3) the theoretical risk of hepatitis that may result from the addition of human serum albumin to prevent binding of Insulin to glassware. (Additional information is available from the manufacturer.)

Desensitization may be completed within eight to ten hours or extended over three to four days. The shorter time is recommended, according to the following procedure.

1. The dilutions as shown in Table 22 (0.1-ml. volumes of Insulins from the Insulin Allergy Desensitization Kit) should be administered at thirty-minute intervals. The vials are labeled A through N and must be used in alphabetical order.

2. If positive reactions occur, administer the same dilution of Insulin given two doses prior to the one causing the reaction.

3. Orange juice or other sources of carbohydrate should be available to treat hypoglycemia that may occur after the last (thirteenth) dose.

4. Following the thirteenth dose, at least 4 units of Insulin should be administered every four to six hours for the next day or, if possible, two days. Thus, if the thirteenth dose is given between 2:00 and 3:00 p.m., Regular Insulin in a dose of at least 4 units should be given every four to six hours until at least 7:00 or 8:00 a.m. the next day.

5. After one or two days of treatment with subcutaneous doses of Regular Insulin, therapy with Lente® Insulin or Lente and Regular Insulin combinations may be initiated. A few patients will lose desensitization if not maintained on two doses of Insulin daily.

6. In patients who repeatedly demonstrate reactivity to a given dilution of Insulin, isotonic saline can be used to further dilute the materials

in the desensitization kits so that the lowest dose given in a 0.1-ml. volume is 1/100,000, or 1,000,000th of a unit. The desensitization procedure will then include as many as fifty to sixty doses in gradually increasing concentrations. In such patients, a new dilution is given every two hours; consequently, desensitization may take a week or longer to accomplish.

In a series of 300 patients with systemic allergy to Insulin,[10B] eighteen (6 percent) could not be desensitized. The majority of these were overweight and could be managed on diet alone. Unfortunately, the rest either have had to tolerate hyperglycemia and its complications or endure the symptoms of a chronic low-grade allergy.[17] If antihistaminic agents are ineffective in such cases, low-dose steroid therapy may be considered.[18]

Table 22. Doses and Dilutions of Regular Insulins for Desensitization (as Contained in the Insulin Allergy Desensitization Kit)

DOSE NUMBER	BOTTLE LABEL LETTER	DILUTION	UNIT/0.1 ML.	
1	A	U-0.01	1/1,000	Administer Intradermally Only
2	B	U-0.02	1/500	
3	C	U-0.04	1/250	
4	D	U-0.1	1/100	
5	E	U-0.2	1/50	
6	F	U-0.4	1/25	
7	G	U-1	1/10	
8	H	U-2	1/5	Administer Subcutaneously Only
9	J	U-5	1/2	
10	K	U-10	1	
11	L*	U-100	2	
12	M*	U-100	4	
13	N*†	U-100	8	

*These doses are withdrawn from 10-ml. vials used for therapy.
†If the possibility of hypoglycemia following this dose is suggested by the blood glucose response to 4 units (the twelfth dose), then a dose of 4 instead of 8 units may be used here. Furthermore, for patients who have demonstrated any evidence of systemic allergy during the desensitization procedure, the thirteenth dose should consist of 4 rather than 8 units.

As indicated by Dolovich *et al.*[19] and other investigators,[20,21] Insulin resistance may coexist with or follow Insulin allergy.

Prognosis is good in the great majority of patients, although the allergic potential may be lifelong. Consultation with an allergist experienced in dealing with this type of reaction is recommended.

INSULIN RESISTANCE‡

Insulin resistance is a rare complication of Insulin therapy. It is customarily defined as "hyporesponsiveness to or a tolerance for at least 200 units of Insulin daily over a period of time in the absence of infection and coma."[22] However, the mechanisms thought to be responsible for Insulin resistance may be present in patients who require considerably less than 200 units of

‡The term "Insulin resistance" may denote any situation in which Insulin requirements are elevated or may mean specifically that the high Insulin dosage is necessitated by antibodies to insulin. In this discussion, the term is used in its broader sense.

Insulin daily. This is suggested by differences between the estimates of Insulin needed and the actual Insulin used by many diabetic patients.

For instance, individuals who have been made diabetic by pancreatectomy require only 40 to 50 units of Insulin daily, but a significant number of hereditary diabetics need 80 to 100 units of Insulin daily to control the blood glucose, even when adhering to proper dietary therapy. Furthermore, there is a wide variation in Insulin requirements among diabetic patients. These findings indicate that Insulin resistance is undoubtedly a multifaceted problem, the mechanisms of which cannot be defined or quantitated on the basis of Insulin dosage alone. Fortunately, published clinical experience makes it possible to classify certain factors that account for most cases of Insulin resistance.

Insulin Resistance Due to Antibody (Immune Insulin Resistance)

This type of Insulin resistance results from the binding of exogenous Insulin by antibodies in the serum. By means of their radioimmunoassay system (see page 50), Yalow and Berson[23] have confirmed the findings of previous investigators which show that six weeks to three months after beginning treatment with Insulin, *all* patients develop antibodies that bind Insulin.

Antibody binding

Their method shows that the serums of diabetic subjects usually bind less than 10 units of Insulin per liter; no binding is found in subjects who have not received Insulin. Serums from patients with chronic Insulin resistance, however, may bind from 6 to 1,000 times this amount of Insulin. Although the serums from diabetic patients react with both pork and beef Insulin, the affinity of antibody is usually greater for beef Insulin than for pork Insulin. This is attributed to the fact that beef Insulin has greater antigenicity because it is more unlike human insulin than is pork Insulin. The following order of reaction was found in diabetic antiserums when examined in the radioimmunoassay system of Yalow and Berson:

$$beef = sheep > pork > horse$$

The relationship of structural differences to antigenicity and the binding of Insulin by antibodies constitute the rationale for treatment of antibody-type Insulin resistance.

Nonimmune Insulin Resistance

Obesity—Perhaps the most common cause of Insulin resistance is obesity. Well known in clinical practice is the markedly overweight individual who often tolerates larger doses than 100 units of Insulin daily. When a weight reduction program is successful, however, Insulin therapy may no longer be required, and the blood sugar may be controlled by diet therapy alone. Boshell *et al.*[24] have demonstrated that when a sample of fat taken from an obese, Insulin-resistant patient is incubated in the epididymal fat pad system of the rat, there is evidence of Insulin antagonism. When the experiment is repeated after the same patient has lost even as little as ten to twenty pounds, Insulin antagonism is often markedly reduced.

Other Medical Disorders—Several medical disorders have been reported to result in or to be associated with resistance to Insulin. These include endocrinopathies such as acromegaly, hyperthyroidism, Cushing's disease, hemochromatosis, chronic lymphocytic leukemia, and liver disease. Also included in this group of disorders is lipoatrophic diabetes. The spectrum of diseases associated with Insulin resistance has been covered in depth by Smelo.[22]

Miscellaneous—Two new types of Insulin resistance have recently been elucidated. Fortunately, the incidence of each is extremely low. In one, there is presumably marked enzymatic destruction of Insulin at the injection site, as evidenced by tolerance to exceedingly high doses of Insulin when given subcutaneously or intramuscularly in comparison with the response to conventional doses given intravenously. This condition has been reported in young adolescent girls but may also be observed in boys.[25]

The other type of Insulin resistance is due to impairment of Insulin action on fat-cell receptors. Adults with this disorder frequently have acanthosis nigricans. A definitive diagnosis requires evaluation of the patient's serum for antibodies to insulin receptors.[26] The clinical course of both types of Insulin resistance is variable.

Diagnosis

The diagnosis of Insulin resistance rests upon establishing the existence of an excessive Insulin requirement (after the exclusion of infection, the use of improper injection technics, and improper storage and agitation of the vial of Insulin before use). Inspection of the patient may readily reveal that obesity is the principal factor leading to the resistance. The endocrinopathies, hemochromatosis, lipoatrophic diabetes, and other causes may be suspected and eliminated by a careful history and physical examination and by appropriate endocrine and blood studies. The diagnosis of immunologic resistance may be confirmed by measuring the concentration of antibodies to Insulin in the patient's serum. (Since cross-reaction between beef antibody and pork Insulin in the assay system may lead to a spuriously high pork titer, elevated pork titers do not rule out the use of pork Insulin in patients with immunologic resistance.) When facilities are not available for the determination of insulin antibodies, the diagnosis of Insulin resistance due to immune factors is made by the exclusion of the above disorders. However, Insulin resistance in some patients may be the result of both obesity and immune factors.

Treatment

The treatment of Insulin resistance depends upon the severity of the diabetic state and the urgency for establishing diabetic control. It is a general principle in medical therapeutics that the simplest, safest, and most convenient mode of therapy should be selected first. The treatment of choice for Insulin resistance due to obesity is, as indicated above, weight reduction. In some obese patients who do not have ketoacidosis, the use of sulfonylurea drugs will, in time, occasionally permit a decrease in the exogenous Insulin requirement. When endocrinopathies, chronic lymphocytic leukemia, or other disorders are associated with Insulin resistance, specific treatment is indicated but may not necessarily be expected to reduce the Insulin requirement. Intermediate-acting or Regular Insulin may be used in the management of lipoatrophic diabetes. Therapy of patients in the miscellaneous category constitutes a unique problem which is best handled in centers where facilities are available for making individual studies and providing special services.

The therapy of Insulin resistance due to antibody depends upon the metabolic state of the patient. When ketoacidosis is absent, a trial of diet or diet and sulfonylurea therapy may be made.

Management of Insulin resistance

The use of a sulfonylurea is based on the assumption that the antibodies present in the serum of the patient and causing resistance to exogenous Insulin have little affinity for endogenous insulin, and it, therefore, is free to exert its metabolic effect.[27] Oral therapy is of no value in persons whose beta cells are incapable of responding to sulfonylurea agents, as indicated by the presence of ketoacidosis. When sulfonylureas are used—e.g., Dymelor® (acetohexamide, Lilly), 1.5 Gm. daily—it may be necessary to continue dosage for one to two weeks before a diminution in the hyperglycemia is observed.

When immunologic Insulin resistance is associated with marked hyperglycemia (with or without ketoacidosis) and more vigorous treatment is needed, pork Insulin and possibly intensive corticosteroid therapy are required. Because steroids are diabetogenic and have other undesirable metabolic effects, pork Regular Insulin is usually tried first. Modified Insulins (Lente® or NPH) are not needed in patients with immunologic resistance because the serum antibodies bind Insulin and impart to it a time action comparable to that of repository Insulin. Therefore, Regular Pork Insulin, U-100 or U-500, is administered in two divided doses before breakfast and supper. Ordinarily, the first day's dose is equal to that of the long-acting Insulin the patient has been receiving and is given in two or three divided doses. Thus, a resistant patient who has been receiving 200 units of NPH or Lente Insulin daily may be given 100 units of Regular Pork Insulin before breakfast and again before supper. Doses are usually increased by 25 to 50 units until control is achieved. When pork Insulin is used for the first time, a dramatic reduction in Insulin requirement may occur within twenty-four hours. Once the blood glucose is brought to normal levels, the resistance often "breaks," and further intensive Insulin treatment is no longer needed.

Steroid therapy, as suggested above, is ordinarily reserved for patients who have not responded to a change in the species source, particularly those who have not reacted satisfactorily to concentrated Insulin (U-500) in doses higher than 300 units daily. When a steroid is used, however, concentrated Insulin is still employed as indicated above.

An adequate dosage of steroid, administered daily, is critically important if such treatment is to succeed. Although large amounts of Insulin may be required for a week or so after appropriate doses of corticosteroid, steroid therapy should not be continued for more than a month. There may be a dramatic reduction in Insulin dosage at any time after steroid treatment, and this may be followed by a period of diminished or no need for exogenous Insulin, a phenomenon presumably related to decreased antibody production and the unbinding of insulin from existent and decaying antibodies.

Fish Insulin,[28] sulfated Insulin,[29] and modified pork Insulin[30] (de-alaninated pork Insulin) have been recommended for the treatment of immunologic Insulin resistance. None are currently available commercially, and careful crossover studies comparing them with unmodified "single peak" pork Insulin have not been reported.

Regardless of the method of treatment, Insulin resistance due to immune factors should be recognized as a rare condition which is subject to spontaneous exacerbations and remissions.

INSULIN LIPODYSTROPHY

One of the distressing, although therapeutically harmless, complications of Insulin administration in the diabetic is the occurrence of changes in subcutaneous fat at the site of injection. These changes, called "lipodystrophy," may take the form of atrophy or hypertrophy (Figures 23 and 24). Occasionally, both types are observed in the same patient.

Atrophy   The etiology of Insulin lipoatrophy was totally obscure until Watson and Calder[31] reported the filling in of atrophic sites by injection of several-times-recrystallized Insulin directly into the affected areas. On the assumption that multiple recrystallizations or other processes yielding Insulin preparations of greater purity remove substances which might be related to the development of lipoatrophy, the Clinical Research Division of Eli Lilly and Company undertook an extensive study of the efficacy of "single peak" and "single component" Insulins.[10D,32]

This effort disclosed that over 80 percent of patients with Insulin lipoatrophy improved if commercially available mixed beef-pork "single peak" Insulin was injected into the affected areas. The remainder failed to respond to this Insulin. About half of the second group noted improvement if pork Insulin was injected into the affected areas. The rest responded only to "single component" Insulin, now officially designated as "purified pork" (see Table 10, Chapter 4). Now that purified pork Insulin is commercially available, it is expected that the frequency of Insulin lipoatrophy will diminish markedly. The filling in of atrophic sites that occurs with the use of the purified Insulins is attributed to the natural lipogenic effects of Insulin. Once filling in has occurred, patients should be advised to rotate injection sites; otherwise, the filling in will progress to Insulin hypertrophy.

Hypertrophy   The second type of lipodystrophy takes the form of a spongy localized hypertrophy and is most commonly found on the anterior or lateral thigh. The incidence of this complication of Insulin administration is slightly higher in males than in females. Patients with hypertrophy almost always give a history of prolonged and constant use of the same injection site. The hypertrophic mass consists of fibrous and comparatively avascular scar tissue. Since the skin over the area becomes relatively anesthetic, the use of the site becomes self-perpetuating because of the comparative painlessness of injections into it. This feature apparently is responsible for the high incidence of subcutaneous hypertrophy among children and young adults. Experimentation has shown that absorption is slow and incomplete from these areas. Instances of presumed "Insulin resistance" in such patients have been quickly cured by a change in the site of injection.

The etiology of the hypertrophic form of Insulin lipodystrophy is unknown but unquestionably related, at least in part, to the local effects of insulin lipogenesis. Treatment consists in reassuring patients that the condition is benign, advising them to alternate injection sites, and specifying use of purified pork Insulin, which is efficacious in 50 to 70 percent of cases.[10D]

On the basis of the foregoing remarks, the indications for use of purified pork Insulin are listed in Table 23.

Figure 23. Both Atrophy and Hypertrophy in a Twenty-Eight-Year-Old Woman Whose Use of Insulin Extended over Sixteen Years

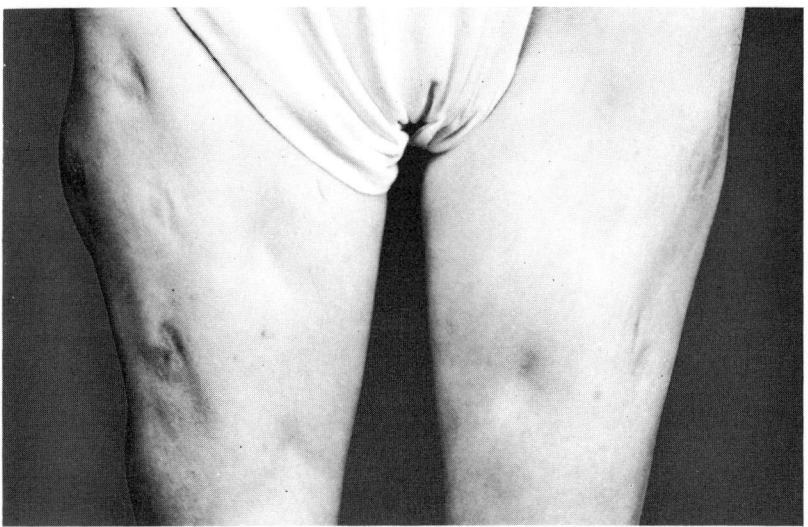

Figure 24. Hypertrophy in a Man Twenty-Two Years of Age Who Had Been Taking Insulin for Six Years

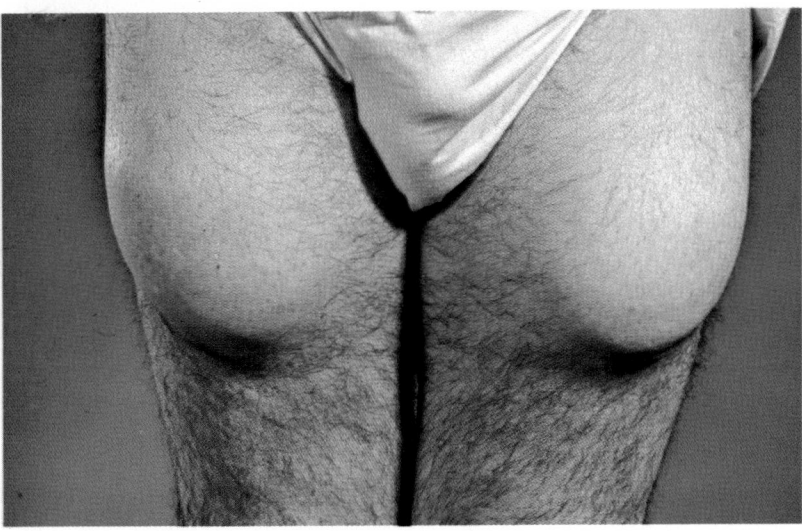

(Photograph courtesy of the Elliott P. Joslin Research Laboratory and Diabetes Foundation)

Table 23. Indications for Use of Purified Pork Insulin[33-37]

1. Patients who are now taking pork Insulin

2. Patients who have persistent local or systemic allergy to mixed beef-pork or beef Insulin

3. Patients now taking mixed beef-pork or beef Insulin who develop Insulin lipoatrophy and/or hypertrophy

There are no conclusive data demonstrating that purified pork Insulin is uniquely effective in the prevention of the complications of diabetes, such as diabetic retinopathy, neuropathy, and nephropathy, or in the treatment of labile diabetes.

EDEMA WITH INSULIN THERAPY

Edema is an infrequently recognized complication of Insulin therapy. It is characterized by generalized retention of fluid and usually appears in association with abrupt restoration of diabetic control in a patient whose disease has been unsatisfactorily managed over a period of time.[38-40] Studies in normal subjects before and after fasting[41,42] and in diabetics before and after restoration of blood glucose control[39] indicate that the edema is due to the inhibition of salt excretion resulting from the immediate increase of available carbohydrate for tissue metabolism. Treatment consists in diuretic therapy and the dietary restriction of salt. If these measures are instituted promptly, the edema will usually subside within three to five days. Awareness that edema may follow the use of Insulin is helpful in making a differential diagnosis in the diabetic patient when there is abrupt improvement in diabetic control.

BIBLIOGRAPHY

1. Galloway, J. A., and Shuman, C. R.: Diabetes and Surgery. A Study of 667 Cases, Am. J. Med., *34:*177 1963.
2. Størvick, W. O.: Personal communication.
3. Størvick, W. O., and Henry, H. J.: Effect of Storage Temperature on Stability of Commercial Insulin Preparations, Diabetes, *17:*499, 1968.
4. Rockwell, D. A., West, K. M., and Wulff, J. A.: Clinical Significance of the Two-Hour Postprandial Blood Glucose in Insulin-Dependent Diabetes, paper presented at the 21st Annual Meeting of the American Diabetes Association, New York, June 24-25, 1961.
5. Duncan, G. G.: Diseases of Metabolism, Ed. 5, p. 1011. Philadelphia: W. B. Saunders Company, 1964.
6. Hallas-Møller, K.: The Lente Insulins, Diabetes, *5:*7, 1956.
7. Bolinger, R. E., Morris, J. H., McKnight, F. G., and Diederich, D. A.: Disappearance of I^{131}-Labeled Insulin from Plasma as a Guide to Management of Diabetes, New England J. Med., *270:*767, 1964.
8. Shuman, C. B.: Diabetes Mellitus in Adults, in Current Therapy (edited by H. F. Conn), p. 295. Philadelphia: W. B. Saunders Company, 1965.
9. Molnar, G. D.: Observations on the Etiology and Therapy of "Brittle" Diabetes, Canad. M. A. J., *90:*953, 1964.
10. Molnar, G. D., Gastineau, C. F., Rosevear, J. W., Helmholtz, H. F., Jr., McGuckin, W. F., and Chenoweth, W. L.: Metabolic Effects of Exercise and of Multiple-Dose Insulin Regimens in Hyperlabile Diabetes Mellitus, Metabolism, *12:*157, 1963.
10A. Wright, A. D., Walsh, C. H., Fitzgerald, M. G., and Malins, J. M.: Very Pure Porcine Insulin in Clinical Practice, Br. Med. J., *1:*25, 1979.
10B. Data on file, Lilly Laboratory for Clinical Research.
10C. Haycock, P.: Personal communication.
10D. Wentworth, S. M., Galloway, J. A., Davidson, J. A., Haunz, E. A., and Willman, R. E.: The Use of the Purified Insulins in the Treatment of Patients with Insulin Lipoatrophy, paper presented at the International Diabetes Federation Meeting, Vienna, Austria, September 13, 1979.
10E. Chance, R. E., Root, M. A., and Galloway, J. A.: The Immunogenicity of Insulin Preparations, Acta Endocrinol. (Copenh.), *83:*185 (S205), 1976.
10F. Galloway, J. A., and Bressler, R.: Insulin Treatment in Diabetes, Med. Clin. North Am., *52:*663, 1978.
11. Dolger, H.: The Management of Insulin Allergy and Insulin Resistance in Diabetes Mellitus, M. Clin. North America, *36:*783, 1952.
12. Kreines, K.: Use of Sheep Insulin in Insulin Allergy, Diabetes, *20:*774, 1971.
13. Davidson, J. A., Galloway, J. A., Petersen, B. H., Wentworth, S. M., and Crabtree, R. E.: The Use of Purified Insulins in Insulin Allergy, paper presented at the 34th Annual Meeting of the American Diabetes Association, Atlanta, Georgia, June 16, 1974.
14. Mattson, J. R., Patterson, R., and Roberts, M.: Insulin Therapy in Patients with Systemic Insulin Allergy, Arch. Intern. Med., *135:*818, 1975.
15. Marble, A.: Allergy and Diabetes, in The Treatment of Diabetes Mellitus, Ed. 10 (edited by E. P. Joslin, H. F. Root, P. White, and A. Marble), p. 395. Philadelphia: Lea & Febiger, 1959.
16. Corcoran, A. C.: Note on Rapid Desensitization in a Case of Hypersensitiveness to Insulin, Am. J. M. Sc., *196:*359, 1938.
17. Ulrich, H., Hooker, S. B., and Smith, H. H.: Allergic Reaction to Insulin, New England J. Med., *221:*522, 1939.
18. Cockel, R., and Mann, S.: Insulin Allergy Treated by Low-Dosage Hydrocortisone, Brit. M. J., *3:*722, 1967.
19. Dolovich, J., Schnatz, J. D., Reisman, R. E., Yagi, Y., and Arbesman, C. E.: Insulin Allergy and Insulin Resistance: Case Report with Immunologic Studies, J. Allergy, *46:*127, 1970.
20. Sherman, W. B.: A Case of Coexisting Insulin Allergy and Insulin Resistance, J. Allergy, *21:*49, 1950.
21. Ezrin, C.: Resistance and Allergy to Insulin, Appl. Therap., *5:*680, 1963.
22. Smelo, L. S.: Insulin Resistance, Proc. Am. Diabetes A., *8:*75, 1948.
23. Yalow, R. S., and Berson, S. A.: Immunologic Aspects of Insulin, Am. J. Med., *31:*882, 1961.
24. Boshell, B. R., Barrett, J. C., Wilensky, A. S., and Patton, T. B.: Insulin Resistance. Response to Insulin from Various Animal Sources, Including Human, Diabetes, *13:*144, 1964.
25. Paulsen, E. P.: An Insulin-Degrading Enzyme in a Diabetic Girl Causing Massive Destruction of Subcutaneous Insulin, Diabetes, *25:*334 (Supplement 1), 1976.
26. Bar, R. S., and Roth, J.: Insulin Receptor Status in Disease States of Man, Arch. Intern. Med. *137:*474, 1977.
27. Segre, E. J.: Diabetes Mellitus with Insulin Resistance: Report of a Case Successfully Treated with Tolbutamide, Metabolism, *11:*562, 1962.
28. Yalow, R. S., and Berson, S. A.: Reaction of Fish Insulins with Human Insulin Antiserums. Potential Value in the Treatment of Insulin Resistance, New England J. Med., *270:*1171, 1964.
29. Davidson, J. K., and Debra, D. W.: Immunologic Insulin Resistance, Diabetes, *27:*307, 1978.
30. Akre, P. R., Kirtley, W. R., and Galloway, J. A.: Comparative Hypoglycemic Response of Diabetic Subjects to Human Insulin or Structurally Similar Insulins of Animal Source, Diabetes, *13:*135, 1964.
31. Watson, B. M., and Calder, J. S.: A Treatment for Insulin-Induced Fat Atrophy, Diabetes, *20:*628, 1971.
32. Wentworth, S. M., Galloway, J. A., Davidson, J. A., Root, M. A., Chance, R. E., and Haunz, E. A.: An Update of Results of the Use of 'Single Peak' (SP) and 'Single Component' (SC) Insulin in Patients with Complications of Insulin Therapy, Presented at the 36th Annual Meeting, American Diabetes Association, June, 1976.
33. Galloway, J. A., and Bressler, R.: Insulin Treatment in Diabetes, Med. Clin. North Am., *62:*673, 1978.
34. Editorial, Lancet, *1:*363 (February 17), 1979.
35. Alberti, K. G. M. M., and Nottrass, M.: Highly Purified Insulins, Editorial, Diabetologia, *15:*77, 1978.
36. Kahn, C. R., and Rosenthal, A. S.: Immunologic Reactions to Insulin: Insulin Allergy, Insulin Resistance, and the Autoimmune Insulin Syndrome, Diabetes Care, *2:*283, 1979.
37. Caterson, I.: New Insulins: Their Role in the Treatment of Diabetes, Drugs, *17:*289, 1979.
38. Kirtley, W. R.: Rapid Correction of Metabolism Defect May Cause Edema in Diabetes. Report of a Case, J. Indiana M. A., *48:*1290, 1955.
39. Saudek, C. D., Boulter, P. R., Knopp, R. H., and Arkey, R. A.: Sodium Retention Accompanying Insulin Treatment of Diabetes Mellitus, Diabetes, *23:*240, 1974.
40. Bleach, N. R., Dunn, P. J., Khalafalla, M. E., and McConkey, B.: Insulin Edema, Br. Med. J., *2:*177, 1979.
41. Bloom, W. L.: Inhibition of Salt Excretion by Carbohydrate, Arch. Int. Med., *109:*26, 1962.
42. Wright, H. K., Gann, D. S., and Albertsen, K.: Effect of Glucose on Sodium Excretion and Renal Concentrating Ability after Starvation in Man, Metabolism, *12:*804, 1963.

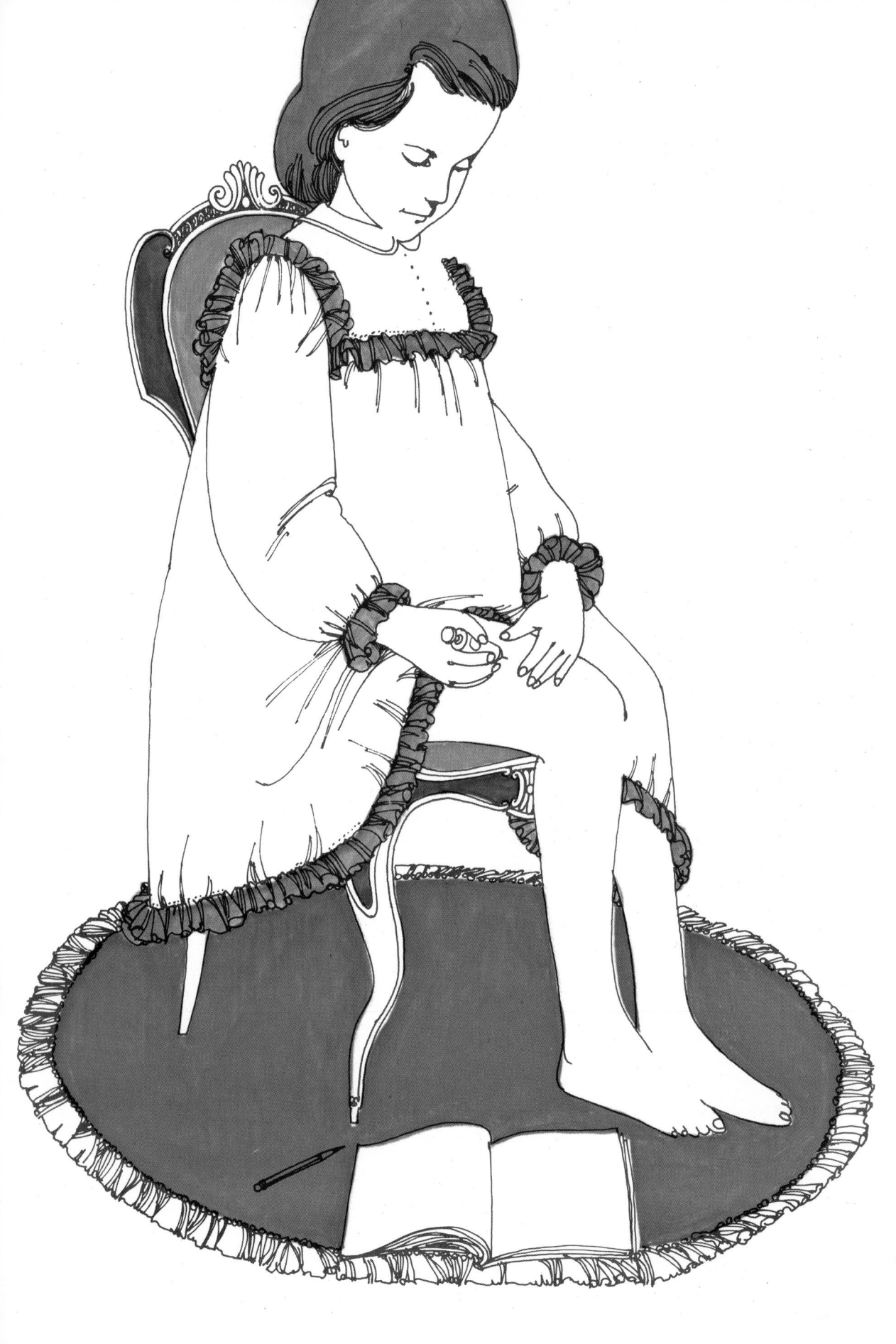

Diabetes Mellitus in Children

8

SYMPTOMS

In children, the onset of diabetes mellitus follows a definite clinical course. After a period of a few months of increased appetite, the child develops unusual thirst, voids frequently, loses weight, strength, and stamina, and often complains of leg cramps or pruritus. Diagnosis is readily made at this juncture. Glycosuria is present, and a single measurement of blood glucose one hour after a carbohydrate meal reveals a value in excess of 200 mg. per 100 ml. Although hyperglycemia usually denotes diabetes mellitus, a glucose tolerance test is indicated when there is doubt. When these symptoms are unrecognized, ketoacidosis may develop at any time. Then the child becomes listless, his appetite wanes, and nausea and vomiting ensue. Headache and weakness occur, followed by abdominal pain and drowsiness and, finally, coma.

INITIAL TREATMENT

When diabetes is diagnosed, hospitalization is indicated to evaluate the response to treatment and to begin education toward a new way of life. The administration of adequate doses of Insulin and the provision of an appropriate diet generally suffice to establish control. The impressions made upon the child during his hospitalization at the beginning of treatment will, to a large extent, determine the attitudes and habits he will hold toward his disease for the rest of his life. Thus, careful instruction by competent persons at this time is mandatory.

OBJECTIVES OF TREATMENT

The major objective of treatment is to maintain control of the diabetic state in a way that sustains the child in his growth and development. Diabetes in the child encompasses not only his physical being but also his person, his family, his entire life, and the community of which he is a part. Therapy which succeeds in a hospital setting may fail at home. Indeed, the long-term course of juvenile diabetes is frequently punctuated by crises in control, severe Insulin reactions, or ketoacidosis. The objective is to allocate medical resources—Insulin, diet, and activity—in order to control the diabetic state.

CRITERIA OF DIABETIC CONTROL

The child who requires Insulin falls far short of physiological control, but the degree of control he strives to achieve is influenced by his physician's objectives. The criteria of White[1] constitute a suitable frame of reference for ascertaining the degree of control of juvenile diabetes (Table 24).

Because children frequently pay more attention to their disease a few days before visits to the physician, blood and urine glucose measurements may indicate better metabolic control than is usually present. Measurement of the glycosylated hemoglobins, which result from the exposure of hemoglobin to long-term hyperglycemia, may improve the assessment of chronic blood glucose control in diabetics.[1A]

Table 24. Standards for Control in Juvenile Diabetes

	PERFECT	GOOD	FAIR	POOR
Hyperglycemia, a.c.	0	0	+ +	+ + + +
p.c.	0	+	+ +	+ + + +
Hypercholesteremia	0	0	0	+ +
Urine glucose (Gm./24 hr.)	0	0 to 25	25 to 50	> 100
Urine acetone	0	0	0 to trace	+ + + +
Growth . . . . Normal	Normal	Satisfactory	Retarded
Activity potential . . . . Normal	Normal	Satisfactory	Diminished

REMISSION—THEN TOTAL DIABETES

Within days or weeks after starting treatment with Insulin and diet, diabetic children develop striking remissions in Insulin requirement. Unless parent and physician are alert to the symptoms of hypoglycemia, which usually herald remission, major Insulin reactions may occur before the dosage is revised downward. After remission, the Insulin requirement may be as little as 1 or 2 units daily. Even though patients may be responsive to sulfonylureas during remission, withdrawal of Insulin is unwise because it would interrupt the formation of lifelong habits, encourage false hopes of total cure, and leave the child unprotected against the abrupt return to total Insulin dependence. After a period of a few months (occasionally longer), the daily requirement of Insulin rises, and the child becomes dependent on it. Five years after the onset of symptomatic diabetes mellitus, the vast majority of children are dependent on Insulin in the sense that its withdrawal would be followed by the onset of keto-acidosis. The mean daily Insulin requirement of Insulin-dependent children is 0.41 unit per pound (s.d. = 0.11 unit/lb.).

LIMITATIONS OF THE INSULINS IN THE MANAGEMENT OF DIABETIC CHILDREN

Although the intermediate-acting Insulins, NPH and Lente®, are usually the first and foremost choices, they possess certain defects in practice, one of which is that the response of blood sugar over the course of twenty-four hours may be uneven.

Three different patterns of response to a single daily dose in the morning were first described by Hallas-Møller[2] (see Figure 22, page 95). The patient with the "B" reaction maintains a normal blood sugar throughout a twenty-four-hour period, whereas the patient with the "C" reaction is hyperglycemic during the day, and the patient with the "A" reaction is hyperglycemic during the early morning, in the evening, and throughout the night. These patterns of response are encountered in diabetic patients[3] frequently enough to provide a useful basis for deciding when a patient needs supplementary short-acting Insulin. For example, patients with "C" reactions to NPH or Lente generally require a supplement of short-acting Insulin before breakfast and supper. Patients with "A" reactions require splitting the NPH or Lente dose into two parts, one before breakfast and one at bedtime, and may require matching supplements of short-acting Insulin before breakfast and supper.

A second defect of single daily dosage of intermediate-acting Insulin stems from day-to-day variation in Insulin requirement. Some of this variability remains unexplained. Some is closely related to the total caloric intake for the day. When dietary intake is erratic, variation in requirement in the face of fixed dosage produces hazards either of Insulin reactions or of sustained hyperglycemia. Unusual activity, another factor affecting Insulin requirement, creates hypoglycemia (see page 141) which demands additional glucose or food. A problem arises when the aftereffect of strenuous exercise persists into the night and the supplement of food given the child is inadequate. Severe Insulin reactions may ensue. Apart from infection, other factors known to alter daily Insulin requirement and deserving special comment are the approach of menstruation, changes in routine, and upheavals in the life pattern. The planning of Insulin dosage needs to be based to some extent on a forecast of diet and activity; the difficulties of forecasting activity often make multiple doses of short-acting Insulin a safer and more effective regimen.

When short-acting Insulins, especially Regular Insulin, are considered, new pitfalls are apparent. Of central importance is the half-life* of Insulin in the plasma, determined by measuring the disappearance of I^{131} or I^{125}-labeled Insulin.[4,5] When the half-life of Insulin is forty to sixty minutes,

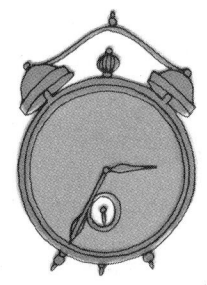

Use of Insulin in children

---

*Half-life is defined as the length of time required for the blood level to fall to one-half the peak concentration.

as in some patients, as few as three or four daily doses of Regular Insulin provide flexible and effective control of hyperglycemia. In patients in whom Insulin has a shorter half-life, rapid decay of the injection demands such frequent doses that therapy is impracticable without supplementary long-acting Insulin. Rapid absorption of Regular Insulin from its injection site creates a sharp transition from the low level in the plasma to which the previous dose has decayed to a critically high level from the present injection. When there is a time lag of three to four hours, the patient experiences a drop from a higher to a lower blood glucose level, and this change will produce symptoms of an Insulin reaction, typically between meals. When such a situation continues day after day, the stimulation of appetite along with the repeated consumption of between-meal feedings may lead to imperceptibly greater caloric intake and therefore undue weight gain. Control of hyperglycemia is replaced by a problem of obesity. Since Semilente® Insulin is absorbed somewhat more gradually, it slows the rate of transition of the patient's blood sugar and thus permits a more physiological Insulin effect.

Because of the difficulties surrounding choice of Insulin type, dosage, and distribution, the day-to-day response of the patient has to be monitored closely, with frequent urine tests for glucose. Glycosuria requires urine tests for acetone as well as checkups by the physician at least monthly. The parent and child together must learn to label the feeling associated with hypoglycemia. From the physician's standpoint, little is gained and much may be lost by underdosage with Insulin; the hyperglycemia that ensues eventually forces recourse to abnormally large doses of Insulin to forestall ketoacidosis.

DIET

Nowhere is communication between physician, dietitian, mother, and child so crucial as in the planning of a diabetic diet. Sound nutritional practice must prevail, and the diet has to be interesting and palatable.

The caloric requirements of a child depend upon such factors as age, weight, height, current rate of growth, sex, exercise, and general condition. The prescription must be adequate to maintain rates of growth normal for the individual child. Obesity is to be discouraged, and body weight should be kept normal. According to White,[1] 1,000 calories should be provided at one year of age, and 100 calories added each year up to 2,000 calories at age eleven. After this, until age fifteen, 100 calories per year are added for girls and 200 calories a year for boys to maximums of 2,400 and 2,800 calories respectively. The prescription is revised up or down according to activity, satiety, body weight, and rate of growth.

Dietary considerations are covered comprehensively in the chapter on diet. Two other instructions must be made regarding the necessity for dietary flexibility in the treatment of children. First, the diet must conform with the eating habits of the family and the patient's tastes. Second, the diet frequently must be adjusted to the Insulin dose. Thus, when a patient on intermediate-acting Insulin develops hypoglycemia in the midafternoon but has otherwise satisfactory control, the borrowing of a fruit, milk, or bread exchange from another meal to be given in the midafternoon is often preferable to changing the type or dose of Insulin.

The most crucial step is the translation of a caloric prescription into *Dietetic* the daily choice of foods. Simplicity of diet in the initial phases is desirable. *principles* With subsequent education, the diet can be made increasingly interesting and palatable. The child is instructed to eat only those foods which are on the diet list, to eat the full amounts prescribed, and never to skip meals. On the occasion of office visits, the mother is encouraged to bring a notation of all those foods she would like introduced into the diet.

Total calories are divided 1/5, 2/5, and 2/5 between breakfast, lunch, and supper. Two 10-Gm. carbohydrate exchanges from breakfast are taken during the morning, one 10-Gm. carbohydrate exchange from lunch during the afternoon, and two 10-Gm. carbohydrate exchanges from supper during the evening and at bedtime. The distribution of between-meal feedings is especially important when crystalline zinc Insulin is used, since its maximum hypoglycemic action occurs three to five hours after administration. The same principle applies with NPH Insulin, and account must be taken of the individual response of the patient.

KETOACIDOSIS

In the course of diabetes mellitus, the child may develop ketoacidosis at any time when dosage lags behind Insulin requirement. By virtue of increasing the child's requirement for Insulin, dietary excess or the onset of an infection may lead to hyperglycemia, ketonuria, then ketonemia, and later ketoacidosis.

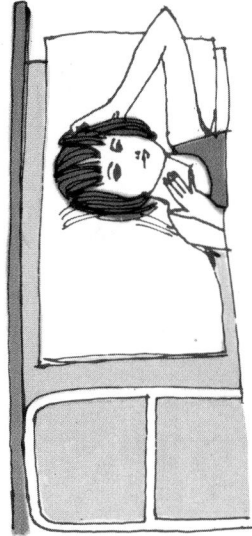

The definition and management of ketoacidosis are closely parallel in diabetic children and adults. Certain special features deserve comment.

1. Ketonuria without ketonemia may be observed in the presence of normoglycemia when a well-controlled diabetic child is starving or vomiting. Such ketonuria will disappear when the child returns to full caloric intake; and as long as normoglycemia is maintained with appropriate Insulin dosage, it should cause no concern.

2. The urgency of giving relatively large doses of crystalline zinc Insulin rapidly to the ketoacidotic child is based on two needs—overcoming mounting Insulin resistance and curtailing dynamic losses of water and electrolytes. Dosage is best calculated in units per pound of body weight; a good starting figure is 0.5 to 1 unit per pound—the lower figure early in ketoacidosis and the higher figure in ketoacidosis marked by coma and Kussmaul's breathing. Because there is a lag of several hours before maximum hypoglycemic response occurs, close observation of clinical and laboratory parameters is required to determine whether the initial Insulin dosage has been adequate, excessive, or insufficient. With excessive initial Insulin dosage, careful monitoring of blood glucose allows prompt institution of parenteral glucose infusion. Without such observation, the comatose patient may develop profound hypoglycemia. On the contrary, mounting resistance to Insulin in the face of inadequate initial dosage

urgently dictates supplementary administration. In either case, the large initial dosage leads to a prolongation of Regular Insulin action beyond the usual five-to-six-hour duration.

3. In parenteral fluid and electrolyte therapy directed at correcting dehydration and static deficits and dynamic losses of sodium and potassium, the usual priority of replacement is that of water and sodium and then of potassium. Occasionally, hypokalemia and characteristic ECG changes develop early in the course of treatment and urgently dictate potassium repletion.

INFECTION

The advent of infection in a diabetic child is usually followed by an increase in the dosage of Insulin needed to maintain normoglycemia. Unless rising Insulin requirements are promptly met by increased Insulin dosage, ketoacidosis ensues.

Each patient responds individually to infection from the standpoint of Insulin requirement, and each demands the greatest attention. Sometimes, diabetic children endure viral infections with little change in diet, Insulin requirement, or diabetic control, whereas infection in others may lead to striking increases in daily Insulin doses. At times, marked glycosuria and hyperglycemia develop immediately with the onset of infection. Close monitoring for urine glucose and acetone is indicated whenever infection is present. When this threatens to lead to glycosuria and hyperglycemia, the usual regimen is immediately supplemented by crystalline zinc Insulin given every three to six hours in a dosage adequate to maintain control of blood glucose. When management of Insulin dosage becomes intricate or the usual caloric intake is threatened, the child should be hospitalized. Strict clinical supervision will reveal whether symptoms of hypoglycemia accompany aglycosuria during periods of peak Insulin action and how diet should be supplemented in the face of hypoglycemic symptoms. When supplementary crystalline zinc Insulin is required, the total caloric intake may be divided equally into twelve feedings every two hours. These feedings may be liquid if so desired.

LONG-TERM HALLMARKS

It is unusual to detect clinical evidence of vascular lesions during the first ten years of diabetes. Thereafter, the appearance of retinopathy (dilated venules and microaneurysms), calcification of arteries, proteinuria, hypertension, nephropathy, and severe retinopathy (hemorrhages, exudates, *Vascular* new vessel formation) correlates with the duration of diabetes mellitus as *complications* shown in Table 25.[6] White states: "In the thirty-year survivors, two trends for the clinical course of angiopathy appear. In the one, more commonly seen in females and those with diabetes onset under ten years, were characteristic retinopathy, dilated venules, preretinal and vitreous hemorrhages, nephropathy, and co-existing azotemia. More commonly seen in males and those with onset after ten years are hypertension, extensive involvement of medium-sized vessels showing calcification in x-ray, minimal evidence of nephropathy and of retinopathy but eventual inclusion of coronary vessels and of the myocardium."[7]

Table 25. Percent of Patients with Vascular Complications among 1,072 Juvenile Diabetics Followed More Than Twenty Years, by Age and by Duration of Diabetes

YEARS	ALBUMIN (%)	ELEVATED BLOOD PRESSURE (%)	RETINITIS (%)	RETINITIS PROLIF-ERANS (%)	CALCIFIED ARTERIES (%)
Age					
0-9	0	0	0	0	0
10-19	4.2	1.8	4.8	0	6.5
20-29	18.5	16.7	63.2	28.7	45.5
30-39	34.7	40.3	84.4	53.1	83.3
40-49	37.0	51.9	88.0	58.4	95.0
Duration of Diabetes					
0-4	0.8	0.5	0	0	0
5-9	1.5	1.2	2.5	0	1.7
10-14	7.0	4.5	19.0	3.0	14.0
15-19	18.0	15.0	59.0	18.0	44.0
20-24	41.0	32.0	82.0	47.0	73.0
25-29	39.0	44.0	88.0	46.0	88.0
30-34	44.0	53.0	93.0	59.0	94.0
35-39	63.0	70.0	—	—	—

HEPATOMEGALY

In poorly controlled diabetic children, the liver may be very much enlarged and extend into the true pelvis. Although hypercholesteremia is generally present, tests for liver function are normal. Liver biopsy reveals infiltration with fat and glycogen. Upon institution of good diabetic control, liver size usually returns to normal over a period of one to several months.

DIABETIC DWARFISM

Retardation of growth is still occasionally encountered in association with poor control of diabetic children. Hepatomegaly is present. Osseous development is delayed. Sexual maturation is retarded, and the child has infantile proportions.

RENAL GLYCOSURIA

Renal glycosuria may coexist with diabetes in children, and the child may be constantly glycosuric despite hypoglycemic levels of the blood sugar.

Under these conditions, treatment must be based on data obtained from the blood sugar.

OBESITY

Obesity in a child should raise suspicion of diabetes. However, obesity may also develop as a consequence of excessive Insulin dosage in the management of diabetes. The hypoglycemic action produced may result in heightened appetite and thus in increased consumption of food. A net positive caloric balance sustained over any considerable period of time will result in obesity.

SKIN AND SUBCUTANEOUS TISSUES

Skin disorders which occur more commonly in diabetic than in nondiabetic children are furunculosis, boils and carbuncles, and pruritus of the external genitalia, all of which are frequently associated with glycosuria. Other dermatologic conditions seen in diabetic children are xanthosis resulting from carotenemia, xanthomas in association with hypercholesteremia, necrobiosis lipoidica, and epidermophytosis. A common disorder of the subcutaneous tissue peculiar to diabetes is lipodystrophy at the site of Insulin injection. Insulin lipodystrophy develops in susceptible persons regardless of the variety of Insulin employed or the pH of the Insulin preparation.

NEUROPATHY

The incidence of neuropathy in diabetic children increases with the duration of diabetes. Diminished vibratory sense, especially of the lower extremities, has been reported in many diabetic children examined between the ages of ten and twelve. After thirty years of diabetes, virtually all juvenile diabetics appear to lose their Achilles tendon reflex. Clinically, neuropathy often, but by no means always, follows a period of poor diabetic control. Consequently, the prognosis for recovery is best following institution of good control.

Clinical picture

The forms that neuropathy may assume are many and varied. The most common one is marked by paresthesia of the lower extremities and dysthesia. Nocturnal burning pain in the feet is very typical. Neurotrophic changes in the skin of the lower extremities may lead to shallow ulcers, commonly of the soles of the feet. Such neurotrophic ulcers may become infected, and cellulitis may result. It will be recalled that nocturnal pain in the thigh and calf muscles may be present at the onset of diabetes. This may recur as part of diabetic neuropathy. Nocturnal diarrhea or symptoms due to gastric atony, as well as postural hypotension and sexual impotence, may develop as a result of autonomic neuropathy. Oculomotor palsies, Argyll Robertson pupils, tabetic bladders, and Charcot's joints occur infrequently. Some authorities regard the loss of the catecholamine-dependent warning symptoms of hypoglycemia as a manifestation of autonomic neuropathy.

VISUAL DISTURBANCES

Transient refractive changes are common when Insulin is first used in treatment. Subsequently, refraction of the eyes should be conducted during periods of stable diabetic control. Cataracts occur in a small number of patients early in the course of diabetes. Subsequently, juvenile diabetics may become susceptible to senile cataracts. Visual symptoms, such as blurring of vision or double vision, are common symptoms of hypoglycemia. Diabetic retinopathy is chief among the complications which may affect vision and lead to blindness.

Retinopathy

In diabetic retinopathy, microaneurysms dot the retina. Venules may be dilated; arterioles may be narrowed and tortuous. Arteriovenous nicking may be noted. Round hemorrhages, hard and waxy exudates, and small flame-shaped hemorrhages may be present. Cotton-wool exudates, areas of edema, and striate hemorrhages suggest attendant renal disease, diabetic nephropathy, or glomerulonephritis. Progression to severe diabetic retinopathy with retinitis proliferans may be heralded by sudden loss of vision from hemorrhage into the retina or the vitreous. Venular dilatation with compression by slender arteries at arteriovenous junctions may give the venules the appearance of sausage links. Strands of dense white fibrous tissue may be noted at the disk and may extend into the vitreous. New blood vessels may form anywhere in the retina. Contraction of scar tissue leads to retinal detachment. Glaucoma, secondary to hemorrhage, may develop.

Early diagnosis and intensive control of diabetes are indicated in order to stay the onset of severe diabetic retinopathy marked by retinitis proliferans. When retinitis proliferans is established, treatment consists in (1) institution of good diabetic control, (2) ophthalmologic consultation in the management of threatened retinal detachment of secondary glaucoma, (3) evaluation of the degree of attendant renal function impairment due to diabetic nephropathy, and (4) exploration of a patient's adjustment to the threat of blindness. Benefit may be derived by use of the Kempner rice diet. The results of hypophysectomy are still being evaluated. Certainly if hypophysectomy is being considered, it should be planned or timed before renal failure develops.

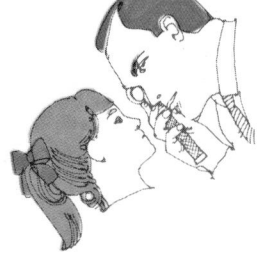

NEPHROPATHY

Diabetic nephropathy is a complex of diabetic glomerulosclerosis, arteriosclerosis, atherosclerosis, and acute and chronic pyelonephritis. Typically, the victim of diabetic nephropathy has been poorly controlled throughout part of his diabetic life. After the onset of diabetes during childhood, control is achieved with diet and Insulin. Following remission, the onset of total diabetes often creates a need for increased reliance on multiple doses of crystalline zinc Insulin. When this requirement is not fully met, recurrent glycosuria becomes a part of daily life, and poor or indifferent control becomes accepted as an outcome of labile diabetes. Dietary adherence is gradually relaxed. After ten or fifteen years of indifferent control, signs and symptoms of diabetic nephropathy begin to appear. On physical examination, diabetic retinopathy is nearly always noted. Mild hypertension and proteinuria are present. There may be swings in body weight, and gradually recurrent edema develops. Proteinuria becomes constant, and microscopic examination of the urine sediment reveals doubly refractile fatty cells and casts at all times. Red blood cells are few or absent, in contradistinction to the urine of acute and subacute glomerular nephritis. Bouts of fever and bacteriuria occur as a result of acute pyelonephritis. The patient may complain of easy fatigability or attacks of nausea. Now, despite increasing attention to diabetic control, renal insufficiency progresses. Massive proteinuria leads eventually to hypoproteinemia, and anemia and azotemia become constant. The terminal weeks or months are marked by persistent hypertension, uremia, and cardiac failure.

Renal involvement

PATIENT, PHYSICIAN, AND PARENT

The diabetic child needs the support of his parents in facing the demands of life as a diabetic. The effort of the physician to listen, inform, and encourage serves to dispel fears and misgivings and helps the parents to assist their child. Several diabetic manuals containing valuable information are available, but this reading has to be supplemented by an exchange of information between parent, child, and physician during every office visit. There is much that parents and, ultimately, children must learn about every facet of diabetes. Sometime after onset, the advent of a remission in the diabetic state, marked by a sharp decrease in Insulin requirements, is encouraging to most parents. Unrealistic ideas about permanent cure often crop up at this time. Above all, the habit of taking Insulin should be preserved.

As children get older, they are encouraged to take an increasing hand in the management of their condition, a process which in fact began when the patient assumed responsibility for recognizing and treating reactions to Insulin on his own. The child perceived and acted upon the need for extra food in the face of unusual activity. Before adolescence, the child should be measuring and giving his own Insulin doses. The promotion of self-management at an early age aims at removing overtones of parental authority prior to the advent of adolescence, a time when the negativism associated with growth and development may imperil diabetic management. At every juncture, the diabetic child should be treated as any other child and encouraged to participate fully in all forms of school life, sports, and recreation. As long as he is not hypoglycemic as a result of excessive Insulin or activity without supplementary food, the diabetic child has normal strength and stamina. Dietetic skill assumes increasing importance during adolescence in the face of the complexities of teen-age social life.

When diabetic control appears to be slipping away from criteria of excellence, the choice of Insulin and its dosage should be reexamined. Increasing need for reliance on crystalline zinc Insulin may develop as a result of alterations in the plasma binding of Insulin. The hyperglycemia typical of poor control may lead to hyperphagia. The child appears to be "breaking diet," and breach of diet seems to be impairing diabetic control when actually the choice of Insulin and its dosage are at fault. Poor diabetic control despite optimal choices of Insulin and dosage usually suggests a problem of dietary indiscretion which may be part of a behavioral reaction. In the experience of most physicians concerned with the care of diabetic children, rejection of medical care occurs commonly in adolescence, but this rarely lasts for more than two years. Psychiatric evaluation is especially indicated in the face of persistent rejection of medical care. Occasional faked urine charts or substitution of a friend's normal urine should not be considered abnormal in the child. Such infantile behavior usually reflects an incomplete acceptance by the child of the realities and exigencies of his disease.

BIBLIOGRAPHY

1. White, P.: The Child with Diabetes, M. Clin. North America, *49:*1074, 1965.

1A. Gonen, B., and Rubenstein, A. H.: Haemoglobin A_I and Diabetes Mellitus, Diabetologia, *15:*1, 1978.

2. Hallas-Møller, K.: The Lente Insulins, Diabetes, *5:*7, 1956.

3. Marler, E., Bressler, R., and Styron, C.: The Use of Insulin in Unstable Diabetes Mellitus, South. M. J., *57:*1447, 1964.

4. Bolinger, R. E., Morris, J. H., McKnight, F. G., and Diederich, D. A.: Disappearance of I[131]-Labeled Insulin from Plasma as a Guide to Management of Diabetes, New England J. Med., *270:*767, 1964.

5. Bressler, R., and Marler, E.: Unpublished data.

6. White, P.: Natural Course and Prognosis of Juvenile Diabetes, Diabetes, *5:*445, 1956.

7. White, P.: Childhood Diabetes. Its Course, and Influence on the Second and Third Generations, Diabetes, *9:*435, 1960.

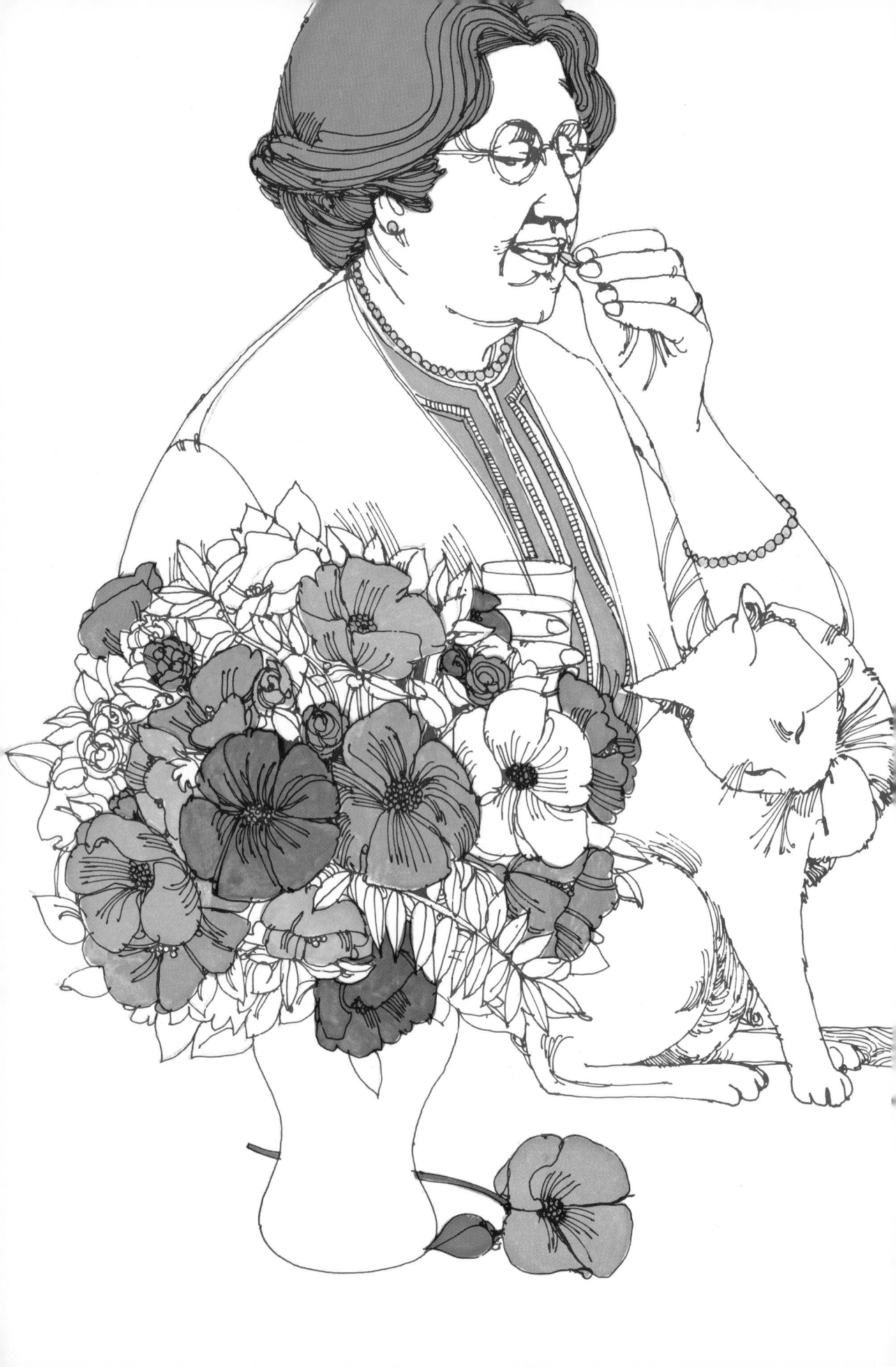

Oral Hypoglycemic Agents

9

Since the discovery of Insulin, innumerable attempts have been made to find a satisfactory means of maintaining a normal blood sugar and controlling diabetes without the inconvenience of parenteral injections. Insulin has been given rectally, orally, and by aerosol, but because of irregular absorption by these routes (and degradation in the gastro-intestinal tract), such forms of administration have been impractical.

SULFONYLUREAS

Although hypoglycemia was observed in malnourished patients receiving the isopropylthiadiazole derivative of sulfanilamide as early as 1942, it was not until 1954 that a sulfonylurea compound was introduced for broad clinical trial in the oral treatment of diabetic patients.[1] The first preparation to be investigated by Eli Lilly and Company was BZ-55, or carbutamide. It had hypoglycemic activity but was withdrawn from further trial in this country because it manifested significant side-effects. Metahexamide and chlorpropamide, more potent drugs, likewise were withdrawn from clinical trial by Eli Lilly and Company because of their relative toxicity.

Four sulfonylurea agents are now widely prescribed. The structural formulas for these drugs are shown in Figure 25.

Phenformin, an oral antidiabetic agent with an entirely different mode of action than that of the sulfonylureas, was removed from the United States market in late 1977 because of a number of deaths reportedly due

Figure 25. Oral Agents Used in the Treatment of Diabetes Mellitus

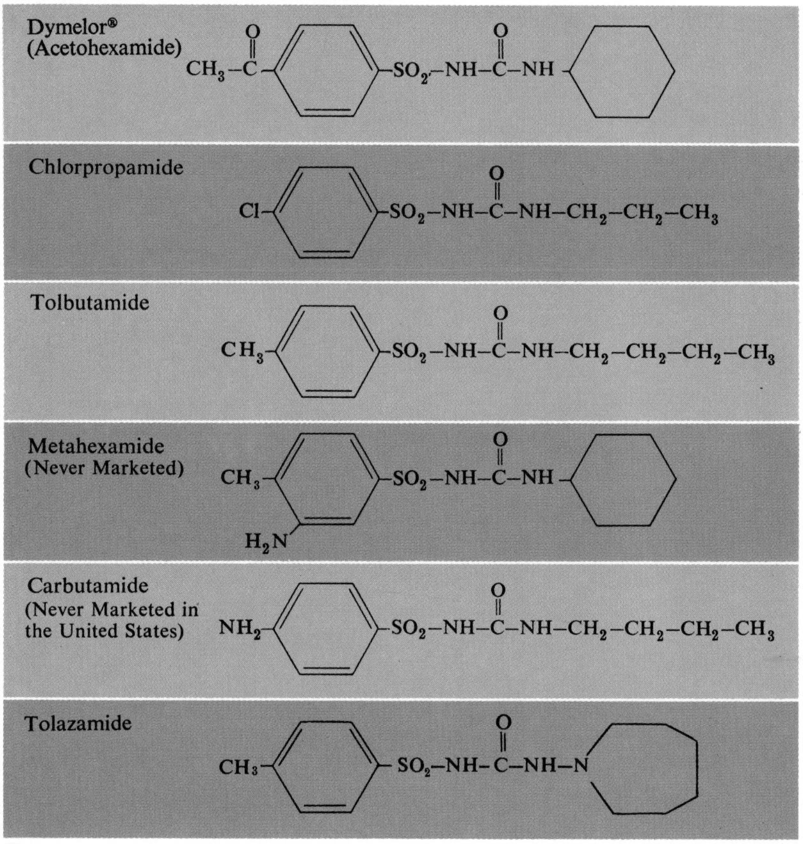

to the development of lactic acidosis ensuing from its use. Therefore, further discussion of phenformin is not deemed appropriate.

Most of the pharmacologic data published on this class of agents concerns tolbutamide. It has been used because of its availability as the first sulfonylurea compound to be marketed in the United States, its high solubility as a sodium salt, and its suitability for intravenous injection. A limited number of comparative studies indicate that the basic information derived from experience with tolbutamide generally is applicable to the other sulfonylureas. The principal differences are related to the metabolism, potency, and duration of action. The latter two are illustrated in Table 26.[2]

PHARMACOLOGY

The primary action of the sulfonylurea compounds, as elucidated by acute experiments, is the stimulation of the pancreatic beta cells to secrete endogenous insulin. The sulfonylureas increase the amount of assayable insulin in the blood, and beta-cell degranulation occurs following their administration. In the totally depancreatized dog, some exogenous Insulin must be present to demonstrate any hypoglycemic action of these drugs.

Table 26. Currently Available Oral Hypoglycemic Compounds

	USUAL DAILY DOSE	MAXIMUM RECOMMENDED DAILY DOSE	DURATION OF ACTION
Sulfonylureas			
Dymelor® (Acetohexamide)	0.25-1.5 Gm. (single or divided doses)	1.5 Gm.	12-24 hours
Chlorpropamide	0.1-0.5 Gm. (single dose)	0.5 Gm.	up to 60 hours
Tolbutamide	0.5-3 Gm. (usually divided doses)	2-3 Gm.	6-12 hours
Tolazamide	0.1-0.25 Gm. (single or divided doses)	0.75 Gm.	12-24 hours

Similarly, in cross-circulation experiments, the blood from a pancreatic vein of an intact animal treated with sulfonylurea produces hypoglycemia in the recipient animal whether it is normal or diabetic. (Because insulin is diluted by the systemic blood and degraded by the liver, a hypoglycemic effect is not observed when the blood supply is received from the mesenteric or femoral vein.) A secondary action of the sulfonylurea drugs is thought to be the inhibition of glucose release from liver glycogen (Figure 26).[3] This and other mechanisms of action of the sulfonylurea agents have been reviewed in detail by Feldman and Lebovitz.[4]

Clinical studies measuring both blood glucose and plasma insulin have yielded data which suggest that, as treatment with the sulfonylureas continues, the detectable mechanism of action may change from insulin stimulation to nonbetacytotropic effects. When Sheldon, Taylor, and Anderson[5] measured glucose tolerance and insulin output before, during, and after three months' treatment with acetohexamide, thirteen of twenty patients had dramatic improvement in glucose tolerance. This improvement was associated with increased insulin output from subnormal to normal levels during the first two months of therapy. However, during the third month, although glucose tolerance was maintained or improved, there was a diminution of insulin output.

Patients on a metabolic ward who were fed standard meals and treated with chlorpropamide for five days showed increase in plasma insulin and reduction in blood glucose over those values observed during a similar period without sulfonylurea treatment.[6] After five weeks of therapy, the hypoglycemic effects persisted but plasma insulin levels were reduced.

METABOLISM OF THE SULFONYLUREA AGENTS

Tolbutamide is converted to and excreted as carboxytolbutamide, a compound which is metabolically inert. Chlorpropamide, after being bound

Figure 26. Suggested Actions of Sulfonylurea Agents

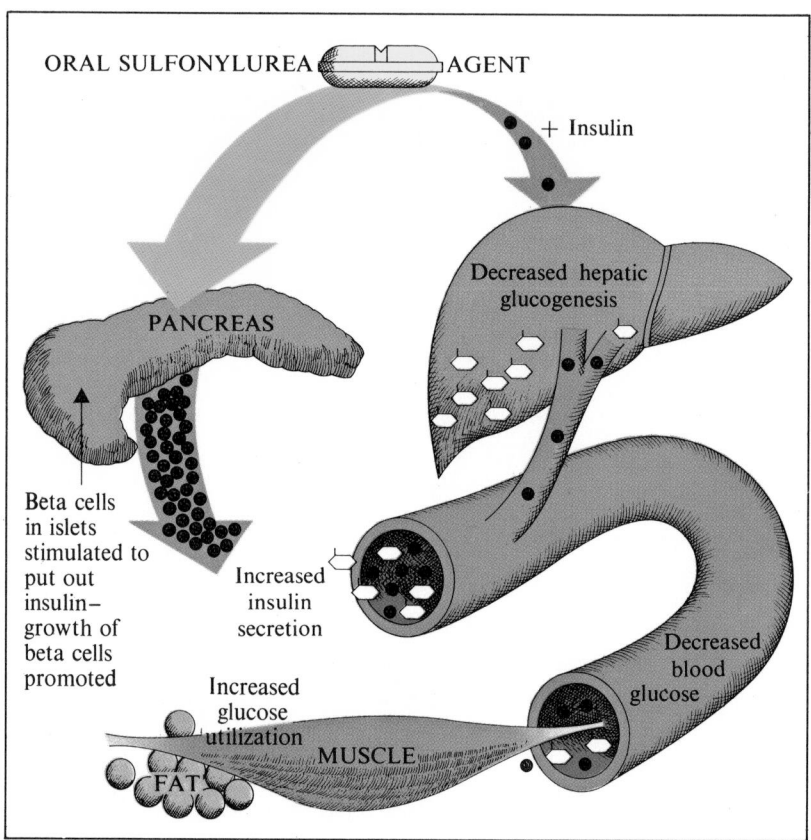

by serum proteins (a phenomenon which apparently accounts for its long duration of action), is excreted without change. The metabolism of Dymelor® (acetohexamide, Lilly) has been elucidated by the use of acetohexamide-C^{14}.

Studies on the nature of the urinary metabolites of Dymelor[7,8] show that the principal metabolic product is hydroxyhexamide and more specifically the levorotatory isomer, L-(—)-hydroxyhexamide. Approximately 10 percent of the metabolites were found to be 4′-trans-hydroxyacetohexamide and 10 percent were 4′-trans-hydroxyhydroxyhexamide. The chemical structures of these compounds are portrayed in Figure 27. Present in small quantities were the 4′-cis, 3′-cis, and 3′-trans isomers of the metabolic products. By means of the methods of Root *et al.*,[9] the hypoglycemic activity of acetohexamide and its principal metabolic product, L-(—)-hydroxyhexamide, has been found to be substantially greater than that of tolbutamide.

Blood levels of Dymelor and L-(—)-hydroxyhexamide have been determined by isotopic technics following the oral administration of 1 Gm. of the drug. These levels indicate that Dymelor is rapidly absorbed from

Figure 27. Metabolic Products of Dymelor® (Acetohexamide) Found in Urine of Human Subjects

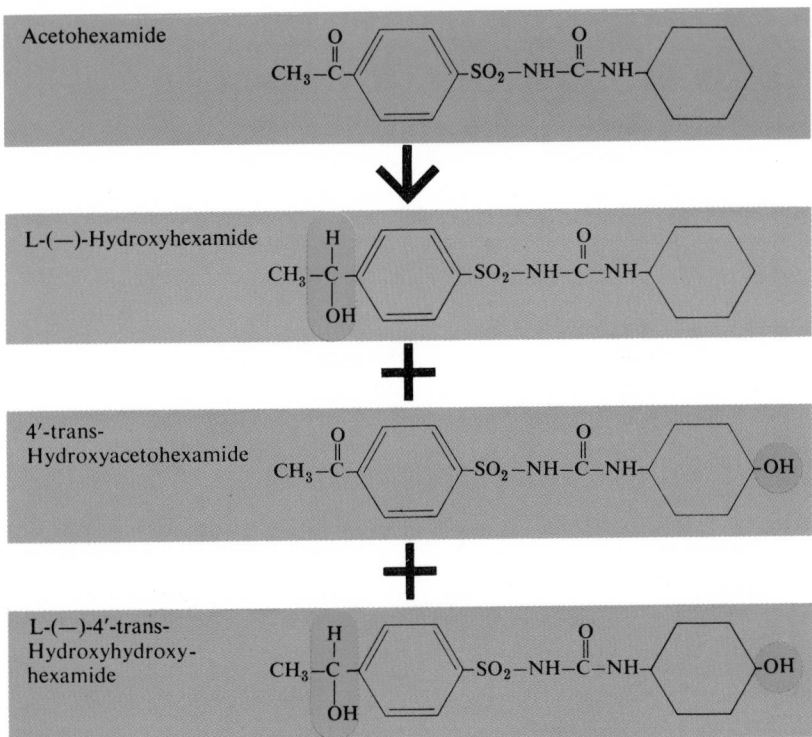

the gastro-intestinal tract and converted to its *active* principal metabolite, L-(—)-hydroxyhexamide (Figure 28). The half-life of the total drug levels of Dymelor and its metabolic product is in the range of 4.7 to 5.3 hours, which is essentially the same half-life as reported for tolbutamide.[10] Although tolbutamide and chlorpropamide show some correlation in duration of action and half-life, data for acetohexamide and hydroxyhexamide and the clinical efficacy[11-14] of once-daily dosage regimens with Dymelor indicate a dissociation between blood levels and time activity. Sheldon, Anderson, and Stoner[15] observe that a therapeutic response may be obtained with substantially smaller quantities of acetohexamide and hydroxyhexamide than of tolbutamide.

INSULIN OR ORAL THERAPY?

The availability of the oral hypoglycemic agents often presents the physician with a dilemma regarding the selection of therapy for his patient. In most instances, the situation can be resolved by a study of the following four questions:

1. What Type of Patient Responds Best to Oral Therapy?

The principal consideration in the selection of therapy depends upon whether the patient is resistant or prone to ketoacidosis. Sulfonylurea agents are the treatment of choice for properly selected patients who are

Figure 28. Blood Levels of Acetohexamide and Its Principal Metabolic Product, L-(—)-Hydroxyhexamide, after 1 Gm. Orally

Mean total

Hydroxyhexamide mean

Acetohexamide mean

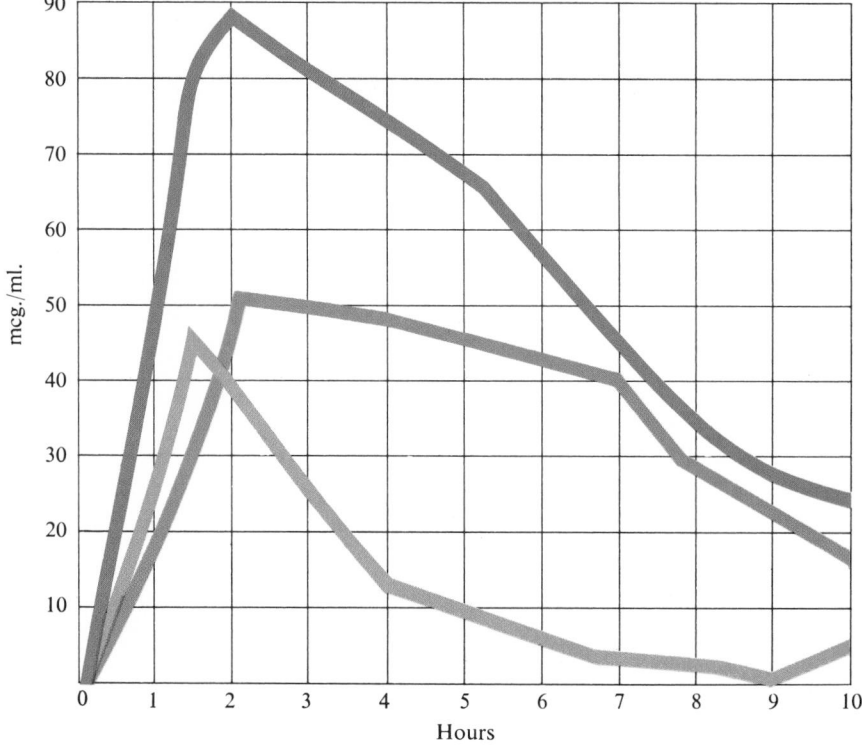

resistant to ketoacidosis and whose diabetes had its onset after adolescence. These drugs may also be used in an attempt to forestall the onset of islet-cell decompensation in young nonobese subjects who have only mild abnormalities in glucose tolerance and who, on the basis of family history, are likely to develop overt diabetes.[16]

2. What Are the Advantages and Disadvantages of Oral Therapy in Properly Selected Patients?

The obvious advantages are ease of administration and patient acceptance. Occasionally, the latter consideration may be of profound importance to the well-being of the patient. For instance, control of nonketotic diabetics with oral agents has permitted some patients to continue in their jobs who otherwise (if on Insulin) may have been forced to give up their occupations (e.g., construction workers, railroad workers, and other types of mechanics in hazardous occupations as well as patients whose working hours are highly irregular).

Another compelling advantage of the sulfonylurea agents lies in the fact that the adult-onset diabetic patient is not truly insulin deficient but has a sluggish insulin response to a glucose load. Thus, instead of resorting to replacement treatment with exogenous Insulin, it is better presumably to correct such a deficiency. When this is done, the beta cells of the pancreas are stimulated to secrete insulin. The insulin then enters the liver by way of the portal vein (the physiological pathway) and, after metabolism and degradation by the liver, reaches the systemic circulation.

Finally, the use of the sulfonylurea agents with the resultant stimulation of endogenous insulin obviates the need for exogenous Insulin, which is antigenic.[17-20] However, the significance of these antibodies in humans has not yet been fully defined.

The main disadvantage of oral therapy is that the convenience and ease of treatment all too often are deceptive, and patients are disinclined to maintain a proper regard for the potential dangers of diabetes and the rules of sound management. The principal transgression is, of course, failure to follow the prescribed diet. Unfortunately, many patients on oral therapy consider the medication not a convenient means for maintaining metabolic control but a crutch for frequent, if not chronic, dietary indiscretion. Finally, although low in incidence, adverse reactions and hypoglycemia must be considered as potential disadvantages to the use of sulfonylurea compounds.

3. Should the Oral Agents Be Used in Patients with Neuropathy, Retinopathy, and Nephropathy?

When the oral agents were first introduced, medical opinion was nearly unanimous that the oral agents were contraindicated in the presence of such chronic complications. The basis for this view, of course, was a lack of adequate data showing the quality of control of the blood sugar that could be achieved with these agents as compared with Insulin. As experience has demonstrated the safety and efficacy of the oral agents in maintaining satisfactory control, the pendulum of opinion has swung toward the view that the hypoglycemic agent of choice for a patient with a given complication of diabetes is that which produces the *best* control of the blood sugar. This is particularly true in cases of neuropathy, in which improvement of the disorder is most likely to be associated with control of the blood sugar. There are, however, some clinicians who prefer to use Insulin for patients with any of the complications of chronic diabetes.

4. What Long-Term Effects Are Produced by the Oral Agents and Insulin?

The most famous effort directed to this question is the University Group Diabetes Program (UGDP) which, in the early 1960's, undertook one of the most ambitious clinical trials ever attempted. This study compared Type II diabetics randomly assigned to one of four regimens: (1) tolbutamide (fixed dose of 0.5 Gm. t.i.d.), (2) placebo (these two treatments were administered double-blind), (3) Insulin in a fixed dose, and (4) Insulin in a variable dose to control diabetes. Phenformin was added later. There were approximately 200 adult-onset diabetic patients in each treatment group. In a report after eight years of study, the death rate due to cardiovascular disease was said to be higher in the tolbutamide-treated group than among the Insulin or placebo-treated patients.[21] The reasons for this are not clear. The authors concluded: "The findings suggest that in the population at risk, tolbutamide plus diet may be less effective than diet alone, insofar as cardiovascular mortality is concerned."

Further clinical evidence suggesting that sulfonylurea agents have a direct effect on the heart is contained in a report by Soler *et al.*[22] In a retrospective study of diabetics with acute myocardial infarction who were monitored in a coronary care unit, these investigators found the frequency of ventricular fibrillation to be higher in patients receiving oral agents than in those treated with Insulin (12 percent versus 3 percent). In-vitro studies have further suggested a direct effect of tolbutamide on the heart.[23]

Conclusions contradictory to those of the UGDP have been reported by others. A study by Keen[24] of 124 borderline diabetics treated with tolbutamide (0.5 Gm. b.i.d.) and 124 treated with placebo found that, after five years, the incidence of worsening of cardiovascular disease (e.g., "probable" evidence, such as myocardial infarction, onset of angina pectoris, onset of intermittent claudication) was less in the tolbutamide-treated group (22 percent) than in the other group (33 percent).

Similarly, Paasikivi[25] compared the effect of tolbutamide, 0.5 Gm. b.i.d., with that of placebo in both controls and patients who had survived a first acute myocardial infarction. At the end of a mean follow-up time of three years, there was little difference in the total mortality between the tolbutamide group and the controls.

Recently, the UGDP reported on the mortality of the Insulin-treated groups and concluded that its findings provide no evidence that Insulin or any other drug which lowers blood glucose will alter the course of the vascular complications of adult-onset diabetes.[26]

Since the UGDP findings run counter to the observations of many specialists in diabetic care, this study has sparked one of the major controversies in American medicine.[27] In spite of confirmation by the Biometric Society[28] of the statistical methods used in the study, critics and commentators[29-33] have pointed out a number of sources of error in its design, execution, results, and conclusions. These include, to list a few, inadequate dietary treatment of all patients in the study, failure to establish drug compliance, increase in cardiovascular risk factors in the tolbutamide-treated group, inappropriate treatment of patients (patients needing more vigorous hypoglycemic treatment did not receive it, and patients with diabetes too mild to be treated received hypoglycemic therapy), inadequate follow-up periods (conclusions on eight years of data have been drawn, yet many of the complications of diabetes do not appear until the disease has been present for ten years or longer). Finally, for purposes of mortality analysis, patients were frequently assigned to treatment groups when, in fact, they had not received that treatment for several months. Clearly, it will be a long time before the UGDP controversy and its relationship to the treatment of patients with adult-onset diabetes are resolved. In the meantime, practitioners and patients alike are left with an alternative that will reduce blood glucose—strict dietary adherence—including attainment of normal body weight and avoidance of concentrated carbo-hydrates.

5. What Are The Effects of Oral Agents and Insulin on the Complications of Diabetes and on Islet-Cell Function?

Studies of the effect of extended sulfonylurea treatment on beta-cell function indicate that plasma insulin levels after several years of therapy are comparable to those found after one year. In addition, in the majority (but not all) of patients who are taken off sulfonylureas[34] (as during a period of stress), the Insulin requirement is equal to or lower than that before the initial use of a sulfonylurea.

ADVERSE REACTIONS TO SULFONYLUREAS

Considering the widespread use of sulfonylurea agents, the reported incidence of side-effects is extremely small (in less than 5 percent of patients).

Several systems may be involved in adverse reactions to sulfonylurea compounds. The severity of a given reaction is determined largely by "patient factors," such as the severity of the diabetes, the presence of non-diabetic disease, and, more important, past and current treatment with other medications, including sulfonylurea agents. Equally significant is individual patient idiosyncrasy. This may be the principal determinant of whether a given side-effect does or does not occur in a specific patient and, if it does appear, of the severity of the reaction. Included in the adverse reactions discussed below are not only the most serious types encountered but also those which may be disturbing to the patient or which may possibly obscure the diagnosis of other conditions.

HYPOGLYCEMIA

Because reduction of the blood sugar is the goal of hypoglycemic therapy, hypoglycemia actually does not fall into the category of adverse reactions. Therefore, this effect is discussed in full in the following chapter, "Hypoglycemia Due to Insulin and the Sulfonylurea Agents."

SKIN REACTIONS

Skin disorders may occur in patients receiving sulfonylurea agents. They may be simple papular or maculopapular eruptions limited to the arms and legs or, rarely, a generalized urticaria. Because diabetics, particularly the poorly controlled, have a high incidence of skin disorders (e.g., fungus and bacterial infections and, less frequently, necrobiosis lipoidica diabeticorum or xanthoma diabeticorum), it is often difficult to determine whether the dermatosis is due to diabetes or to the drug. If skin eruptions should result from a hypoglycemic agent, they usually develop within the first three to six weeks of treatment. Previous therapy with a sulfonylurea or sulfa drug may or may not result in later sensitivity to the same or another sulfonylurea compound. However, for patients with a history of allergy to any drug (particularly of the sulfa or sulfonylurea type), a sulfonylurea is always prescribed with caution. When drug eruption occurs, the offending medication should be discontinued. Usually this will be done by the patient without instruction from the physician. There are, of course, case reports of spontaneous remission with persistence in the treatment.

VISUAL DISTURBANCES

The most common side reaction affecting the eyes is refractive change. It may also occur in patients treated with diet alone or with Insulin. In most instances, such changes are attributable to alterations in accommodation from differences in the osmolarity of the lens as well as to metabolic changes in the ciliary body. These, in turn, are related to hyperglycemia.[35,36] Ordinarily, the refractive errors due to poor diabetic control subside spontaneously after six to eight weeks of satisfactory blood sugar levels. The presence of visual signs and symptoms also suggests the possibility of diabetic retinopathy.

THYROID DYSFUNCTION

Although short-term investigations have revealed no statistically significant changes in thyroid function due to Dymelor® (acetohexamide, Lilly),[37] long-term studies[38] show a marked increase in the incidence of clinical hypothyroidism in patients treated with other sulfonylureas as compared with those given Insulin. For this reason, the possibility of an antithyroid effect from sulfonylureas should be considered in diabetic patients who develop signs or symptoms of hypothyroidism. The precise mechanism by which sulfonylureas may interfere with thyroid function is not known.

EFFECTS ON RENAL CONSERVATION OF WATER

In a few elderly patients, the use of chlorpropamide has been associated with hyponatremia, serum hypo-osmolality, and water intoxication.[39] The mechanism postulated is that the sulfonylurea drug enhances the activity of antidiuretic hormone. No documented cases have been reported with Dymelor or other sulfonylureas. Because this condition may result in both edema and confusion, it needs to be included in the differential diagnosis of elderly patients presenting with signs of heart failure or hypoglycemia.

GASTRO-INTESTINAL AND HEPATIC DISORDERS

Gastro-intestinal symptoms may occur as a result of treatment with sulfonylurea compounds; the reported incidence is perhaps 1 to 3 percent among new patients. Symptoms may be mild and may involve only nausea and occasional vomiting or diarrhea. Rarely, there may be gastro-intestinal bleeding.[40] Although the mechanisms responsible for these complaints are not definitely known, local irritation is strongly suspected.

Liver function studies   Of great interest and importance is the occurrence of abnormal liver function tests in some diabetics, particularly those receiving sulfonylurea compounds. Liver dysfunction in these patients may range from mild elevations of the alkaline phosphatase to jaundice. For instance, Camerini-Dávalos et al.[41] found a significant rise in alkaline phosphatase following treatment with tolbutamide except for the period from the seventh to the

Figure 29. Liver Function Test Values in Diabetic Patients (After L. G. McArthur, M.D., Ph.D.)

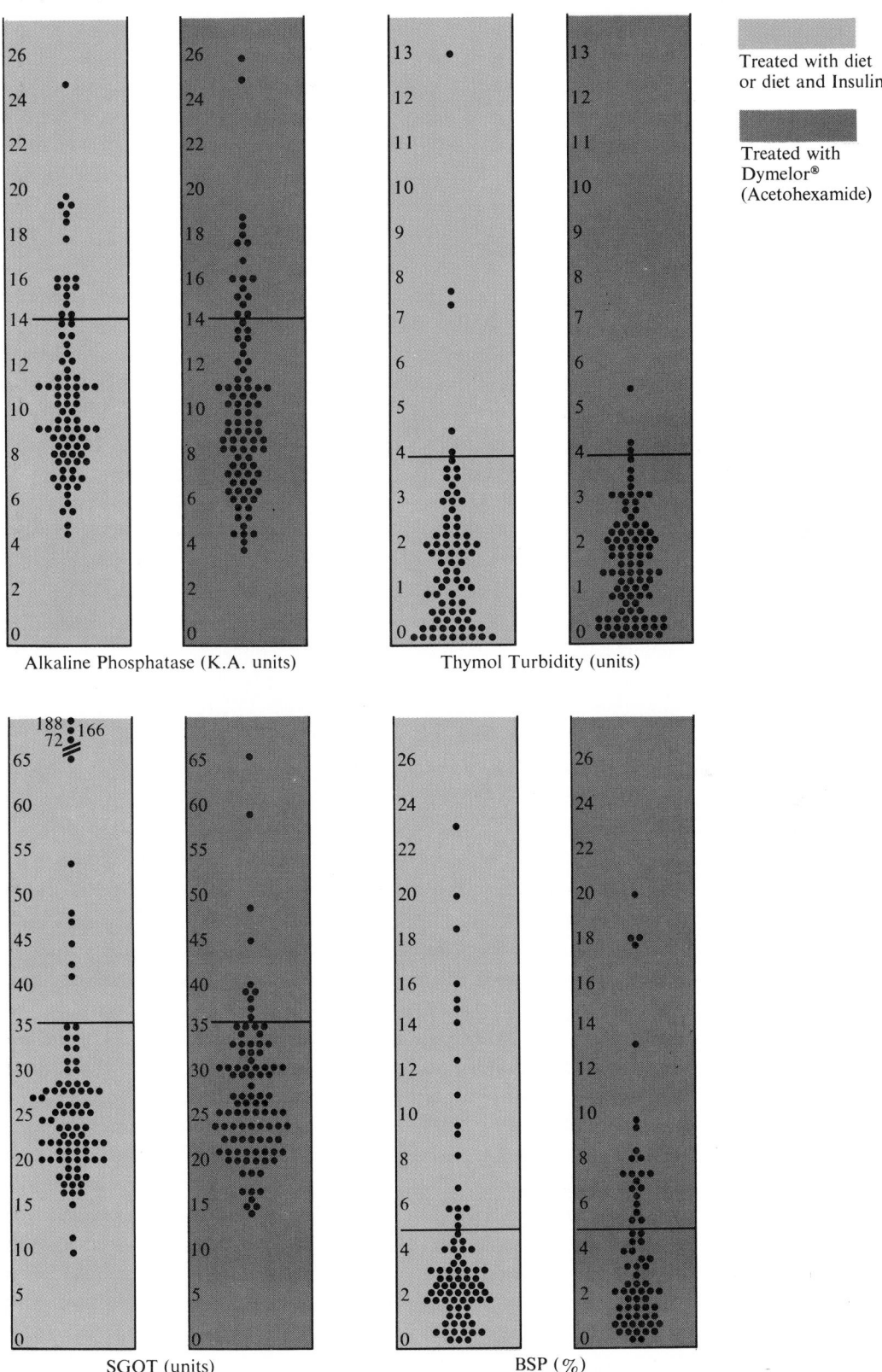

Treated with diet or diet and Insulin

Treated with Dymelor® (Acetohexamide)

Alkaline Phosphatase (K.A. units)

Thymol Turbidity (units)

SGOT (units)

BSP (%)

twelfth month and also after thirty-seven months of treatment. They are unable to explain the increase.

Montgomery et al.[42] reported a statistically notable rise in the level of serum alkaline phosphatase three and six months after initiation of treatment with Dymelor® (acetohexamide, Lilly). They were unable to correlate the finding with any other clinical disturbance or other hepatic toxic effects; therefore, the cause was not understood. However, there was no mention of other medications the patients may have been taking.

It is not known whether abnormal liver function is a part of the diabetic syndrome. Many authors believe that liver function is often impaired in diabetes.[43-45] On the other hand, others[46,47] believe that liver function is normal in those who have uncomplicated, well-controlled diabetes. In comparing their results with those of other workers who reported on healthy nondiabetic subjects, Camerini-Dávalos et al.[48] found elevated bromsulfalein retention, alkaline phosphatase, and thymol flocculation in their diabetic patients. An attempt to discover a correlation between the abnormal values and the patients' age, body weight, duration of diabetes, control of the diabetes, type of treatment, and blood cholesterol levels revealed no relationship except that there was a somewhat higher bromsulfalein (BSP) retention in those who were overweight and/or had elevated serum cholesterol levels. There also was an elevation of bromsulfalein in patients with gastro-intestinal abnormality, especially hepatomegaly.

The problem of variation in liver function among diabetics, particularly those on sulfonylurea compounds, is illustrated in Figure 29, where the liver function of one hundred patients who had received Dymelor is compared with that of one hundred who had never been given sulfonylurea agents. The incidence of abnormal values for thymol turbidity, BSP, alkaline phosphatase, and serum glutamic oxalacetic transaminase (SGOT) is practically identical in both groups. Thus, although the mechanism for mild alterations in laboratory values is unknown, the available evidence indicates that, when liver function in the diabetic is evaluated, the possibility of nondiabetic disease and the effects of other drugs the patient may be receiving should be considered.

Jaundice with the sulfonylurea compounds is a rare complication; its incidence appears to be related to the potency of the compound being used. The fewest cases have been reported with tolbutamide and the most with chlorpropamide. On the basis of reports received by Eli Lilly and Company, the incidence of jaundice with Dymelor is estimated to be in the range of one case in 20,000 patients treated. When it occurs, jaundice ordinarily develops within one to three months after initiation of treatment and may or may not be associated with a skin rash. The chemical and histopathologic findings show that sulfonylurea jaundice may be mixed hepatocellular or cholestatic in type.[49] Drerup et al.[50] indicate the difficulties in determining the cause of jaundice because of the number of therapeutic agents the diabetic patient often is taking. Because diabetes may be one of the first signs of carcinoma of the pancreas, jaundice attributed to sulfonylurea therapy has unfortunately turned out to be due to cancer on more than one occasion.

BLOOD DYSCRASIAS

Blood dyscrasias have been reported with the sulfonylurea compounds.[51] These differ in severity from patient to patient, and the manifestations range from transient leukopenia to thrombocytopenic purpura, agranulocytosis, and aplastic anemia. Fortunately, the incidence is very low, and the prognosis for recovery is usually good if the diagnosis is made promptly and the drug is stopped immediately.

ALCOHOL SENSITIVITY

A peculiar reaction to alcohol has been reported in a few patients receiving sulfonylurea compounds. Apparently this may occur with any of the sulfonylurea agents available in the United States. The reaction consists in flushing, a feeling of facial warmth, and occasionally a pounding headache, dyspnea, nausea, giddiness, and tachycardia. In severe cases, there may be injection of the conjunctivae. The reaction, which may be an idiosyncrasy, comes on three to ten minutes after ingestion of only small amounts of alcohol and may last an hour or longer.[52] Patients taking sulfonylurea compounds should be advised of the possibility of this type of reaction if they ingest alcohol.

PORPHYRIA

Although diabetes and porphyria rarely occur together, sulfonylurea compounds, like the sulfa drugs and barbiturates, aggravate the abdominal symptoms of hepatic porphyria.[53]

CRITERIA FOR CONTROL OF DIABETES

Various clinicians have different definitions for control of diabetes. The criteria of the Joslin Clinic,[54] representing stricter control than many others, are shown in Table 27.

Table 27. Criteria Used by the Joslin Clinic to Assess Degree of Control of Blood Glucose in Diabetic Patients Receiving Sulfonylurea Therapy*

	HIGHEST ACCEPTABLE BLOOD GLUCOSE LEVELS (MG./100 ML.)		
RESPONSE	FASTING OR 3 OR MORE HOURS P.C.	1 HOUR P.C.	2 HOURS P.C.
Good	110	150	130
Fair	130	180	150
Poor	———— All other cases ————		

*Based on 70 percent of the blood glucose determinations (by the Autoanalyzer method).

Less stringent criteria of control are used by other authorities. For instance, the criteria of Montgomery et al.[42] are indicated in Table 28.

Table 28. Criteria for Judging Response to Treatment with Acetohexamide in Diabetes Mellitus

RESPONSE	BLOOD GLUCOSE LEVELS (MG./100 ML.) MEAN—2 1/2 TO 3 HOURS P.C.	GLYCOSURIA
Good	< 150	None
Fair	150-200	Occasional; always < 2 Gm./100 ml.
Poor	> 200	Considerable; usually > 2 Gm./100 ml.

Good or fair response within one month after initiation of treatment indicates primary success. This may be achieved in approximately 60 percent of newly diagnosed, properly selected, adult-onset diabetic patients treated with a given sulfonylurea compound. Secondary failures are individuals who initially qualified as primary successes but subsequently failed to meet the criteria for control. The secondary failure rate ranges from 3 to 30 percent. The probable incidences are summarized in Table 29. The

Table 29. Probable Incidence of Success and Failure among Patients Who Have Been Properly Selected for Sulfonylurea Therapy

Primary success	60-65%
Secondary failure	3-30%
Success with another sulfonylurea agent after secondary failure with a previous agent	20%

Table 30. Probable Causes of Secondary Failures in Sulfonylurea Therapy (Tolbutamide)

	PERCENT OF 1,965 PATIENTS
Poor initial selection of patients	5.6
Poor adherence to diet	3.5
Inadequate dosage or failure of patient to take drug.	8.3
Temporary failure due to metabolic stress	0.9
True drug failure	3.7
Total	22.0

causes of secondary failure with tolbutamide are shown in Table 30.[34] Undoubtedly, the relative importance of these factors varies with the type and dose of the agent being used and the criteria of the individual clinician. However, each factor should be considered in any patient in whom diabetic control becomes less satisfactory. Secondary failure may result because some patients neglect to take the drug.[15,55] Those who do not respond to one sulfonylurea have a 20 percent chance of good control with another one of the agents.[56]

ADMINISTRATION AND DOSAGE

Three conditions should be satisfied before treatment with the sulfonylurea compounds is instituted. First, diagnosis of true diabetes must be established. Nondiabetic conditions which may produce chemical findings of diabetes, such as renal glycosuria, liver disease, and kidney disease, should be ruled out.

Second, the effects of dietary therapy should be evaluated before initiation of treatment with the sulfonylurea agents. In many instances, dietary adherence alone will result in satisfactory control of the blood sugar, and use of a sulfonylurea may result in hypoglycemia.

Third, in the case of women, it should be established that the patient is not pregnant.

Since the severity of diabetes is subject to fluctuation, patients should be seen regularly after sulfonylurea treatment is started. Blood sugar levels should be determined at each visit so that the dosage of the hypoglycemic agent may be adjusted. This procedure will obviate periods of undertreatment and overtreatment.

Dosage of Dymelor® (Acetohexamide)

The daily dosage of Dymelor may range from 125 mg. to 1.5 Gm.; the majority of patients can be controlled with 750 mg. or less daily. Patients who require 1 Gm. or less ordinarily can be satisfactorily controlled with one dose a day. When two daily doses are needed, the usual procedure is to divide the amount equally.

In mild, stable diabetics, after dietary regulation has been established and its results evaluated, therapy is usually initiated with 250 mg. daily before breakfast. Then, dosage is adjusted by increments of 250 to 500 mg. every five to seven days, as necessary.

Because of the hyperresponsiveness of some elderly patients to sulfonylureas, a daily dose of 250 mg. of Dymelor before breakfast is used, and the blood and urine sugars are checked during the first twenty-four hours of treatment. If control is satisfactory, the dose is continued at 250 mg. However, if an increase is required, 250 to 500 mg. are added daily. If there is a tendency toward hypoglycemia on 250 mg. daily, the dose may be reduced to 125 mg. or discontinued.

For patients who demonstrate persistent hyperglycemia (4+ glycosuria) in spite of adherence to diet, two treatment procedures are suggested. (1) The patient may be started on a dosage of 500 mg. daily and checked at the end of seven days for response to the drug. (2) A daily dose of 10 to 15 units of Lente® or NPH Insulin for three to seven days may be used until the blood sugar is brought down to the normal level. The patient may then be transferred to 250 mg. of Dymelor daily, with adjustment of dosage as indicated below.

When the patient has been receiving other oral agents

When a patient is transferred from tolbutamide, the initial dose of Dymelor ordinarily should be about half of the tolbutamide dose. Thus, a patient controlled with 500 mg. of tolbutamide would be given 250 mg. of Dymelor. If the patient is receiving 3 Gm. or more of tolbutamide daily, the dose of Dymelor should not exceed 1.5 Gm.; this is usually administered as 750 mg. twice daily or as 1 Gm. before breakfast and 500 mg. before supper.

When transfer is made from chlorpropamide, the initial dose of Dymelor® (acetohexamide, Lilly) is ordinarily about twice that of chlorpropamide; that is, a patient who was receiving 250 mg. of chlorpropamide is given 500 mg. of Dymelor.

In neither instance is it necessary to allow for a transition period. Subsequent adjustment of the doses of Dymelor following the transfer from chlorpropamide or tolbutamide, of course, is made on the basis of clinical response.

Patients maintained on 20 units of Insulin daily may be transferred directly to Dymelor, 250 mg. daily. When patients receiving larger doses of Insulin are transferred to Dymelor, the dose of Insulin ordinarily is reduced 20 to 30 percent daily and the initial dose of Dymelor is 250 mg. This procedure is carried out with particular care, however, in elderly patients. During the period of Insulin withdrawal, patients should test their urine for sugar and acetone at least three times daily and report the results to their physicians so that appropriate dosage adjustments of both Insulin and Dymelor can be made.

BIBLIOGRAPHY

1. Janbon, M., Chaptal, J., Vedel, A., and Schaap, J.: Accidents hypoglycémiques graves par un sulfamidothiodiazol (le VK 57 ou 2254 RP), Montpellier méd., 21-22:441, 1942.

2. Ferguson, B. D.: The Oral Hypoglycemic Compounds, M. Clin. North America, 49:929, 1965.

3. Williams, R. H., Pollen, R. H., Tanner, D. C., and Barnes, R. H.: Oral Antidiabetic Therapy, Ann. Int. Med., 51:1121, 1959.

4. Feldman, J. M., and Lebovitz, H. E.: Appraisal of the Extrapancreatic Actions of Sulfonylureas, Arch. Int. Med., 123:314, 1969.

5. Sheldon, J., Taylor, K. W., and Anderson, J.: The Effects of Long-Term Acetohexamide Treatment on Pancreatic Islet Cell Function in Maturity-Onset Diabetes, Metabolism, 15:874, 1966.

6. Chu, Ping-Chi, Conway, M. J., Krouse, H. A., and Goodner, C. J.: The Pattern of Response of Plasma Insulin and Glucose to Meals and Fasting during Chlorpropamide Therapy, Ann. Int. Med., 68:757, 1968.

7. Galloway, J. A., McMahon, R. E., Culp, H. W., Marshall, F. J., and Young, E. C.: Metabolism, Blood Levels and Rate of Excretion of Acetohexamide in Human Subjects, Diabetes, 16:118, 1967.

8. McMahon, R. E., Marshall, F. J., and Culp, H. W.: The Nature of the Metabolites of Acetohexamide in the Rat and in the Human, J. Pharmacol. & Exper. Therap., 149:272, 1965.

9. Root, M. A., Sigal, M. V., Jr., and Anderson, R. C.: Pharmacology of 1-(p-chlorobenzenesulfonyl)-3-n-propylurea (Chlorpropamide), Diabetes, 8:7, 1959.

10. Smith, D. L., Vecchio, T. J., and Forist, A. A.: Metabolism of Antidiabetic Sulfonylureas in Man. I. Biological Half-Lives of the p-Acetylbenzenesulfonylureas, U-18536 and Acetohexamide and Their Metabolites, Metabolism, 14:229, 1965.

11. Krall, L. P., and Bradley, R. F.: The How, When and Where of the Oral Hypoglycemic Compounds, Postgrad. Med., 37:75, 1965.

12. Lozano-Castaneda, O., Camerini-Dávalos, R. A., Krall, L. P., and Marble, A.: Two Years' Experience with Acetohexamide, Metabolism, 13:99, 1964.

13. Breidahl, H. D., Martin, F. I. R., and Taft, H. P.: The Treatment of Diabetes Mellitus with Acetohexamide, a New Sulphonylurea, M. J. Australia, 1:688, 1963.

14. Montgomery, D. A. D.: Acetohexamide, Practitioner, 193:555, 1964.

15. Sheldon, J., Anderson, J., and Stoner, L.: Serum Concentration and Urinary Excretion of Oral Sulfonylurea Compounds. Relation to Diabetic Control, Diabetes, 14:362, 1965.

16. Fajans, S. S., and Conn, J. W.: The Use of Tolbutamide in the Treatment of Young People with Mild Diabetes Mellitus. A Progress Report, Diabetes, 11 (Supplement):123, 1962.

17. Arquilla, E. R., and Finn, J.: Genetic Differences in Antibody Production to Determinant Groups on Insulin, Science, 142:400, 1963.

18. Berson, S. A., Yalow, R. S., Bauman, A., Rothschild, M. A., and Newerly, K.: Insulin-I131 Metabolism in Human Subjects. Demonstration of Insulin-Binding Globulin in the Circulation of Insulin-Treated Subjects, J. Clin. Invest., 35:170, 1956.

19. Lockwood, D. H., and Prout, T. E.: Isoantibodies to Insulin, Clin. Res., 10:401, 1962.

20. Renold, A. E., Soeldner, J. S., and Steinke, J.: Immunological Studies with Homologous and Heterologous Pancreatic Insulin in the Cow, in Aetiology of Diabetes Mellitus and Its Complications, Ciba Foundation Colloquia on Endocrinology, 15:122, 1964.

21. Meinert, C. L., Knatterud, G. L., Prout, T. E., and Klimt, C. R.: The University Group Diabetes Program: A Study of the Effects of Hypoglycemic Agents on Vascular Complications in Patients with Adult-Onset Diabetes. II. Mortality Results, Diabetes, 19(Supplement):789, 1970.

22. Soler, N. G., Pentecost, B. L., Bennett, M. A., Fitzgerald, M. G., Lamb, P., and Malins, J. M.: Coronary Care for Myocardial Infarction in Diabetics, Lancet, 1:475, 1974.

23. Roth, J., Prout, T. E., Goldfine, I. D., Wolfe, S. M., Muenzer, J., Grauer, L. E., and Marcus, M. L.: Sulfonylureas: Effects in Vivo and in Vitro, Ann. Intern. Med., 75:607, 1971.

24. Keen, H.: Minimal Diabetes and Arterial Disease: Prevalence and the Effect of Treatment, in Early Diabetes (edited by R. A. Camerini-Dávalos and H. S. Cole), p. 437. New York: Academic Press, Inc., 1970.

25. Paasikivi, J.: Long-Term Tolbutamide Treatment after Myocardial Infarction, Acta med. scandinav., Supplementum 507, 1970.

26. Knatterud, G. L., Klimt, C. R., Levin, M. E., Jacobson, M. E., and Goldner, M. G.: Effect of Hypoglycemic Agents on Vascular Complications in Patients with Adult-Onset Diabetes. VII. Mortality and Selected Nonfatal Events with Insulin Treatment, J.A.M.A., 240:37, 1978.

27. Ingelfinger, F. J.: Editorial: Debates on Diabetes, N. Engl. J. Med., *296:*1228, 1977.

28. Observers from the Biometric Society (Armitage, P., and Schneider, B.): Report of the Committee for the Assessment of Biometric Aspects of Controlled Trials of Hypoglycemic Agents, J.A.M.A., *231:*583, 1975.

29. Feinstein, A. R.: Clinical Biostatistics—VIII. An Analytic Appraisal of the University Group Diabetes Program (UGDP) Study, Clin. Pharmacol. Ther., *12:*167, 1971.

30. Schor, S.: The University Group Diabetes Program—A Statistician Looks at the Mortality Results, J.A.M.A., *217:*1671, 1971.

31. Krall, L. P., and Chabot, V. A.: Oral Hypoglycemic Agent Update, Med. Clin. North Am., *62:*681, 1978.

32. Editorial: The UGDP and Insulin Therapy, Diabetes Care, *1:*328, 1978.

33. Kilo, C., Williamson, J. R., Choi, S. C., and Miller, J. P.: Letter to the Editor, J.A.M.A., *241:*26 (January), 1979.

34. Camerini-Davalos, R. A., and Marble, A.: Incidence and Causes of Secondary Failure in Treatment with Tolbutamide, Experience with 2,500 Patients Treated up to Five Years, J.A.M.A., *181:*1, 1962.

35. Chodos, J. B., and Habegger-Chodos, H. E.: Cataract Formation in Human and Experimental Diabetes. I, Surv. Ophthal., *5:*129, 1960.

36. Kapetansky, F. M.: Refractive Changes with Tolbutamide, Ohio M. J., *59:*275, 1963.

37. Johnson, P. C.: Personal communication.

38. Hunton, R. B., Wells, M. V., and Skipper, E. W.: Hypothyroidism in Diabetics Treated with Sulphonylurea, Lancet, *2:*449, 1965.

39. Weissman, P. N., Shenkman, L., and Gregerman, R. I.: Chlorpropamide Hyponatremia, N. Engl. J. Med., *284:*65, 1971.

40. Gelfand, M. L.: Gastrointestinal Bleeding during Tolbutamide Therapy, J.A.M.A., *171:*258, 1959.

41. Camerini-Dávalos, R., Lozano-Castaneda, O., and Marble, A.: Five Years' Experience with Tolbutamide, Diabetes, *11* (Supplement):74, 1962.

42. Montgomery, D. A. D., Rastogi, G. K., and Weaver, J. A.: Acetohexamide in Treatment of Diabetes Mellitus, Brit. M. J., *1:*868, 1964.

43. Leevy, C. M., Ryan, C. M., and Fineberg, J. C.: Diabetes Mellitus and Liver Dysfunction. Etiologic and Therapeutic Considerations, Am. J. Med., *8:*290, 1950.

44. Popper, H., and Schaffner, F.: Liver: Structure and Function, p. 642. New York: McGraw-Hill Book Company, Inc., 1957.

45. Schneider, T., and Bersohn, I.: Liver Function Tests in Diabetes Mellitus. Their Correlation with Late Clinical Manifestations and Complications of Disease, Med. Proc. (Johannesb.), *3:*375, 1957.

46. Bradley, R. F., Sagild, U., and Schertenleib, F. E.: Diabetes Mellitus and Liver Function, New England J. Med., *253:*454, 1955.

47. Brown, H.: Liver Function in Diabetes Mellitus, Am. J. M. Sc., *218:*540, 1949.

48. Camerini-Dávalos, R., Marble, A., and Muench, H.: Liver Function in Diabetes Mellitus, New England J. Med., *266:*1349, 1962.

49. Zimmerman, H. J.: Drugs and the Liver, in Disease-a-Month (edited by H. F. Dowling). Chicago: Year Book Medical Publishers, Inc., May, 1963.

50. Drerup, A. L., Alexander, W. A., Lumb, G. D., Cummins, A. J., and Clark, G. M.: Jaundice Occurring in a Patient Treated with Chlorothiazide, New England J. Med., *259:*534, 1958.

51. Huguley, C. M., Jr.: Drug-Induced Blood Dyscrasias, in Disease-a-Month (edited by H. F. Dowling). Chicago: Year Book Medical Publishers, Inc., October, 1963.

52. Editorial: Alcohol Sensitivity to Sulphonylureas, Brit. M. J., *2:*586, 1964.

53. Schlesinger, F. G., and van Gastel, C.: Possible Aggravation of Abdominal Symptoms by Tolbutamide in a Patient with Diabetes and Hepatic Porphyria, Acta med. scandinav., *169:*433, 1961.

54. Marble, A., and Camerini-Dávalos, R.: Clinical Experience with Sulfonylurea Compounds in Diabetes, Ann. New York Acad. Sc., *71:*239, 1957.

55. Handelsman, M. B., Levitt, L., and Calabretta, M. F.: A Laboratory and Clinical Study of Chlorpropamide in Ambulatory Diabetics, Ann. New York Acad. Sc., *74:*632, 1959.

56. Boshell, B. R., Wilensky, A. S., Barrett, J. C., and Almon, J. V.: Acetohexamide: Comparison with Other Sulfonylurea Compounds in the Treatment of Diabetes Mellitus, Clin. Pharmacol. & Therap., *3:*750, 1962.

Hypoglycemia Due to Insulin and the Sulfonylurea Agents

10

DEFINITION

The term "hypoglycemia" usually refers to the clinical condition resulting from an abnormally low blood glucose. It is characterized by varying degrees of neurological dysfunction, may occur with or without signs resembling epinephrine overactivity, and is responsive to the administration of glucose. Fever is not uncommon.

During a hypoglycemic reaction, the blood sugar is usually less than 50 mg. per 100 ml., but typical hypoglycemic reactions may occur even in the presence of a higher-than-normal blood sugar level. The occurrence of hypoglycemic reactions in diabetics has been reported[1] when the blood sugar ranged between 82 and 472 mg. per 100 ml. forty to one hundred minutes following the intravenous administration of Regular Insulin. The clinical picture during these reactions was identical to that found in patients with blood glucose at levels classically defined as "hypoglycemic." On the other hand, when the concentration of blood glucose is 25 to 30 mg. per 100 ml., occasionally there may be no obvious clinical findings of hypoglycemia.

Although a number of factors apparently are responsible for this paradox, probably the most important one is the rate of fall in blood glucose, as determined by the plasma insulin concentration.[1A] It becomes readily apparent that the glucose level in the blood does not necessarily reflect its level in the brain cell; therefore, the term "hypoglycemic reaction" cannot be limited to those reactions in which the blood glucose is below a certain value. (Furthermore, all episodes of neurological dysfunction in the diabetic should not be attributed solely to derangements in cerebral glucose metabolism. Fabrykant[2] has called attention to the syndrome of pseudohypoglycemic reactions. These episodes are characterized by clinical findings identical to those found in true hypoglycemia, but there is no depression of the blood glucose and also no response to the administration of carbohydrate. Patients in this category must be studied for the presence of other disorders, such as arteriosclerosis and hypoparathyroidism, which may interfere with normal cerebral function.)

HYPOGLYCEMIA IN THE CHILD

In a diabetic child, the signs and symptoms of a hypoglycemic reaction are especially variable. He may have a voracious appetite, a feeling of heaviness in the extremities, unsteadiness of gait, and a tremor of the hands and may fatigue easily or become faint. Early cerebral cortical signs may include confusion, somnolence, apathy, nervousness, and, sometimes, delusions and hallucinations.

Somnolence is a particularly deceptive symptom. Instead of waking and getting up in the morning, the child may seem sleepy, and the mother may think her child simply wants to sleep late. Therefore, it is vitally important that the young diabetic adopt a rigid schedule with regard to time for going to bed, rising, taking Insulin, and eating meals. Once he is up in the morning, he should not return to bed after taking his Insulin, and rest periods during the day should be closely supervised. A child who fails to arise on time in the morning should be suspected of having a hypoglycemic reaction until it is proved otherwise.

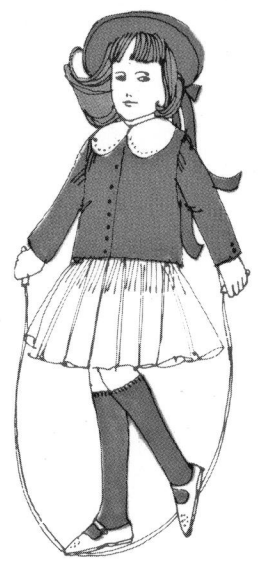

The diabetic child must learn to eat everything that is placed before him—or ask for substitutions. However, a rigid attitude toward diet should be avoided, because a child having a hypoglycemic reaction may develop an unusual appetite and yet may be hesitant about meeting the need for extra food. He should always carry a source of concentrated sugar with him to treat reactions which may come on when he is alone.

ETIOLOGY

The most common causes of hypoglycemia are the hypoglycemic agents— namely, Insulin and the sulfonylurea compounds. Numerous conditions may be associated with or may be responsible for the hypoglycemia due to these drugs. Some are common to both treatments; others are observed exclusively or more frequently with one or the other. Hypoglycemia may result from therapy with Insulin and the sulfonylureas in connection with (1) dietary change or nutritional inadequacy; (2) weight reduction; (3) exercise; (4) removal of stress, i.e., septic, emotional, or surgical; (5) termination of pregnancy; (6) correction of hyperendocrinopathies (thyrotoxicosis, Cushing's syndrome, acromegaly); (7) onset of diseases associated with hypoglycemia (hypoadrenalism, pituitary insufficiency, liver disease); and (8) factitious hypoglycemia.

FACTORS ASSOCIATED WITH HYPOGLYCEMIA DUE TO INSULIN

Causes of hypoglycemia associated with the use of Insulin are (1) errors in injection technic, such as failure to agitate the vial before use, improper measurement of Insulin, injection into an area of hypertrophic lipodystrophy, and the use of Insulin in which the precipitate has become clumped or granular; (2) reduction of Insulin requirement as a result of a spontaneous change in the course of diabetes; and (3) chronic use of excessive dosage.

Although errors in the technic of Insulin injection appear to be an unimportant factor in producing hypoglycemia, they probably account for a significant number of such reactions. Therefore, when hypoglycemia occurs, one must consider the possibility of faulty technic, even in the diabetic patient whose skill in Insulin injection has apparently been established. Hypoglycemic reactions in patients with hypertrophic lipodystrophy usually result from injection of an increased dose of Insulin into a normal site after the previous injection into the anesthetic hypertrophic areas.

Hypoglycemic reactions may occur when Insulin is injected into the leg and the extremity is then exercised.[2A] This phenomenon is the result of increased rate of absorption of Insulin by the exercised limb and has been attributed to increased subcutaneous and lymphatic blood flow.

Insulin hypoglycemia due to spontaneous improvement in carbohydrate tolerance may occur at any time after the discovery of diabetes. In early juvenile diabetes, there may be spontaneous remissions during which the need for Insulin may vary from 0 to 6 or 8 units. The average periods of diminished need for Insulin last approximately eighteen months.

A common cause of Insulin hypoglycemia late in the course of diabetes is the onset of renal insufficiency associated with Kimmelstiel-Wilson disease, also known as diabetic glomerulosclerosis. Although the mechanisms for the reduction in Insulin requirement with the onset of this complication are unknown, the improvement may be related to a diminished rate of degradation and/or excretion of administered Insulin which occurs secondarily to involvement of the renal parenchyma.[3] Occasionally, hypoglycemia may appear during the course of diabetes as a result of the spontaneous changes in the patient's response to the Insulin he is using. These changes may be viewed on the basis of the A, B, and C types of reaction (see pages 93 and 94).[4]

Finally, hypoglycemia may result from an excessive dose of Insulin. Usually, such a situation is readily identifiable by the presence of the classic symptoms and signs of hypoglycemia. However, hyperglycemia, glycosuria, and, in some instances, ketosis may occur occasionally as a result of the epinephrine response to a low blood sugar.[5] These, in turn, may lead to an increase in the Insulin dosage, which sets off a vicious circle of more marked hyperglycemia and further increase in the Insulin dosage. Therefore, the persistence of poor diabetic control in the presence of satisfactory dietary intake and successive increases in Insulin may indicate the need for a paradoxic reduction in dosage. Often, a 25 to 30 percent reduction will lead to improvement in the control of the diabetes except in the labile diabetic, in whom reduction of Insulin dosage should be carried out with restraint, e.g., 1 to 2 units per dose.

FACTORS ASSOCIATED WITH HYPOGLYCEMIA DUE TO ORAL AGENTS

1. INAPPROPRIATE DOSAGE

Sulfonylurea compounds may cause hypoglycemia in nondiabetic patients, in new patients whose initial dose is greater than needed, and in those transferred from Insulin to oral therapy. Such situations may be averted if the need for sulfonylurea therapy is firmly established before these agents are used and if patients are carefully monitored during the first few days of treatment. The sulfonylurea compounds are contraindicated in nondiabetic individuals. Therefore, when a family history of diabetes or other historical findings consistent with this diagnosis are lacking and when the fasting blood sugar is less than 120 mg. per 100 ml., tests to determine glucose tolerance, blood urea nitrogen level, and liver function may be needed before therapy with sulfonylureas is initiated.

Dosage may also be excessive if the effects of dietary therapy alone are not fully evaluated before sulfonylurea treatment is begun. Following the patient for several weeks with diet regulation alone before starting medication will prevent such a situation. Then, if a sulfonylurea is indicated, start with a small dose of the drug, e.g., 250 mg. of Dymelor® (acetohexamide, Lilly). Once treatment has been instituted, the patient should be seen by the physician at least every three months. During the visits, the patient should be questioned directly for evidence of hypoglycemia. Fasting and/or postprandial blood sugar levels should be obtained. This procedure may detect spontaneous fluctuations in carbohydrate tolerance and permit adjustment in sulfonylurea dosage.

2. IMPAIRED RENAL FUNCTION

This impairment may be associated with a hyperresponsiveness to the hypoglycemic activity of the sulfonylurea compounds. The result may be a severe and prolonged hypoglycemia which requires intensive treatment. The occurrence of this reaction in patients with end-stage renal disease may be attributed, in part, to abnormal retention of the sulfonylureas (or the possibility that the patients are not true diabetics).

The basis for prolonged hypoglycemia from these agents in cases of mild renal impairment is less clear. In patients with prolonged hypoglycemia in whom the blood urea nitrogen level was reported, the BUN concentration was elevated to some extent in about a third of the cases treated with tolbutamide and in 25 percent of those treated with acetohexamide. Because blood levels of acetohexamide and insulin in many of the patients studied often are not strikingly elevated,[6] other abnormalities deserve consideration. Patients with azotemia frequently have diminished capacity to recover from an Insulin-induced hypoglycemia[7] and show an increased responsiveness to tolbutamide.[8] In addition, other mechanisms, such as those observed in the Insulin-dependent patients with Kimmelstiel-Wilson disease, may be operative.

3. POTENTIATION BY CONCURRENT ADMINISTRATION OF OTHER DRUGS

Certain drugs, such as the antimicrobial sulfa agents and phenylbutazone, have been reported to potentiate the hypoglycemic activity of the sulfonylurea agents. Soeldner and Steinke[9] noted the slight elevation of plasma insulin levels in two patients who received a sulfa drug in combination with a sulfonylurea. The mechanism of potentiation of these two types of drugs is apparently related to several phenomena which have been reviewed by Bressler.[10] In spite of wide use of drug combinations, relatively few instances of hypoglycemia have been reported. This suggests that hypoglycemia due to drug therapy is in part related to individual patient idiosyncrasy.

4. USE IN THE ELDERLY

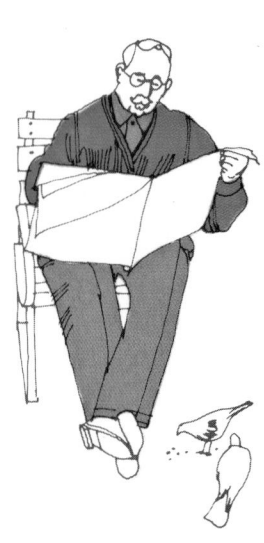

Elderly patients occasionally appear to be unusually responsive to the sulfonylurea compounds. The reason is not known, but it is conceivable that mild to moderate abnormalities in glucose tolerance which occur in the elderly may actually represent a physiological aging process and not true diabetes mellitus.

Such patients treated orally for mild glycosuria or hyperglycemia without establishment of the diagnosis actually represent cases of inappropriate dosage. In addition, the tendency of elderly patients to eat improperly may enhance their susceptibility to hypoglycemia from the sulfonylurea compounds.

5. ACCIDENTAL INGESTION

Rare instances of severe hypoglycemia have been reported in children who have ingested a parent's or grandparent's sulfonylurea medications. Because such patients may be subject to prolonged hypoglycemia, therapy must be vigorous and sustained until recovery is complete.

6. MISCELLANEOUS

There have been a few cases of severe and/or prolonged hypoglycemia in which the cause does not appear to fit any of the above categories. These included instances in which the metabolism of the drug may have been atypical or in which the patient was extremely responsive to the effect of the drug. Fortunately, the number of such patients reported has been small. However, it has not been possible to predict which patients will be hyperresponsive.

CLINICAL FINDINGS

The clinical picture of hypoglycemia is quite varied, for the symptoms and signs differ not only from patient to patient but also in the same patient from episode to episode. Nevertheless, careful clinical studies have made it possible to describe a typical, fully developed Insulin reaction. Such a reaction has two components—response of the autonomic nervous system and response of the central nervous system. Sussman et al.[11] described four phases of an Insulin-induced hypoglycemic reaction: (1) parasympathetic phase—characterized by hunger, nausea, eructation, and possibly bradycardia and mild hypotension; (2) diminished cerebral function—signified by the presence of lethargy, lassitude, frequent yawning, decreased spontaneity of conversation, and inability to do simple calculations; (3) sympathetic phase—during which signs of epinephrine activity occur, including increased systolic and mean blood pressure, sweating, and tachycardia; and (4) hypoglycemic coma, with or without convulsions.

These findings have been correlated with the specific brain sites involved with the neurological manifestations observed in hypoglycemia.[12]

Some patients are aware of the autonomic response; others may have clinical signs of an autonomic response but may not be aware of it; and still others may progress from a state of alertness to frank coma without an awareness of the symptoms or objective signs of hypoglycemia.[11]

Although the pathophysiology of hypoglycemia due to Insulin and to the sulfonylurea compounds is identical, three points concerning these agents should be noted.

First, physicians generally are less aware that serious hypoglycemia may occur with the sulfonylurea agents.

Second, the onset of hypoglycemia with Insulin can usually be predicted on the basis of the peak action of the Insulin being used, whereas the sulfonylurea-caused hypoglycemia may occur at any time from thirty to sixty minutes after ingestion of the drug to many hours later. However, unexpected exercise or omission of food may hasten the onset or augment the intensity of effect of both Insulin and the oral agents.

Finally, in contrast to the hypoglycemic reactions following Insulin, autonomic signs are frequently diminished or absent in reactions due to sulfonylurea compounds. The basis for this is unclear.

THE TREATMENT OF HYPOGLYCEMIA

Prevention

The best treatment of hypoglycemia is prevention. Except for the rare patient who is acutely responsive to sulfonylurea compounds, prevention can be accomplished satisfactorily by carefully evaluating the patient *before* the initiation of sulfonylurea treatment, by being aware of the various factors associated with Insulin and sulfonylurea hypoglycemia, and by seeing the patient frequently once treatment has begun.

When prevention has failed, the treatment of hypoglycemia depends upon the cause, duration, and severity of the hypoglycemic episode as well as upon the age and general health of the patient, particularly with respect to renal, hepatic, and cardiovascular function. It also depends upon the facilities and modes of therapy that are available. Satisfactory results of treatment may be expected if the diagnosis is made promptly, proper therapy is selected and immediately instituted, and the program is continued until a normal or elevated blood sugar can be maintained without further treatment. The choice of agents for combating hypoglycemia depends upon whether or not the patient is conscious and upon his response to treatment. Beverages, syrups, juices, and food with high carbohydrate content, intravenous hypertonic glucose solution, glucagon, and, in special situations, epinephrine and hydrocortisone may all be effective.

The carbohydrate content and types of sugars present in beverages, syrups, and foods which are commonly used in treating hypoglycemia are listed in Table 31.

Parenteral glucose

Parenteral sugar solutions are available in concentrations of 5, 10, and 50 percent (either as pure glucose or as glucose and fructose). However, the quantity of sugar in the 5 percent sugar solutions is usually insufficient for the treatment of hypoglycemia. When parenteral glucose is needed, 10 to 50 percent glucose solutions must be used. The latter is preferred.

Table 31. Nature and Concentration of Sugars in Carbohydrate-Containing Substances Commonly Used for the Oral Treatment of Hypoglycemia Due to Insulin and Sulfonylurea Agents

SYRUPS	APPROXIMATE CARBOHYDRATE PER TABLESPOON (GM.)	APPROXIMATE CONCENTRATION (%)	PRINCIPAL SUGARS
Corn syrup	14.8	74	Sucrose
Honey	16.4	78	Glucose and fructose
Maple syrup	12.8	64	Sucrose
Molasses (light)	13.0	65	Sucrose
Table syrup	14.8	74	Sucrose

BEVERAGES	APPROXIMATE CARBOHYDRATE PER 8-OUNCE GLASS (GM.)	APPROXIMATE CONCENTRATION (%)	PRINCIPAL SUGARS
Whole milk	12.4	20	Lactose
Orange juice	24.0	10	Glucose
Cola beverage	20.4	11	Sucrose
Ginger ale	20.7	9	Sucrose
Soft drinks in general	25.0	8	Sucrose

SOLID FOODS	APPROXIMATE CARBOHYDRATE (GM.)	APPROXIMATE CONCENTRATION (%)	PRINCIPAL SUGARS
Sugar (tsp.)	5.0	100	Sucrose
Average candy bar (1 oz.)	21.6	60	Sucrose
Piece of fudge (1 1/4 sq. in.— 30 Gm.)	23.7	79	Sucrose

Glucagon

Glucagon, a polypeptide hormone of known amino acid structure,[13] is produced in the pancreas (alpha cells of the islands of Langerhans). Upon injection, it causes a rapid breakdown of glycogen to glucose in the liver. It has been purified and crystallized by scientists at the Lilly Research Laboratories.[14]

Glucagon has no sympathomimetic activity. It increases the activity of phosphorylase, the enzyme which acts on the first step in glycogenolysis. It is a supremely safe agent. The principal side-effect is nausea, and this occurs only after large doses.

Another advantage of glucagon is that its effect is due to utilization of endogenous glucose, and thus there is considerably less fluctuation of the blood glucose level than after the intravenous administration of 50 percent dextrose solutions. Moreover, glucagon has practically unlimited stability in dry powder form before mixture and can be given subcutaneously, intramuscularly, or intravenously. Therefore, it is an ideal agent for the outpatient treatment of hypoglycemia. Its safety and efficacy have led most physicians who treat diabetics to keep glucagon in their medical bags at all times and to instruct all new patients on Insulin and/or their families in its use.

In doses as low as 1 or 2 mg., glucagon is highly effective in treating the great majority of cases of hypoglycemia; however, the hyperglycemic response following its use may be reduced in emaciated or undernourished patients with uremia[7] or liver disease.[15]

In a study of forty-one induced and spontaneous Insulin reactions in eighteen adult diabetic patients, Elrick et al.[16] found that 1 or 2 mg. of glucagon administered intramuscularly or subcutaneously resulted in complete recovery in all but one patient within five to twenty minutes after administration. A comparison was made of the response of hypoglycemic diabetic campers to 1 or 2 mg. of glucagon injected subcutaneously and 20 Gm. of glucose administered orally.[17] In all instances, a measurable increase in the glucose concentration was found within five minutes, and the blood sugar level was in normal range within fifteen minutes. There was relief from the hypoglycemia within ten minutes.

Most studies used 1 or 2-mg. doses administered subcutaneously. An important factor, however, in the efficacy of glucagon is the promptness with which it is given. Satisfactory response occurred in only forty of 100 patients with Insulin-induced hypoglycemia who had been comatose for forty-five to sixty minutes before the glucagon was given.[18]

At the Lilly Clinic, Wishard Memorial Hospital, Indianapolis, 1 mg. of glucagon is administered parenterally to the hypoglycemic patient. The dose is repeated if no response is elicited in ten to fifteen minutes. When the patient recovers, he is given a fruit or bread exchange from the next meal, 10 to 25 Gm. of carbohydrate, or the full contents of a 25-Gm. tube of glucose paste in order to prevent relapse into hypoglycemia caused by depleted stores of liver glycogen.

Use of glucagon

Glucagon has also been used to terminate Insulin-shock hypoglycemic episodes in the treatment of mental disorders. Laqueur and LaBurt[19] reported success with glucagon in 92 percent of a series of 375 psychiatric patients. Of interest is the fact that the patients received only 0.33 mg. of glucagon intramuscularly; the usual dose is 1 to 2 mg.

Epinephrine may be used for the symptomatic treatment of hypoglycemic coma in the absence of either parenteral glucose or glucagon. The maximum initial dose is 0.5 ml. of a 1:1,000 solution; not more than 0.3 ml. of this solution should be administered to children who weigh less than fifty pounds. The dose may be repeated in fifteen minutes if no response is observed.

The ability of hydrocortisone to increase gluconeogenesis makes it a useful *adjunct* in the management of prolonged hypoglycemia. It is particularly useful in patients with azotemia. However, hydrocortisone should never be used as the sole treatment in hypoglycemic coma.

SPECIFIC PLAN FOR TREATMENT

There are many methods of treating hypoglycemia. The choice of therapy depends upon the patient's state of consciousness, the cause of his hypoglycemia, and his previous response to hypoglycemic agents. The scheme presented here[20] is one of many that may be used.

The Alert Patient—Oral carbohydrate is the treatment of choice for the alert patient with signs and symptoms of hypoglycemia. Orange juice or high-carbohydrate beverages, such as cola beverages, ginger ale, or juices (see Table 31), should be given in 3 or 4-ounce doses every five to ten minutes until there are no further signs of hypoglycemia. An alternative treatment is the administration of 1 or 2 mg. of glucagon. This may be repeated in fifteen minutes if necessary.

The patient should be observed for at least one hour or until the next meal is taken. Although the alert patient may recognize the appearance of hypoglycemia and treat himself, he should be certain that there is someone on hand who is aware of his condition.

*The more
serious case*

The Patient Who Failed to Respond Satisfactorily to Oral Carbohydrate and Is in a Coma or Who Will Not Co-operate in Taking Carbohydrate Orally—If glucagon has not been administered previously, 1 or 2 mg. may be given intramuscularly or subcutaneously, but not intravenously, to patients whose hypoglycemia is due to sulfonylurea agents.[21] As an alternate, or if glucagon has failed, 50 ml. of 50 percent dextrose in water should be given intravenously.

It is advisable to determine the degree of hypoglycemia by obtaining a blood sugar level, but this procedure should not delay treatment.

If the patient is unconscious, care must be taken to keep the airway open and to prevent tongue-biting. Pillows should be removed.

Recovery should occur within five to ten minutes after the injection of intravenous glucose and within fifteen minutes after glucagon is given. Then, if possible, the cause of the hypoglycemia should be ascertained.

When neither glucagon nor hypertonic glucose is available, a subcutaneous dose of 0.5 ml. of a 1:1,000 solution of epinephrine may be given and repeated in fifteen minutes. If honey is available, this may be applied with the finger to the buccal mucosa and the process repeated if necessary. Care must be taken to avoid aspiration.

If the hypoglycemia is an isolated episode, the Insulin dosage need not be changed, but it usually must be reduced if two reactions have occurred in a forty-eight-hour period.

*The emergency
case*

The Patient Who Failed to Respond to Previous Treatment; Is Known to Have Renal Disease with Mild to Marked Azotemia; Has a History of Treatment with Sulfonylurea Compounds; Has Evidence of Heart, Liver, or Cerebrovascular Disease; or Is a Nondiabetic Who Accidentally Ingested a Sulfonylurea Agent in Large Quantities—Such a patient must be hospitalized promptly and, if possible, initial treatment carried out in an emergency or intensive care unit. The following program is recommended.

1. Check blood glucose, blood urea nitrogen, and hematocrit immediately. Blood for electrolytes and C.B.C. may be drawn at this time for determinations as necessary.

2. Give an intravenous injection of 100 ml. of 50 percent dextrose solution immediately.

3. Follow this with a continuous drip (20 drops per minute) of a 10 percent dextrose solution in water.

4. Place the patient in a lateral recumbent position, and use restraints if necessary. Bed rails should be up.

5. Administer 100 mg. of hydrocortisone immediately and every eight hours thereafter.

6. Record fluid intake and output.

7. Check vital signs every thirty minutes.

If the patient relapses into hypoglycemia when being given 10 percent dextrose at 1.33 ml. per minute (i.e., 2,000 ml. containing 200 Gm. glucose per twenty-four hours), either the rate of infusion should be raised to 2 ml. per minute, or it should be left the same and 100 to 200 Gm. dextrose added to the 10 percent dextrose solution. The choice depends upon the nutritional and cardiovascular status of the patient. Since the hypoglycemic tendency often persists for several days, the constant infusion of hypertonic glucose should not be discontinued until there is evidence that the blood sugar will be maintained at a satisfactory level for at least three hours without the addition of glucose. A recommended practice is to keep the vein open by using a slow drip of isotonic saline and to observe the patient carefully during the period when carbohydrate is withheld. Before the intravenous feeding is discontinued, there should be no clinical signs of hypoglycemia, and the blood sugar should be normal or elevated.

BIBLIOGRAPHY

1. Bolinger, R. E., Stephens, R., Lukert, B., and Diederich, D.: Galvanic Skin Reflex and Plasma Free Fatty Acids during Insulin Reactions, Diabetes, *13*:600, 1964.

1A. DeFronzo, R. A., Andres, R., Bledsoe, T. A., Boden, G., Faloona, G. A., and Tobin, J. D.: A Test of the Hypothesis That the Rate of Fall in Glucose Concentration Triggers Counterregulatory Hormonal Responses in Man, Diabetes, *26*:445, 1977.

2. Fabrykant, M.: Pseudohypoglycemic Reactions in Insulin-Treated Diabetics: Etiology, Laboratory Aids and Therapy, J. Am. Geriatrics Soc., *12*:221, 1964.

2A. Koivisto, V. A., and Felig, P.: Effects of Leg Exercise on Insulin Absorption in Diabetic Patients, N. Engl J. Med., *298*:79, 1978.

3. Ricketts, H. T., Wildberger, H. L., and Regut, L.: The Role of the Kidney in the Disposal of Insulin in Rats, Diabetes, *12*:155, 1963.

4. Hallas-Møller, K.: The Lente Insulins, Diabetes, *5*:7, 1956.

5. Somogyi, M.: Exacerbation of Diabetes by Excess Insulin Action, Am. J. Med., *26*:169, 1959.

6. Cohen, B. D., Galloway, J. A., McMahon, R. E., Culp, H. W., Root, M. A., and Henriques, K. J.: Carbohydrate Metabolism in Uremia: Blood Glucose Response to Sulfonylurea, Am. J. M. Sc., *254*:608, 1967.

7. Cohen, B. D.: Abnormal Carbohydrate Metabolism in Renal Disease. Blood Glucose Unresponsiveness to Hypoglycemia, Epinephrine, and Glucagon, Ann. Int. Med., *57*:204, 1962.

8. Westervelt, F. B., Jr., and Schreiner, G. E.: The Carbohydrate Intolerance of Uremic Patients, Ann. Int. Med., *57*:266, 1962.

9. Soeldner, J. S., and Steinke, J.: Hypoglycemia in Tolbutamide-Treated Diabetes. Report of Two Cases with Measurement of Serum Insulin, J.A.M.A., *193*:398, 1965.

10. Bressler, R.: Editorial: Combined Drug Therapy, Am. J. M. Sc., *255*:89, 1968.

11. Sussman, K. E., Crout, J. R., and Marble, A.: Failure of Warning in Insulin-Induced Hypoglycemic Reactions, Diabetes, *12*:38, 1963.

12. Himwich, H. E.: Brain Metabolism and Cerebral Disorders, p. 306. Baltimore: The Williams & Wilkins Company, 1951.

13. Bromer, W. W., Sinn, L. G., Staub, A., and Behrens, O. K.: The Amino Acid Sequence of Glucagon, Diabetes, *6*:234, 1957.

14. Staub, A., Sinn, L., and Behrens, O. K.: Purification and Crystallization of Hyperglycemic Glycogenolytic Factor (HGF), Science, *117*:628, 1953.

15. Van Itallie, T. B., and Bently, W. A. B.: Glucagon-Induced Hyperglycemia as an Index of Liver Function, J. Clin. Invest., *34*:1730, 1955.

16. Elrick, H., Witten, T. A., and Arai, Y.: Glucagon Treatment of Insulin Reactions, New England J. Med., *258*:476, 1958.

17. Shipp, J. C., Delcher, H. K., and Munroe, J. F.: Treatment of Insulin Hypoglycemia in Diabetic Campers. A Comparison of Glucagon (1 and 2 mg.) and Glucose, Diabetes, *13*:645, 1964.

18. MacCuish, A. C., Munro, J. F., and Duncan, J. P.: Treatment of Hypoglycaemic Coma with Glucagon, Intravenous Dextrose, and Mannitol Infusion in a Hundred Diabetics, Lancet, *2*:946, 1970.

19. Laqueur, H. P., and LaBurt, H. A.: Experiences with Low-Zinc Insulin, with Semi-Lente Insulin, with Glucagon and Adrenalin-Thiamine in Insulin Coma Treatment, J. Neuropsychiat., *2*:86, 1960.

20. Galloway, J. A.: Treatment of Hypoglycemia Secondary to Hypoglycemic Agents, Mod. Treat., *3*:412, 1966.

21. Galloway, J. A.: Glucagon in Sulphonylurea Hypoglycaemia? (Letters to the Editor), Lancet, *1*:815, 1968.

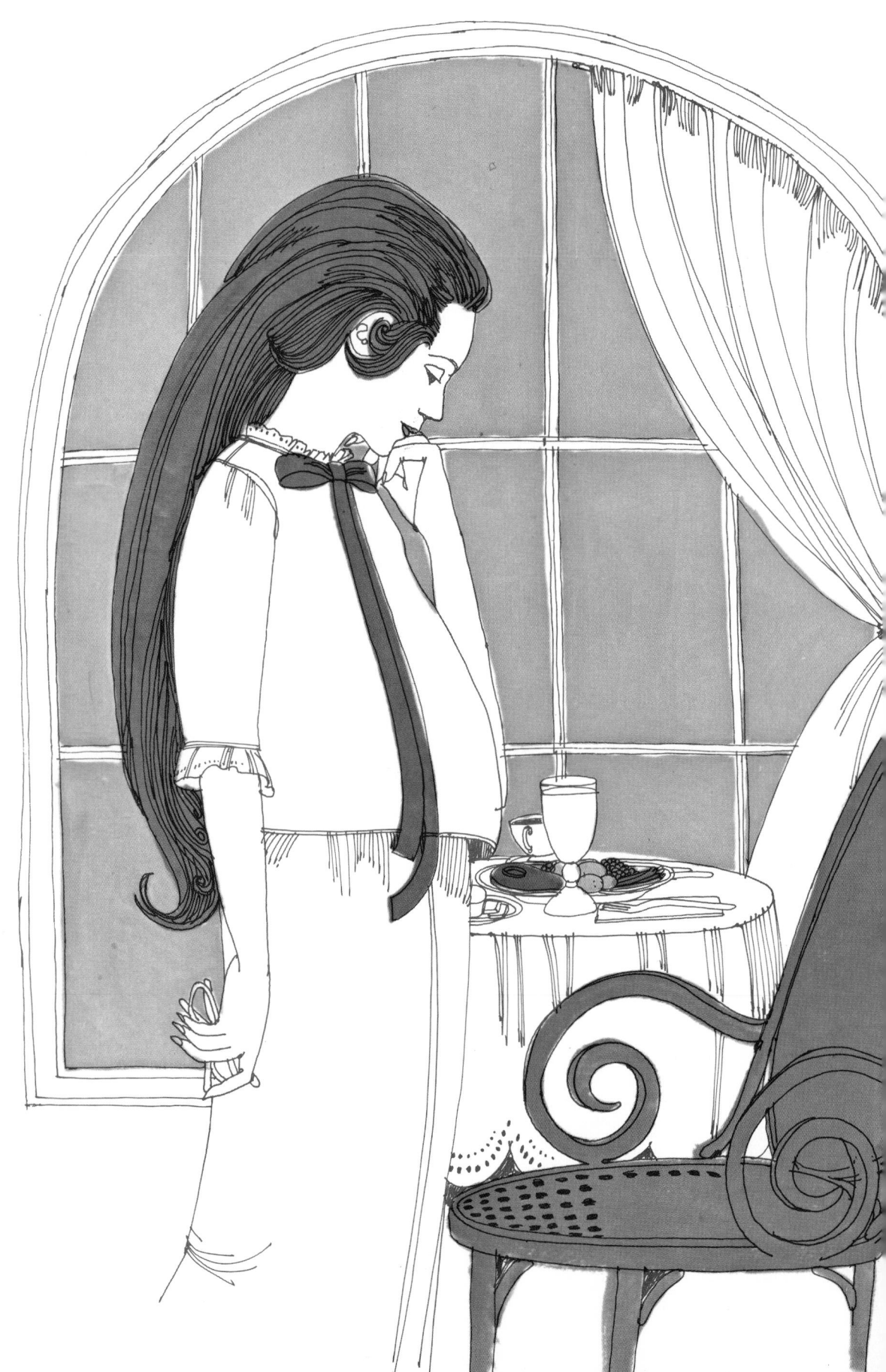

Diabetes and Pregnancy

11

The management of the diabetic during pregnancy and delivery has been reviewed by Mintz et al.[1] and Gabbe[2] as well as by many others.[3-8] The comments which follow are intended to provide an outline for practical management; the references given may be consulted for more detailed information.

Advances in medical care have conferred on the diabetic female a reproductive capacity which approaches that of her nondiabetic counterpart. This heightens the likelihood that general physicians, internists, and obstetricians will encounter diabetes during pregnancy. White[5] states that pregnancy occurs at one time or another in approximately 10 percent of the diabetic population. About one in one thousand of all pregnancies involves a diabetic woman. The interpretation of these figures must take into account the type of diabetes. The statistics of the Joslin Clinic include a high proportion of well-established, Insulin-dependent, growth-onset patients.[5] Another study has reported the incidence of mild diabetes in pregnancy to be one in 116.[9]

EFFECTS OF PREGNANCY ON THE DIABETIC STATE

Even in the normal individual, pregnancy exerts a diabetogenic effect. For instance, during normal pregnancy, an elevation occurs in plasma insulin levels (Figure 30) and, in some instances, in blood glucose levels in the postabsorptive state.[10-12] These changes have been attributed to increased degradation of insulin in the placenta[13] and to the elaboration of growthlike hormone substances by the placenta.[12,14] Although pregnancy did not elevate the fasting blood sugar in a large series of selected patients, postabsorptive levels during tolerance testing showed a general rise with the progression of the pregnancy.[15] On the basis of a retrospective study (Table 32), O'Sullivan and Mahan have suggested the limits within which diabetes is likely to develop.[16]

Because of the diabetogenic effects of pregnancy, Insulin requirements usually, but not always, increase significantly at this time. An important effect of pregnancy on diabetes is that occasionally there is an increased concentration of reducing substances in the urine which will give positive tests when the copper-reduction methods are used.[17] It is essential, therefore, to determine whether such a positive test is due to glucose or some other sugar. If it is caused by glucose, this could indicate poor diabetic control and/or renal glycosuria. The latter condition may be seen in pregnancy even in nondiabetic subjects, a phenomenon that has been attributed to increased glomerular filtration[18,19] and, to a lesser extent, to a relative

Figure 30. Mean Values of Plasma Insulin in Twenty Nondiabetic Pregnant Women (After Spellacy and Goetz[10])

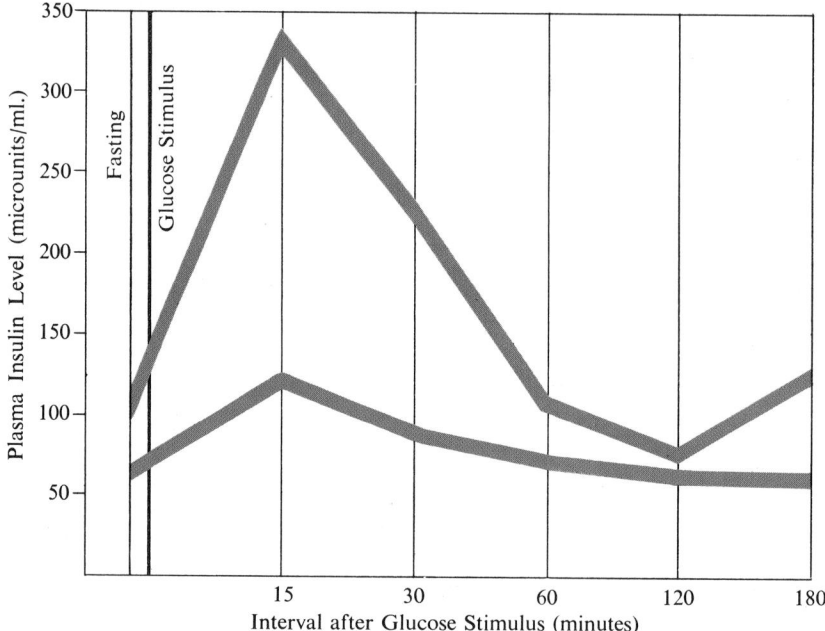

Pregnant

Postpartum

reduction in tubular reabsorption of glucose. The principal nonglucose reducing sugar that may be present in the urine of pregnant patients (diabetics and normals alike) is lactose. It may appear during the last six weeks of pregnancy[1] and often persists after parturition until lactation has ceased. Lactosuria and glycosuria may be differentiated by Tes-Tape, which is specific for glucose.

Table 32. Levels of Blood Glucose during Pregnancy above Which the Risk of Eventual Development of Diabetes Is Significantly Increased*

TIME	FASTING	ONE HOUR	TWO HOURS	THREE HOURS
Blood sugar† (mg./100 ml.)	90	165	145	125

Note: A positive test is said to occur when any two or more of the above values are met or exceeded.

*Twenty-nine ± 4.5 percent became diabetic on the average of two years and five months after a positive test during pregnancy.

†Somogyi-Nelson method was used on venous samples.

EFFECTS OF DIABETES ON PREGNANCY

In the diabetic, there is increased rate of toxemia, hydramnios, lethal congenital defects, and large babies. The incidence of the first three of these defects has been compared by Miller and Black (Table 33).[6]

The fact that pregnant diabetics have large babies takes on special significance because this may be one of the first manifestations, or prodromes, of the development of diabetes (see page 9). In a retrospective study,[20] it was noted that babies over ten pounds were born to 12.6 percent

Table 33. A Comparison of the Incidence of Three Complications of Pregnancy in Nondiabetic and Diabetic Women

	NONDIABETIC (%)	DIABETIC (%)
Toxemia	4.4	20.0
Hydramnios	0.3	20.4
Lethal congenital defects	0.5	2.0

of diabetic women but to only 5 percent of nondiabetic controls. Apparently, diabetes in the father has no effect on the occurrence of large offspring. White[5] points out that an inverse relationship exists between fetal size and duration of the diabetes. Thus, growth-onset diabetics seldom have large babies, especially in the presence of complications such as hypertension and nephropathy, which may be associated with placental dysfunction. On the other hand, patients with the mild, nonketotic, adult-onset type of the disease frequently do. Despite the high incidence of diabetes in women who have large babies, it should be pointed out that another cause of large children is large parents.

MANAGEMENT OF THE GROWTH-ONSET DIABETIC DURING PREGNANCY

OUTPATIENT CARE

During the patient's initial visit, the physician attempts to assess the severity of the diabetes and the amount of success the patient has had in controlling it (diet, type of Insulin, and frequency of doses). In addition, careful attention is paid to the course and outcome of previous pregnancies. For instance, the occurrence of preeclampsia or toxemia, hypertension, edema, glycosuria, hydramnios, stillbirths, and miscarriages is noted. In addition, there should be a study of neonatal morbidity and mortality and their causes, such as immaturity, birth trauma, congenital malformations, and respiratory distress syndrome. Attention is also given to changes in the Insulin requirement, ketoacidosis, and hypoglycemia during previous pregnancies.

In the physical examination, it is necessary to view the retina carefully, not only to assess the degree of diabetic retinopathy but also to establish a base line on which to judge the progression of hypertensive changes (arteriolar narrowing, sclerosis, and focal spasm) in the event that they occur in preeclampsia. The remainder of the physical examination is directed toward checking the nutritional status (whether the patient is obese, normal in weight, or undernourished), height, blood pressure (both arms), and vascular insufficiency (as indicated by palpation of the radial, popliteal, and posterior tibial pulses). Neurological examination is also carried out, with extra attention being paid to peripheral neuropathy. Finally, sources of focal infection are sought.

The initial laboratory testing includes the determination of fasting and postprandial blood sugars, a complete blood count, urinalysis, and

Clinical work-up

blood urea nitrogen. Albuminuria is of special concern, particularly if it is found on successive examinations and along with hypertension, because this combination plus retinopathy often denotes diabetic glomerulosclerosis. Any evidence of urinary tract infections or previous pyelonephritis should lead the physician to obtain a urine specimen for bacterial culture and susceptibility studies. In order to avoid the introduction of organisms into the bladder, catheterization is not done; instead, the specimen is taken from a cleansed midstream sample. A colony count is carried out to determine quantitatively the degree of bacteriuria. A value of over 100,000 per ml. usually indicates infection. Coliform organisms are more likely than cocci to indicate significant infection.

On the basis of these findings and the classification of White,[21] the risk of pregnancy to the mother may be determined and a general estimate made of the chances of a viable child (Table 34).[22]

Table 34. Classifications of Diabetes in Pregnant Women and Expected Fetal Salvage

CLASS A	CLASS B	CLASS C
By glucose tolerance only 100%	Diabetes onset after 20 years of age Duration less than 10 years No vascular lesions 67%	Onset between 10 and 19 years of age Duration 10 to 19 years No vascular lesions 48%

CLASS D	CLASS E	CLASS F
Diabetes onset before 10 years of age Diabetes over 20 years Retinitis or calcified vessels in legs 32%	Calcified pelvic arteries 13%	Nephropathy 3%

Clinical management

The proper diabetic program is established as follows:

1. Diet. This is established in accordance with the methods indicated in the chapter on "Dietary Treatment." In addition, it is important to recognize that, since ketonuria may have lifelong effects on the conceptus,[23] starvation diets are contraindicated and weight reduction diets rarely used in pregnancy.

2. Antidiabetic therapy. Insulin dosage is adjusted to meet the requirements of the patient. Strict control of the diabetes is mandatory to the delivery of a normal, healthy child.

3. Diuretics. Thiazide diuretics are withheld until they are needed for the treatment of edema and/or hypertension. Their use for such indications more than offsets the diabetogenic effect they may exert.

The pregnant diabetic is usually checked at two-week intervals from the time of the initial visit until the seventh month, and then weekly unless complications occur, e.g., hyperemesis gravidarum, ketoacidosis, or signs of preeclampsia. (If these complications develop, immediate hospitalization is required.) The visits may be alternated between the medical and the obstetric physician; however, regardless of which one the patient sees, fasting and/or postprandial blood sugars should be obtained. In addition, the patient should present an up-to-date record of her urine tests.

If renal glycosuria is severe in the diabetic, weight loss and ketonuria may occur. If these happen, it is important to determine the total glucose lost in a twenty-four-hour period and add this amount to the diet.

WHEN TO HOSPITALIZE

Most medical experts agree that diabetic patients should be hospitalized at about the thirty-fifth week of pregnancy and delivered no later than the thirty-seventh or thirty-eighth week. The purpose of hospitalization is to bring about maximum control of the diabetes and to obtain information essential for ascertaining the correct time and mode of delivery (e.g., the size of the fetus and detection of hydramnios, early manifestations of preeclampsia, or urinary tract infection). When possible, base-line urinary estriol determinations are made.

Hospitalization may be indicated at any time before the thirty-fifth week for the diabetic who has demonstrated a tendency toward preeclampsia, who has vascular complications, or who, for other reasons, has failed to deliver a viable child. Admission to the hospital, of course, may be necessary whenever poor diabetic control occurs during pregnancy.

Time of Delivery

Estimation of the time of delivery must be made by the medical and obstetric physicians, particularly the latter. The hazard of delivery before the optimal time is neonatal death due to prematurity. If delivery is too late (after the thirty-eighth week), there is an increased likelihood of death *in utero*. Of course, in the event of fetal distress (as indicated by a diminishing heart rate, reduced intrauterine movement, diminishing urine estriol levels)[24] or toxemia of pregnancy, there is no alternative to immediate delivery. Kahn *et al.*[25] and Gabbe[2] have reviewed and assessed a number of procedures used in evaluating diabetic pregnancy.

Fetal maturity, formerly evaluated by radiographic technic,[26,27] is now ascertained by ultrasound procedures. However, the suspicion of fetal abnormality may be confirmed by an abdominal film.

Mode of Delivery

Many elements influence the mode of delivery. If the patient has not previously had a cesarean section and there are no nondiabetic obstetric indications for such a procedure, an attempt is made to induce labor with Pitocin® (oxytocin) in order to accomplish vaginal delivery. On the other hand, if the cervix is not soft or if after six to ten hours an induction fails, a cesarean section is carried out.

Diabetic Management during Delivery

There are several methods of management during delivery. Some physicians prefer to transfer the patient to Regular Insulin, which is administered in association with intravenous glucose solutions. Others[28] give one-half to two-thirds of the predelivery intermediate-acting Insulin and

Delivery

follow this with Regular Insulin as needed. When half of the dose is given before delivery, the second half is administered postpartum. Regardless of the method used, great care is given to prevent hypoglycemia in the infant and mother immediately after delivery. Continuous low-dose infusions of Insulin, as recommended by Mintz et al.,[1] are replacing the foregoing methods of Insulin administration in many centers.

CARE OF THE INFANT

At the time of delivery, diabetic mothers, particularly those with growth-onset diabetes, are always attended by a pediatrician. The principal problems of infants of diabetic mothers have been reviewed.[29] A direct relationship has been shown to exist among prematurity, the respiratory distress syndrome, hyperbilirubinemia, and neonatal mortality. Although the severity of maternal diabetes has a great influence on the occurrence of stillbirth, it apparently is unimportant in the prognosis of the live-born infant. The methods of Hubbell and Drorbaugh[29] for delivery room care are outlined in Table 35.

Table 35. Check List for Postnatal Care of Infants of Diabetic Mothers

Delivery Room

1. Presence of a clear airway established.
2. Umbilical cord clamped 3 to 4 cm. from its base.
3. Apgar scores* recorded at one, two, five, and ten minutes after delivery.
4. Infant moved to observation nursery.

Observation Nursery

1. Infant weighed and examined.
2. Placed in Isolet®, with temperature set between 86° and 94°F. and relative humidity at 40 to 60 percent.
3. For first two to three days of life, respiratory rate, degree of effort, color, and activity of infant are recorded every two hours.
4. When oxygen is used, measurement of concentration must be noted.
5. Aqueous colloidal solution of phytonadione given intramuscularly.
6. Anteroposterior and lateral chest x-rays taken as soon as possible.
7. Measurement of blood glucose, hematocrit, and bilirubin.
8. Suctioning of nasopharynx as needed.

---

*Apgar scores[30] are based on a rating of ten points for the best possible condition. Two points each are allowed for respiratory effort, reflex irritability, muscle tone, heart rate, and color.

Subsequent attention is directed toward the complications usually observed in the newborn infants of diabetic mothers. These are listed in Table 36.

MANAGEMENT OF THE MILD, NONKETOTIC DIABETIC

There are two schools of thought regarding the need for vigorous treatment of the mild, nonketotic diabetic whose impaired carbohydrate metabolism is discovered during pregnancy. Some believe that control as effective as that obtained in the growth-onset, Insulin-dependent patient can be

Table 36. Neonatal Complications of Infants of Diabetic Mothers

Respiratory distress
Hyperbilirubinemia
Increased neuromuscular excitability
Apneic spells
Congenital malformations
Hypoglycemia
Sepsis
Combined respiratory and metabolic acidosis[31]

achieved with dietary restriction. On the other hand, others[32,33] have pointed out that there is a reduction in the incidence of large babies when mild diabetes is treated with Insulin. Pedersen[34] has shown a correlation between the level of the maternal blood sugar in the last six to seven weeks of pregnancy and the birth weight of the offspring. Carrington and others[7,35] noted reduced perinatal mortality in the infants of mildly diabetic mothers whose blood glucose was well controlled. Therefore, they recommend the following treatment program for all prenatal patients.

Management of the adult-onset diabetic

1. A two-hour blood sugar determination on the initial examination. If this is borderline, a standard three-hour glucose tolerance test.

2. Glucose tolerance test for all patients with a family history or obstetric record (large babies, preeclampsia, hydramnios) that suggests diabetes.

3. Diabetic diet if glucose tolerance test is abnormal. If diet alone is unsuccessful in reducing two-hour postprandial blood sugars below 150 mg. per 100 ml. (when true blood glucose methods are used), then intermediate-acting Insulin is used. Initial doses of 8 to 10 units of NPH or Lente® Insulin will usually bring the fasting and postprandial blood sugars to acceptable levels without hypoglycemia. (Larger doses may often be required.)

4. In general, obstetric and prenatal care as described for the growth-onset pregnant diabetic.

Sulfonylurea agents have been used in mild, nonketotic diabetics by several investigators.[36-38] Ordinarily, the results in terms of maternal blood sugar control and fetal salvage have been favorable;[38] however, when the dosage of chlorpropamide was 500 mg. daily, only five of nineteen fetuses survived.[39] Most workers believe that until more extensive data are available concerning the effect of these agents on metabolic and developmental patterns in infants, Insulin is the antidiabetic agent of choice in managing even mild diabetics during pregnancy.

BIBLIOGRAPHY

1. Mintz, D. H., Skyler, J. R., and Chez, R. A.: Diabetes Mellitus and Pregnancy, Diabetes Care, *1:*49, 1978.

2. Gabbe, S. G.: Diabetes in Pregnancy: Clinical Controversies, Obstet. Gynecol., *21:*443, 1978.

3. Shlevin, E. L., and Pedowitz, P.: Pregnancy and Diabetes, in Clinical Diabetes Mellitus (edited by M. Ellenberg and H. Rifkin), p. 280. New York: The Blakiston Division, McGraw-Hill Book Company, Inc., 1962.

4. Goodner, C. J.: Newer Concepts in Diabetes Mellitus, Including Management, in Disease-a-Month (edited by H. F. Dowling). Chicago: Year Book Medical Publishers, Inc., September, 1965.

5. White, P.: Pregnancy and Diabetes, Medical Aspects, M. Clin. North America, *49:*1015, 1965.

6. Miller, M., and Black, M. E.: Pregnancy, in Diabetes Mellitus: Diagnosis and Treatment (edited by T. S. Danowski), p. 137. New York: American Diabetes Association, Inc., 1964.

7. Carrington, E. R., and Messick, R. R.: Diabetogenic Effects of Pregnancy. A 10 Year Survey, Am. J. Obst. & Gynec., *85:*669, 1963.

8. Molnar, G. D.: Management of Diabetes Mellitus during Pregnancy, Clin. Obst. & Gynec., *5:*333, 1962.

9. O'Sullivan, J. B.: Gestational Diabetes. Unsuspected Asymptomatic Diabetes in Pregnancy, New England J. Med., *264:*1082, 1961.

10. Spellacy, W. N., and Goetz, F. C.: Plasma Insulin in Normal Late Pregnancy, New England J. Med., *268:*988, 1963.

11. Bleicher, S. J., O'Sullivan, J. B., and Freinkel, N.: Carbohydrate Metabolism in Pregnancy. V. The Interrelations of Glucose, Insulin and Free Fatty Acids in Late Pregnancy and Post Partum, New England J. Med., *271:*866, 1964.

12. Kalkhoff, R., Schalch, D. S., Walker, J. L., Beck, P., Kipnis, D. M., and Daughaday, W. H.: Diabetogenic Factors Associated with Pregnancy, Tr. A. Am. Physicians, *77:*270, 1964.

13. Freinkel, N., and Goodner, C. J.: Insulin Metabolism and Pregnancy, Arch. Int. Med., *109:*235, 1962.

14. Kaplan, S. L., and Grumbach, M. M.: Studies of a Human and Simian Placental Hormone with Growth Hormone-Like and Prolactin-Like Activities, J. Clin. Endocrinol., *24:*80, 1964.

15. Wilkerson, H. L. C., and O'Sullivan, J. B.: A Study of Glucose Tolerance and Screening Criteria in 752 Unselected Pregnancies, Diabetes, *12:*313, 1963.

16. O'Sullivan, J. B., and Mahan, C. M.: Criteria for the Oral Glucose Tolerance Test in Pregnancy, Diabetes, *13:*278, 1964.

17. Flynn, F. V., Harper, C., and DeMayo, P.: Lactosuria and Glycosuria in Pregnancy and the Puerperium, Lancet, *2:*698, 1953.

18. Welsh, G. W., III, and Sims, E. A. H.: The Mechanisms of Renal Glycosuria in Pregnancy, Diabetes, *9:*363, 1960.

19. Christensen, P. J.: Tubular Reabsorption of Glucose during Pregnancy, Scandinav. J. Clin. & Lab. Invest., *10:*364, 1958.

20. Malins, J. M., and FitzGerald, M. G.: Childbearing Prior to Recognition of Diabetes. Recollected Birth Weights and Stillbirth Rate in Babies Born to Parents Who Developed Diabetes, Diabetes, *14:*175, 1965.

21. White, P.: Pregnancy Complicating Diabetes, in The Treatment of Diabetes Mellitus, Ed. 10 (edited by E. P. Joslin, H. F. Root, P. White, and A. Marble), p. 690. Philadelphia: Lea & Febiger, 1959.

22. Crampton, J. H.: Pregnancy in the Diabetic, in Diabetes (edited by R. H. Williams), p. 655. New York: Paul B. Hoeber, Inc., 1960.

23. Churchill, J. A., and Berendes, H. W.: Intelligence of Children Whose Mothers Had Acetonuria during Pregnancy, in Perinatal Factors Affecting Human Development, Scientific Publication No. 185, p. 30. Washington, D.C.: Pan American Health Organization, 1969.

24. Kyle, G. C., Yalcin, S., Green, J. W., Jr., and Smith, K.: Urinary Oestriol Excretion in the Pregnant Diabetic, in On the Nature and Treatment of Diabetes (edited by B. S. Leibel and G. A. Wrenshall), p. 700. New York: Excerpta Medica Foundation, 1965.

25. Kahn, C. B., White, P., and Younger, D.: Laboratory Assessment of Diabetic Pregnancy, Diabetes, *21:*31, 1972.

26. Berman, R.: Obstetric Roentgenology, in Obstetrics, Ed. 13 (edited by J. P. Greenhill), p. 443. Philadelphia: W. B. Saunders Company, 1965.

27. Driscoll, J. J., and Gillespie, L.: Obstetrical Considerations in Diabetes in Pregnancy, M. Clin. North America, *49:*1025, 1965.

28. Pedersen, J., Osler, M., and Brandstrup, E.: Caesarian Section in Diabetics, Acta obst. et gynec. scandinav., *38:*631, 1959.

29. Hubbell, J. P., Jr., and Drorbaugh, J. E.: Infants of Diabetic Mothers. Neonatal Problems and Their Management, Diabetes, *14:*157, 1965.

30. Apgar, V.: A Proposal for a New Method of Evaluation of the Newborn Infant, Anesth. & Analg., *32:*260, 1953.

31. Reardon, H. S., Field, S., Vega, L., Carrington, E., Arey, J., and Baumann, M. L.: Treatment of Acute Respiratory Distress in Newborn Infants of Diabetic and "Prediabetic" Mothers, A. M. A. J. Dis. Child., *94:*558, 1957.

32. Wilkerson, H. L. C.: Pregnancy and the Prediabetic State, Ann. New York Acad. Sc., *82:*219, 1959.

33. Wilkerson, H. L. C., and Remein, Q. R.: Studies of Abnormal Carbohydrate Metabolism in Pregnancy. The Significance of Impaired Glucose Tolerance, Diabetes, *6:*324, 1957.

34. Pedersen, J.: Weight and Length at Birth of Infants of Diabetic Mothers, Acta endocrinol., *16:*330, 1954.

35. Carrington, E. R., Shuman, C. R., and Reardon, H. S.: Evaluation of the Prediabetic State during Pregnancy, Obst. & Gynec., *9:*664, 1957.

36. Dolger, H., Bookman, J. J., and Joelson, R. H.: Diabetes Mellitus. I. The Pregnant Diabetic and Prediabetic, in Medical, Surgical, and Gynecological Complications of Pregnancy (edited by A. F. Guttmacher and J. J. Rovinsky), p. 457. Baltimore: The Williams & Wilkins Company, 1960.

37. Dolger, H., Bookman, J. J., and Nechemias, C.: The Diagnostic and Therapeutic Value of Tolbutamide in Pregnant Diabetics, Diabetes, *11* (Supplement):97, 1962.

38. Jackson, W. P. U., Campbell, G. D., Notelovitz, M., and Blumsohn, D.: Tolbutamide and Chlorpropamide during Pregnancy in Human Diabetics, Diabetes, *11* (Supplement):98, 1962.

39. Campbell, G. D.: Chlorpropamide and Foetal Damage, Brit. M. J., *1:*59, 1963.

Surgery in Diabetic Patients

12

A surgical operation is one of the most formidable stresses diabetic patients may face. Even well-controlled, relatively mild diabetes may be thrown out of control by the multiple strains of anesthesia, surgical trauma, fluid and nutritional imbalance, and altered physical activity. Because diabetic patients approach surgery in such a variety of clinical states and because of the nature of the particular operation, no standard procedure for regulating all diabetics is possible. The following general principles should be of value to the clinician in meeting this challenge. Each patient must be considered as an individual problem in the application of these principles.

PREOPERATIVE CONSIDERATIONS

INITIAL EVALUATION

Preoperative evaluation of the diabetic patient must include a thorough history and physical examination. Some of the laboratory procedures performed routinely are a complete blood count, urinalysis, blood sugar, blood urea nitrogen, electrocardiogram, and chest x-ray. It is important to remember that there is a significant incidence of abnormalities in the results of these examinations in diabetics (Figure 31).[1,2] Admission of a "nondiabetic" to the hospital for surgery frequently reveals the presence of diabetes; the stress of surgery (or even the anticipation of it) often has a diabetogenic effect. In fact, more than 20 percent of a large group of patients were found to be diabetic only on the occasion of their admission to surgery.[1,2] Table 37 shows that in 70 percent of these individuals, their histories or physical examinations suggested the possibility of diabetes.

Admission laboratory tests

Figure 31. Incidence of Abnormalities Revealed by Examination of 487 Surgical Patients

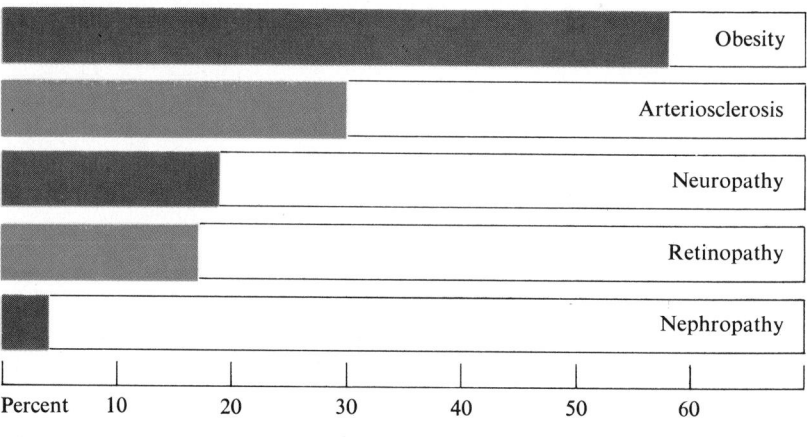

Obesity

Arteriosclerosis

Neuropathy

Retinopathy

Nephropathy

Percent   10   20   30   40   50   60

Table 37. Findings Associated with Diabetes Detection in 100 of 487 Surgical Patients Discovered to Be Diabetic on the Occasion of Their Admission to Surgery

FINDINGS	NUMBER OF PATIENTS
Found in initial survey of patients	47
Carcinoma of the pancreas	3
Pancreatitis	4
Diabetic retinopathy	7
Significant lower-extremity disease	8
Polyneuropathy	7
Infection (carbuncle or abscess, genito-urinary tract)	14
"Female, fat and over forty," with gall-bladder disease	4
Found in review of remaining fifty-three charts	23
History of polydipsia, polyphagia, and polyuria	10
Family history of diabetes	13
No history or physical findings to suggest diabetes mellitus	30
Total	100

PREMEDICATION AND ANESTHESIA

Agents selected for premedication and anesthesia of the diabetic patient are the same as those for the nondiabetic, with two exceptions. First, because of the hazards of nausea, special measures should be taken to avoid this side-effect. Therefore, the dosage of meperidine, morphine, and other preanesthetic drugs is generally only 50 to 75 percent of that given to nondiabetic subjects. Second, agents (e.g., ether) which have potent glycogenolytic effects can upset diabetic control and should be avoided if possible. During the operation, the anesthesiologist must take special care to prevent acidosis[3] that may occur because of carbon-dioxide retention, hypoxia, or direct effect of the anesthetic agent, since acidosis may lead to inhibition of Insulin effect[4] and result in loss of metabolic control.

PRINCIPLES OF MANAGEMENT DURING SURGERY

The selection of management of the diabetic patient during surgery requires the consideration of many factors, the most important of which are (1) whether the surgery is emergency or elective, (2) whether the surgery is major or minor, (3) the severity of the diabetes, and (4) the presence of complications of diabetic and/or nondiabetic disease. Clinicians differ in their methods of meeting the various combinations of these factors; however, all share the goal of maintaining the patient as free as possible from acetonuria and hypoglycemia. When these goals are achieved, acceptable blood and urine glucose levels usually are obtained also. As a result, predisposition to infection is reduced to a minimum, and glycogenolysis, which diverts protein from its necessary function of tissue regeneration, is averted.

Emergency surgery

Emergency surgery is more common in diabetics than in nondiabetics, probably because of their greater susceptibility to infection. In one study,[1] for example, 80 percent of the operations on diabetics were for infection, with appendectomy as the most common major surgical procedure. Management of diabetic patients undergoing emergency surgery requires especially close co-operation between the medical and surgical physicians. The timing of surgical intervention varies greatly from one situation to another and has a critical bearing on the ultimate result obtained.

Ordinarily, an attempt is made for a period of two to four hours to improve the metabolic control and to hydrate the patient. However, in some instances of sepsis (e.g., abscess formation), delay in operating merely increases the risk to the patient. Insulin resistance and the metabolic decompensation associated with infection will respond only after the source of infection has been treated properly with antibiotics, incision and drainage, or excision.

Major and minor surgery

The designation "major" or "minor" surgery denotes the over-all stress associated with the surgical procedure. The total stress is the sum of such factors as the length of the operation and the type of anesthesia used, the amount of physical trauma in the manipulation of organs and the incision and suturing of tissue, and the patient's psychological reaction. These elements will be reflected in the blood sugar and corticosteroid levels following the operation and are the principal determinants of the amount of Insulin the patient will require during the day of surgery and for several days thereafter. The greatest disturbance in metabolic control probably occurs after major procedures of several hours' duration, such as subtotal gastrectomy, radical mastectomy, thoracotomy, and abdominal perineal resections. Metabolic control is likely to be less deranged during minor procedures, such as dilatation and curettage, cataract removal, and tooth extractions.

The severity of diabetes is usually judged by the patient's treatment and response before surgery. In this context, those who are controlled by diet alone or diet and oral hypoglycemic agents may be considered mild diabetics. These patients are usually able to withstand the stress of

Table 38. Recommended Methods for Treating Diabetes of Different Intensity

CLINICAL SITUATION	TYPE OF PROCEDURE	SPECIFIC METHOD OF MANAGEMENT
For elective and emergency surgery in mild diabetes if infection is not present	Minor	A. Dietary carbohydrate is administered intravenously as 5 and/or 10 percent dextrose in water. Usually, no Insulin or sulfonylurea therapy is needed.*
	Major	B. Same as "A" but 0.16 to 0.2 unit of Regular Insulin per Gm. of glucose[1] is administered with the intravenous infusions.† That is, to a liter of 5 percent dextrose in water containing 50 Gm. of glucose, 8 to 10 units of Regular Insulin would be added. For a liter of 10 percent dextrose solution, 16 to 20 units of Regular Insulin would be used.*
For elective and emergency surgery in moderate diabetes if infection is not present	Minor Major	C. Carbohydrate allowed in preoperative diet is given as 5 and/or 10 percent dextrose in water. Usual preoperative dose of intermediate-acting Insulin (NPH or Lente®) is administered subcutaneously after infusion has been started. Details of this method are listed in Table 39.*
For elective and emergency surgery in severe diabetes and in mild and moderate diabetes when emergency surgery is associated with sepsis	Minor Major	D. Insulin, fluids, and electrolytes are prescribed according to the assessed metabolic situation (urinary glucose, acetone, CO_2, and blood sugar being used as parameters) every one to six hours until the diabetes is stable. The patient's daily carbohydrate requirement is estimated and administered as 5 and/or 10 percent dextrose in water or appropriate electrolyte solutions infused over a six-hour period. After each six-hour infusion has been started, Regular Insulin is given subcutaneously.

*If moderate or strong acetone occurs, additional glucose and Regular Insulin are needed.

†Some workers[6] condemn the use of Regular Insulin in the intravenous infusions because of the alleged tendency for Insulin (since it is heavier than water) to settle to the bottom of the flask and be infused ahead of the glucose instead of as a homogeneous solution with the glucose. Experience[1] has not confirmed that Insulin in intravenous solutions is hazardous. The homeostatic mechanisms of the patient and the tendency for the infusion equipment to adsorb some Insulin[14] are protective factors against hypoglycemia when Insulin is added to the intravenous glucose infusions. (See also review by Galloway and Bressler.[15])

most elective surgical procedures with little or no change in blood sugar. When glycosuria and hyperglycemia occur, Regular Insulin is usually preferred over sulfonylurea treatment.

Moderate diabetics are those who are satisfactorily controlled with one or two daily doses of intermediate-acting Insulin either alone or in combination with short-acting Insulin. Severe diabetics are patients whose control is seldom satisfactory even with two or more doses of Insulin per day. These are labile, brittle diabetics, described in the chapter on "Clinical Use of Insulin."

Management of the Insulin-dependent patient of the moderate type during surgery is subject to great variation. Some workers[5-9] divide the

Table 39. Outline of Management of Moderately Severe Diabetic with Intermediate-Acting (NPH or Lente®) Insulin during Elective Surgery

Fluids, Electrolytes, and Nutrition*

1. Preoperative dietary carbohydrate is replaced with 5 and/or 10 percent dextrose in water. Usually, no allowance is made for the fat and protein in the preoperative diet because these ordinarily can be made up from endogenous stores during the period of surgery. However, some clinicians supply an additional 40 to 60 Gm. of carbohydrate to provide the glucose equivalent of protein in the preoperative diet.

2. Fluids and electrolytes are administered according to the needs and limitations of the patient. Volumes should be restricted in patients having prostatectomy, heart disease, or oliguria and increased if dehydration is present. Potassium salts are added if parenteral fluids are required for more than forty-eight hours. Saline solution is used only if there are extrarenal losses (e.g., nasogastric suction).

3. If parenteral feedings extend over seventy-two hours, the caloric value of the infusion is increased 50 to 100 percent by the use of 10 percent dextrose solutions plus protein hydrolysate or amino acid solutions.

Insulin

1. Intermediate-acting Insulin is given in the usual preoperative dose when administration of glucose is begun. If possible, the operation is scheduled for the first part of the morning.

2. Urine is tested for glucose every four to six hours after the operation. Three to 6 units of Regular Insulin are administered for each "plus" if the copper-reduction methods are used.

3. Blood sugar levels are determined daily before fluids and Insulin are given—more frequently if hypoglycemia is suspected.

4. On the mornings of the first and second (and occasionally third and fourth) postoperative days, intermediate-acting Insulin is given in an amount based on the sum of intermediate-acting Insulin plus two-thirds of the supplemental Regular Insulin doses the day before.

5. Anticipate reduction of the daily Insulin dose three to four days after surgery as the stress of surgery wanes.

*Most workers administer a minimum of one ampoule of a parenteral vitamin supplement each day in the intravenous fluids.

preoperative prescription for Insulin and carbohydrate into four to six equal feedings to be given over a twenty-four-hour period. Others[10,11] give one-half the usual dose of intermediate-acting Insulin on the day of surgery and the remainder as Regular Insulin according to blood and fractional urine sugars throughout the day. Moore[12] withholds Insulin until the operation has been completed and then uses Regular Insulin. Fletcher *et al.*[13] also feel that no preoperative Insulin administration is required. Suitable methods for managing the various types of diabetes are outlined in Table 38. There is extensive published information on one method in which the usual dose of intermediate-acting Insulin is given the day of surgery. The details are reviewed in Table 39.

POSTOPERATIVE CONSIDERATIONS

In the postoperative period, a reduction in Insulin dosage must be anticipated as the stress of surgery wanes, particularly if the source of infection has been removed, such as a chronically infected gall bladder. The high incidence of infection and coronary artery disease in diabetics should keep the physician constantly aware of the possibility of myocardial infarction, genito-urinary tract infection, thrombophlebitis, and other septic complications until recovery is completed. As in the nondiabetic subject, protein must be provided liberally as soon as the patient is able to tolerate oral feedings. If the patient is not able to take nourishment by mouth after the second or third day, the protein must then be supplied as 5 percent amino acid or protein hydrolysate solutions.

Regardless of the severity of the diabetes, patients having minor elective surgery ordinarily can resume their preoperative diet and antidiabetic programs within a day or two. Depending upon the nature and stress of the major elective surgery, patients can usually be returned to their preoperative management programs within four to seven days. After both types of elective surgery, the effects of dietary standardization which occur in the hospital setting must be considered in prescribing Insulin or an oral hypoglycemic agent. Occasionally, a 25 to 50 percent reduction in the daily dose can be accomplished. Because of the many factors which influence the recovery of patients from emergency surgery, no rule can be applied for the rapidity with which preoperative treatment programs can be resumed.

BIBLIOGRAPHY

1. Galloway, J. A., and Shuman, C. R.: Diabetes and Surgery. A Study of 667 Cases, Am. J. Med., *34:*177, 1963.

2. Galloway, J. A., and Shuman, C. R.: Profile, Specific Methods of Management, and Response of Diabetic Patients to Anesthesia and Surgery, Internat. Anesth. Clin., *5:*437, 1967.

3. Brown, S.: Anesthetic Management of the Surgical Diabetic Patient, Missouri Med., *60:*233, 1963.

4. Walker, B. G., Phear, D. N., Martin, F. I. R., and Baird, C. W.: Inhibition of Insulin by Acidosis, Lancet, *2:*964, 1963.

5. Bortz, W. M., II, and Bortz, E. L.: Surgery of the Diabetic Patient. Changing Concepts, Am. J. Clin. Nutrition, *3:*494, 1955.

6. Ralli, E. P., and Standard, S.: The Case of the Surgical Diabetic. A Report of Two Hundred and Two Cases, Surg. Gynec. & Obst., *58:*228, 1934.

7. Duncan, G. G.: Diabetes Mellitus, Principles and Treatment, p. 221. Philadelphia: W. B. Saunders Company, 1951.

8. Duncan, G. G.: Diseases of Metabolism, Ed. 4, p. 897. Philadelphia: W. B. Saunders Company, 1959.

9. Izzo, J. L.: Treatment of the Diabetic Undergoing Surgery, Mod. Treat., *2:*681, 1965.

10. Wheelock, F. C., Jr., and Root, H. F.: Surgery and Diabetes, in Treatment of Diabetes Mellitus, Ed. 10 (edited by E. P. Joslin, H. F. Root, P. White, and A. Marble), p. 595. Philadelphia: Lea & Febiger, 1959.

11. Forsham, P. H.: Management of Diabetes during Stress and Surgery, in Diabetes (edited by R. H. Williams), p. 511. New York: Paul B. Hoeber, Inc., 1960.

12. Moore, F. D.: The Metabolic Care of the Surgical Patient, p. 643. Philadelphia: W. B. Saunders Company, 1959.

13. Fletcher, J., Langman, M. J. S., and Kellock, T. D.: Effect of Surgery on Blood-Sugar Levels in Diabetes Mellitus, Lancet, *2:*52, 1965.

14. Bay, J., and Hallund, O.: Glukose-insulin drop. Undersøgelse over insulins adhaesion til infusionsmateriel, Nord. med., *74:*841, 1964.

15. Galloway, J. A., and Bressler, R.: Insulin Treatment in Diabetes, Med. Clin. North Am., *62:*663, 1978.

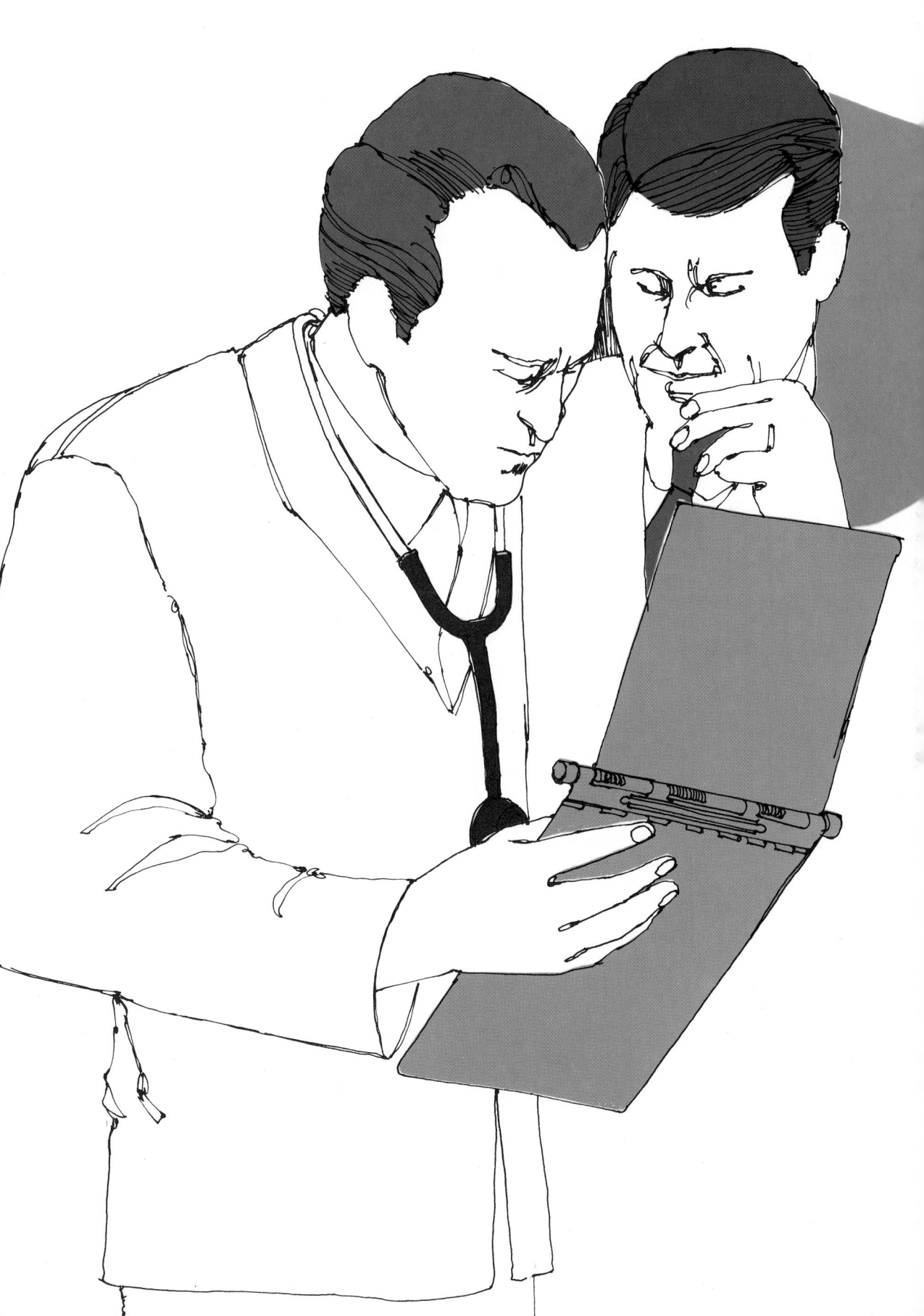

Diabetic Acidosis and Coma

13

The most common cause of ketoacidosis and coma in the diabetic patient is the complex derangement of glucose metabolism resulting from a critical reduction in insulin activity. With the general advancement of medical knowledge, however, there has been an increased recognition of several other causes. These include lactic acid acidosis and nonketotic hyperosmolar coma. The high incidence of diabetes adds to the likelihood of its coexistence with other disorders that may result in the development of metabolic acidosis or lead to coma. These are listed in Table 40.[1]

Diabetic acidosis and coma are the most important of the acute complications of diabetes. The abnormal biochemical changes associated with insulin deficiencies leading to acidosis have been presented in Chapter 3. The clinical picture is related to the sequelae of insulin deficiency, namely, mobilization of fatty acids, accumulation of ketone bodies, hyperglycemia, impaired cellular uptake of glucose, and deficits in body water and electrolytes. These abnormalities result in nausea, vomiting, abdominal pain, dehydration, circulatory insufficiency, and clouding of consciousness leading to coma and eventually, if untreated, to death. Other findings in ketoacidosis are listed in Table 41.

Lactic acidosis and ketoacidosis may coexist. When this occurs, the nitroprusside test may markedly underestimate the quantities of ketone bodies present.[1A]

The total problem of ketoacidosis and its treatment has been reviewed by many authors.[1-9] The method outlined below, based on programs suggested by Shuman[9] and Bradley,[1] is only one of many which are satisfactory and has been chosen because of the author's personal experience with it.

TREATMENT PROTOCOL

Proper treatment is best conducted with a program based on a standardized protocol, because ketoacidosis is an emergency situation. Furthermore, since its occurrence is relatively infrequent, physicians ordinarily are not able to keep up on the essential details of a correct program. In addition, it is important that one individual physician be assigned to the patient from the time of his admission to the hospital until metabolic control is established. This practice obviates the loss of continuity in treatment—an essential aspect in the successful management of diabetic coma.[10]

FIRST HOUR AFTER ADMISSION

Immediately upon suspicion of ketoacidosis and coma, the patient's urine and blood should be examined.

Table 40. Differential Diagnosis of Altered Consciousness and Acidosis in the Diabetic

	URINE SUGAR	URINE KETONES AND DIACETIC ACID	BLOOD SUGAR	BLOOD CO_2	PLASMA OR SERUM ACETONE
Diabetic coma	++++*	++++*	High	Low	++++ in at least the undiluted specimen
Hyperglycemic coma†	++++	0	High	Normal or slightly low	0 or minimal
Hypoglycemia	0 or +‡	0 or +‡	Low	Normal	0 or minimal
Lowered seizure threshold	0 or +	0	Low, normal, or high	Normal	0 or +
Cerebrovascular accident	0 or +	0	Often high	Normal	0
Uremia	0 or +	0	High or low	Decreased	0 or +§
Lactic acid acidosis	0 or +	0	High or low	Decreased	0 or +§
Other causes of anion gap, such as salicylate intoxication	0 or +	0	High or low	Decreased	0 or +§

*May be absent in markedly oliguric patients.
†Usually in older patients. Often associated with hypernatremia and hyperosmolarity.
‡Urine present in bladder for a number of hours may contain sugar as a result of earlier hyperglycemia. In addition, ketones (but usually *not* diacetic acid) may be present.
§Positive results may be found in association with uncontrolled diabetes but not of the degree found with ketoacidosis.

Urine

So that a urine specimen may be obtained, an indwelling catheter is inserted for the convenience of collecting serial specimens. The initial sample is checked for acetone, diacetic acid, and glucose. An aliquot from this initial sample is sent to the laboratory for an immediate analysis for albumin and microscopic examination as well as for bacterial culture and antibiotic susceptibility tests.

Blood

Specimens of both clotted and unclotted blood are collected. An aliquot from the clotted blood sample is taken for determination of plasma ketone content, which will be markedly elevated in diabetic coma. When this specimen contains acetone, treatment is instituted promptly without a waiting period for the results of further blood studies. Unclotted blood is sent to the laboratory for glucose, carbon dioxide, sodium, chloride, and potassium determinations.

Additional blood tests should include a complete blood count and hematocrit, serum amylase (elevation may indicate the presence of acute pancreatitis), and enzyme studies (lactic acid dehydrogenase and/or SGOT) to detect acute myocardial infarction. If, on the other hand, a diabetic is admitted in a comatose state and *hypo*glycemia is suspected, it may be ruled out by the intravenous administration of 1 mg. of glucagon or 50

Examination of the blood

Table 41. Differential Diagnosis of Diabetic Coma and Hypoglycemic Reactions

| | DIABETIC COMA | HYPOGLYCEMIC REACTIONS | |
		REGULAR INSULIN	MODIFIED INSULIN OR ORAL AGENTS
Clinical Features			
Onset	Slow—days	Sudden—minutes	Gradual—hours
Causes	Ignorance Neglect of therapy Intercurrent disease or infection	Overdosage Omission or delay of meals Excessive exercise before meals	
Symptoms	Thirst Headache Nausea Vomiting Abdominal pain Dim vision Constipation Dyspnea	"Inward nervousness" Hunger Sweating	Fatigue Headache Nausea Sweating (sometimes absent) Dizziness
		Weakness Diplopia Blurred vision Paresthesia Psychopathic behavior Stupor Convulsions	
Signs	Florid face Air hunger (Kussmaul's respiration) Finally, respiratory paralysis	Pallor Shallow respiration	
	Dehydration (dry skin) Rapid pulse Soft eyeballs Normal or absent reflexes Acetone breath	Sweating Normal pulse Eyeballs normal Babinski's reflex often present	Skin may be dry Pulse not characteristic
Chemical Features			
Urine Glucose...............	Positive	Usually absent, especially in second voided specimen	
Acetone................	Positive	Negative	
Diacetic acid............	Positive	Negative	
Blood Glucose...............	> 250 mg./100 ml. ordinarily	60 mg. or less/100 ml.	
CO_2 combining power	<20 volumes/100 ml.	Usually normal	
Leukocytosis............	Present; may be very high		
Response to treatment	Slow	Rapid; occasionally delayed	May be delayed

ml. of 50 percent dextrose. This procedure will not harm the patient with ketoacidosis. The differential diagnosis of the two conditions is listed in Table 41.

If the patient is in vascular shock, measures must be taken to correct it. A history and physical examination are carried out within the limits imposed by the patient's condition. Of particular importance is the necessity for establishing the cause of the coma. The most frequent possibilities are listed in Table 42.

Table 42. Factors and Diseases Responsible for or Associated with the Development of Ketoacidosis and Coma

Undiagnosed or untreated diabetes

Failure to take Insulin and/or food because of the nausea and vomiting of gastroenteritis or because of emotional disturbances

Acute myocardial infarction

Infection (bacterial or viral), such as pneumonia, abscess (furunculosis), cholecystitis, pancreatitis, appendicitis, cystitis, and pyelonephritis

Treatment with steroids or thiazide diuretics

Thrombophlebitis

Hyperthyroidism

The factors to be noted particularly in the physical examination are the state of consciousness of the patient, deep-tendon reflexes, type of respiration, pulse rate, blood pressure, rectal temperature, tonicity of the eyeballs, hydration of the tongue and skin, and the presence of gastric dilatation and possible sources of infection.

EARLY MANAGEMENT

Insulin

Regular Insulin is used exclusively in the treatment of ketoacidosis. The initial Insulin dose ranges from 10 to 200 units, depending upon the severity of the coma and the age and size of the patient. In most instances, the total initial dose is administered intramuscularly in two injection sites. In the presence of shock or in a severely ill patient, half or all of the Insulin may be given intravenously. Adults in coma usually receive 80 to 100 units.

For patients with early ketoacidosis and children over the age of ten, the initial dose of Insulin is in the range of 25 to 50 units. When the blood sugar exceeds 600 mg. per 100 ml., this Insulin dose is doubled. In the rare case of a blood sugar higher than 1,000 mg. per 100 ml., four times the initial values are used. The initial Insulin dosage schedules are summarized in Table 43. Recently, the use of low-dose regimens has become widespread. Methods that have been found successful are those of Fisher *et al.*[10A] (0.33 unit/Kg. intravenous bolus followed by 7 units per hour intramuscularly or subcutaneously) and of Piters *et al.*[10B] (10 units per hour by continuous intravenous infusion). However, if definite metabolic improvement is not seen in four hours, the use of larger (conventional) doses of Insulin intravenously must be considered.

Table 43. Recommended Initial Insulin Doses (Units) for Ketoacidosis

	BLOOD SUGAR RANGE		
TYPE OF PATIENT	LESS THAN 600 MG. PER 100 ML.	600-1,000 MG. PER 100 ML.	1,000 MG. OR MORE PER 100 ML.
Adults in coma	80-100	160-200	320-400
Adults not in coma or children over 10 years old	25-50	50-100	100-200
Children 10 years or less	10-20	20-40	40-80

An alternate method[11] relies on the plasma acetone levels as determined by nitroprusside tablets.* The nitroprusside test measures chiefly, if not exclusively, acetoacetate.[11A] However, the principal source of hydrogen ion and the cause of the acidosis is β-hydroxybutyric acid. Thus, patients in severe diabetic ketoacidosis, with an arterial pH of less than 7.2 and a plasma bicarbonate of less than 9 mEq. per liter, can have small as well as moderate and large nitroprusside reactions. Insulin dosages based on the nitroprusside method are shown in Table 44.[6]

Table 44. Recommended Insulin Doses Based on Serum or Plasma Acetone Test in the Early Phases of Treatment of Ketoacidosis

	UNITS OF REGULAR INSULIN			
IF SERUM OR PLASMA ACETONE IS 4+	ADULTS OR FULLY GROWN ADOLESCENTS	CHILDREN OR ADOLESCENTS NOT FULLY GROWN	CHILDREN 10 YEARS OR LESS	INFANTS
Undiluted specimen	100	50	25	10
1:2 dilution	200	100	50	20
1:4 dilution	300	150	75	30
1:8 dilution	400	200	100	40

Fluids and Electrolytes

There is a diversity of medical opinion regarding what alkalinizing solutions should be used to counteract the acidosis. Except for the most severe cases (arterial pH <7.1 and CO_2 < 8 mEq. per liter), in which bicarbonate therapy is considered,† most workers prefer isotonic saline solution for initiating therapy. One liter should be infused rapidly (i.e., during the first one to one and one-half hours of treatment). In diabetic patients with heart failure, 0.45 percent (half-normal) saline should be used and infused at a somewhat slower rate. In children, the volume of the initial infusion

*The details of this method are as follows: 4 ml. of unclotted blood are centrifuged to yield clear plasma. Dilutions of 1:1, 1:4, and 1:8 are prepared with normal saline or tap water. Three drops of the undiluted plasma and three drops of each of the three dilutions are placed on separate nitroprusside tablets. At the end of sixty seconds, the color is read; the depth of the purple color which develops indicates the concentration of acetone. Unclotted blood containing no anticoagulant may be used. In this case, if coagulation occurs during exposure to the tablet, the blood is merely peeled from the tablet, and the change in color of the tablet's surface is used as an index of ketone formation.

†With bicarbonate therapy, the sensorium of the patient may worsen, a phenomenon attributed to higher hydrogen-ion concentration in the cerebrospinal fluid that results from the more rapid transfer of carbon dioxide than of bicarbonate to the spinal fluid.[12,13]

is 20 ml. per Kg., and the solution of choice is Ringer's lactate.[14] The various solutions that may be used are indicated in Table 45.[7]

Additional Measures

1. In the presence of shock, plasma expanders (such as whole blood, plasma, or dextran) are indicated. Because these agents may need to be administered at a rapid rate, separate infusions may be required. Levophed® (levarterenol bitartrate) may be administered if the peripheral vascular collapse has not responded to other measures.

2. Gastric lavage is performed if the patient is vomiting. For gastric distention, a solution of sodium bicarbonate (approximately 3 percent) may be used. This may be prepared by adding a heaping teaspoonful of sodium

Table 45. Repair Solutions and Additives for Treatment of Diabetic Acidosis

	ELECTROLYTE CONCENTRATION (APPROXIMATE) (MEQ./LITER)	
Repair Solutions	**Each Ion**	**Total**
Glucose: 5, 10, 20, 50%	0	
Isotonic saline (0.9%)	154	
2.5% glucose in 0.45% saline	77	
$\frac{M}{6}$ sodium lactate	167	

Saline-bicarbonate mixture
  Isotonic saline (650 ml.)
  7.5% sodium bicarbonate (50 ml.)
  Distilled water (300 ml.)
		$\begin{cases} 145 \ Na^+ \\ 100 \ Cl^- \\ 45 \ HCO_3^- \end{cases}$

Ringer's lactate
  Sodium chloride
  Sodium lactate
  Potassium chloride
  Calcium chloride
	103
	25
	4
	3.6
		$\begin{cases} 128 \ Na^+ \\ 4 \ K^+ \\ 3.6 \ Ca^{++} \\ 110.6 \ Cl^- \\ 25 \ HCO_3^- \end{cases}$

Commonly Used Additives	**Ampoule Size (ml.)**	**Usual Available Forms and Ionic Content (mEq./Ampoule)**
$NaHCO_3$	50	45 Na^+, 45 HCO_3^-
Potassium chloride	20	40 K^+, 40 Cl^-

Potassium phosphate/
  potassium acid phosphate
	50	Buffered solution
		50 mEq. of K^+ and
		  50 mEq. of PO_4^-

Magnesium sulfate	20	16.2 Mg^{++}, 16.2 SO_4^-
Calcium chloride	10	9 Ca^{++}, 18 Cl^-
Calcium gluconate	10	2.2 Ca^{++}, 4.5 gluconate

These additives permit preparation of any desired electrolyte-containing fluid when used in conjunction with the above repair solutions. Before any additives are used, the manufacturer's directions supplied with each ampoule should be read and followed precisely.

bicarbonate to a pint of water; 250 ml., or 8 ounces (half a pint), of the lavage solution are left in the stomach.

3. In the presence of abdominal distention, a saline enema may be useful. Any fecal impactions should be removed.

4. Cultures of the nasal pharynx, sputum, and blood are obtained when indicated.

5. Most clinicians give penicillin and/or a broad-spectrum antibiotic every eight hours to combat infection or for prophylaxis, but these are withheld in the presence of shock unless obvious infection is present.

6. An hourly record is started for intake and output of fluids and fractional urine determinations for glucose and ketone bodies. These findings may be recorded on special charts which are available for this purpose.

SECOND TO SIXTH HOURS

Insulin

After the initial dose, Insulin is given every one to two hours according to urine sugar and acetone levels (Table 46). In adults, after one to three doses of Insulin, reduction in urine glucose and acetone content usually will permit the administration of 5 units of Regular Insulin for each "plus" of urine glucose.

In the rare event that there is no response, the Insulin dosage should be increased to 80 to 100 units per hour. Doses twice those in Table 46 may be used. If the situation appears critical and no improvement is observed in the urinary or plasma acetone and in blood sugar after four to six doses (i.e., after four to six hours), the dose may be increased to 160 to 200 units per hour.

Table 46. Recommended Regular Insulin Doses (after Initial Dose) for First Twenty-Four Hours of Treatment*—Based on Concentration of Sugar and Acetone in the Urine

	URINE ACETONE							
	STRONGLY POSITIVE†				MODERATELY POSITIVE†			
Adults								
Urine sugar‡	1+	2+	3+	4+	1+	2+	3+	4+
Regular Insulin (units)	10	20	30	40	5	10	15	20
Children								
Urine sugar‡	1+	2+	3+	4+	1+	2+	3+	4+
Regular Insulin (units)	5	10	15	20	0	0	5	10

*Frequently, clinical improvement occurs while acetonuria remains strongly positive. Reduction in Insulin dosage must be based on clinical factors as well as on acetone concentration in the urine.
†Nitroprusside test
‡Copper-reduction methods

Fluids and Electrolytes

Several types of electrolyte solutions may be used to correct the fluid and electrolyte deficits and imbalances that occur in ketoacidosis. The first liter of fluid (isotonic saline) should be infused during the first one to one and one-half hours of treatment; the second is then infused over two and one-half to three hours.

Sodium lactate and bicarbonate can also be used. Solutions of this type are indicated especially in the presence of persistent hyperventilation, extreme acidosis, or low carbon-dioxide content ($<$ 8 mEq. per liter). The approximate fluid and electrolyte deficits seen in diabetic acidosis are indicated in Table 47.[3] After initial treatment with the electrolyte solutions and oral feedings, the use of 5 percent dextrose solution will generally correct water deficits.

Table 47. Fluid and Electrolyte Losses Associated with Ketoacidosis and Coma*

	UNITS PER KG. OF BODY WEIGHT		
	MEAN	RANGE	APPROXIMATE MEAN AMOUNTS FOR A 70-KG. PATIENT
Water	85 ml.	70-100 ml.	6,000 ml.
Na^+	7 mEq.	5.1-13.3 mEq.	500 mEq.
Cl^-	4.5 mEq.	2.5-9.5 mEq.	300 mEq.
K^+	5.5 mEq.	3.9-6.1 mEq.	385 mEq.

*Mg^{++} and PO_4^- losses also occur. Although the necessity for replacing Mg^{++} has not been established, the need for giving PO_4 is being recognized.[15] The potassium salt of phosphate is used as a buffered solution of KH_2PO_4 and K_2HPO_4, available in ampoules containing 50 mEq. of K^+. For instance, after initial K^+ replacement with 50 mEq. of KCl, two 50-mEq. ampoules of KH_2PO_4/K_2HPO_4 are administered. This procedure usually results in replacement of about half the potassium loss in ketoacidosis.

During this second phase of treatment, an assessment is made of total fluid intake in order to anticipate the total requirement for twenty-four hours and to adjust the rate of infusion. So that pulmonary edema may be avoided, the total fluid intake for twenty-four hours should not exceed 5,000 ml. If, after the administration of 3,000 ml., the urinary output exceeds 40 ml. per hour, serious dehydration has been corrected. Ordinarily, an attempt should be made within the first twenty-four hours to replace approximately 50 to 80 percent of the water, sodium, and chloride losses.

If the urinary output, however, is less than 20 ml. per hour and is associated with hypochloremia (serum chloride below 80 mEq. per liter), 50 ml. of 10 percent salt solution should be administered intravenously. If oliguria or anuria is found along with hyperchloremia (serum chloride over 110 mEq. per liter), saline should be discontinued and fluid therapy limited to glucose solutions only. In the presence of anuria, the total volume of fluids may need to be limited to 1,000 ml. in twenty-four hours.

Because infusion of glucose early in the treatment of ketoacidosis merely produces further elevations of the blood sugar and increases the osmolarity of the already hyperosmolar blood, such solutions are not recommended until there is evidence of Insulin response and reduction in the blood sugar level. However, after a period of four to six hours (when the blood sugar is in the range of 300 mg. or less per 100 ml.), a solution of 5 percent dextrose in saline or water is used.

After four to five hours of treatment, careful attention must be given to the restoration of potassium, which is lost from the cells in great quantities during ketoacidosis. The physical signs of potassium deficit may include muscle flaccidity, weakness, rapid and shallow respirations (which will replace Kussmaul's breathing), areflexia, and quadriplegia.

An electrocardiogram may be helpful in detecting low potassium levels. Although a normal tracing does not exclude potassium deficiency, serum potassium levels below 3 mEq. per liter are frequently associated with the following:

1. Lowered or inverted T waves
2. Depressed S-T segments
3. Lengthened Q-T and/or appearance of U wave
4. Prolonged P-R interval

The patient who is alert and can take food by mouth may be given beef broth, cola beverage, skim milk, or orange, tomato, or grapefruit juice, all of which have a high potassium content.

If the patient cannot tolerate potassium by mouth and the urinary output is adequate (50 ml. or more per hour), potassium should be added to the intravenous infusions. This may be administered as 4 Gm. of potassium chloride (approximately 54 mEq. of K^+) in the intravenous infusion. The rate of infusion should not be more than 25 mEq. per hour unless potassium deficits are great; it is wise not to exceed 100 mEq. in twelve hours.

Potassium may also be given by nasogastric tube either as the citrate salt, 15 mEq. per 5 ml., or as 2 Gm. dibasic potassium phosphate and 0.4 Gm. monobasic potassium phosphate in 50 ml. of distilled water. The latter may be added to the infusion being administered and has the advantage of providing phosphate ions. Twenty-five to 50 percent of the potassium deficit is usually replaced in the first twenty-four hours.

Additional Measures

1. Fluids may be given by mouth as tolerated but should be limited to 100 to 120 ml. per hour for adults and to 50 ml. an hour for children. If nausea recurs, fluids should not be administered orally for two to six hours. Antinauseant drugs may be useful.

2. If a cause for ketoacidosis has not been established, a repetition of the history and a physical examination may be revealing at this time; the patient may be more alert and co-operative as a result of proper hydration, and a more accurate examination may be possible. In addition, significant physical findings (of lobar pneumonia, for example) that may not be apparent during severe dehydration may become manifest when fluid losses have been replaced.

SIXTH TO TWENTY-FOURTH HOURS

Every four to six hours, the blood sugar and carbon-dioxide determinations should be repeated and the Insulin dosage schedule adjusted according to the urinary acetone and glucose findings.

At this time, an attempt should be made to give soft or liquid food (such as oatmeal, gruel, orange juice, or milk diluted half-and-half with water) not to exceed 10 Gm. of carbohydrate per hour. If the blood glucose level is approaching normal and the patient is unable to tolerate food by mouth, 5 or 10 percent dextrose in saline may be given at the rate of 200 ml. per hour. The levels of serum potassium should be measured at intervals of eight to twelve hours.

A disturbing but rare complication of diabetic ketoacidosis that begins to manifest itself during the early hours of treatment is cerebral edema. This occurs in young (adolescent and younger) patients. Since the etiology is unknown and the results of treatment (usually mannitol and steroid in the majority of cases) are disappointing, the mortality is high.[16]

SECOND AND SUCCEEDING DAYS

The patient is given an appropriate diet as indicated in the chapter on "Dietary Treatment." In addition, administration of intermediate-acting Insulin is initiated by the methods described in Chapter 7, "Clinical Use of Insulin." The past program of diabetic management is reviewed and reevaluated for possible factors which led to coma. The patient may need to be reeducated in methods of dealing with infectious complications, reminded to avoid the omission of Insulin doses, and instructed in proper diet. It is advisable to arrange a conference with the dietitian.

COMA DUE TO LACTIC ACID ACIDOSIS

Metabolic acidosis due to the production and retention of excessive quantities of lactic acid may cause this form of coma. It may occur in nondiabetic as well as diabetic subjects. The lactic acid level in venous blood seldom increases more than 1 mM per liter, with a corresponding rise in pyruvic acid in normal subjects even during exercise; patients with this form of acidosis, however, may have lactic acid levels which are elevated both absolutely and in relation to the pyruvate level. Lactate-pyruvate ratios of 10:1 may occur. Clinically, these excesses of lactic acid have been reported in association with serious illnesses in which tissue hypoxia exists (e.g., cardiac tamponade, peripheral circulatory collapse, preterminal heart failure, acute hemorrhage, hypotension, and carbon-dioxide retention) and when the use of vasopressor agents results in peripheral vasospasm and the pooling of blood in the tissues.[17-20]

Marked elevations of lactic acid have also been reported in ketoacidosis, in uremic acidosis, and in patients receiving phenformin. Rarely, lactic acidosis may occur with no obvious precipitating factors. The chief biochemical abnormality is apparently related to tissue hypoxia and to the body's inability to convert lactate to pyruvate.

Lactic acid acidosis should be suspected whenever hypoxia coexists with an unexplained acidosis that is characterized by a widening of the anion gap.* Physicians should be aware that coma due to lactic acid aci-

---

*An "anion gap" is said to exist when the sum of the chloride and bicarbonate anions is less than the serum sodium minus 12 (i.e., $[Cl^- + HCO_3^-] < [Na^+ - 12]$).[21]

dosis (particularly in the growth-onset diabetic) may be confused clinically with that resulting from typical ketoacidosis. It may be distinguished by the absence of hyperglycemia and severe ketosis.

Treatment consists in correcting the conditions leading to hypoxia and using an alkalinizing solution (sodium bicarbonate) to alleviate the acidosis. However, the results of the latter procedure may be disappointing even though large amounts of alkali are used. Until the mechanism for lactic acid accumulation is better understood, sodium bicarbonate may be considered the best therapy available.

NONKETOTIC HYPEROSMOLAR COMA

Although this form of diabetic coma was first described by Umber-Berlin in 1924,[22] a significant number of case reports have appeared subsequently.[10,19,20,23-25] Nonketotic coma occurs in patients with ketosis-resistant-type diabetes; in fact, in a substantial number of the cases reported, there was no previous awareness that the patients had diabetes. Frequently, especially in elderly diabetics, there is a history of an intercurrent illness during which hyperglycemia and polyuria (resulting from osmotic diuresis) are present. Such an illness, often in conjunction with arteriolar nephrosclerosis, leads to a failure to retain water. Eventually, glomerular filtration becomes reduced, and, in turn, hyperglycemia and hypernatremia leading to hyperosmolarity develop. Osmotic forces cause extraction of water from the cells, including the cerebral cells; in many cases, the function of such cells is already compromised by preexisting vascular disease. The end result is coma.*

Laboratory findings   Although laboratory data are incomplete in many cases, patients with nonketotic hyperosmolar coma generally have very high blood sugars, frequently in excess of 1,000 mg. per 100 ml. In addition, the serum sodium levels usually exceed 150 mEq. per liter (normal is under 142), and osmolarities have ranged from 330 to as high as 460 mOsm per Kg. of body water (normal range is 275 to 295). The carbon dioxide may be elevated, normal, or depressed; its depression may indicate the presence of respiratory alkalosis, metabolic acidosis due to hypercapnia, or retention of unmeasured anions (as in renal failure or lactic acid acidosis). Evidence of ketosis is characteristically minimal or absent.

The most important aspect of treatment is the provision of water to correct the dehydration. Water is usually administered as 0.45 percent (half-normal) saline. In addition, Insulin is given; however, the total quantity needed ordinarily is less than that required in the coma associated with ketoacidosis. Improvement in the state of consciousness is best correlated with correction of the water deficit, the total quantity of which may approach ten to fifteen liters. During this period of treatment, renal excretion of water is minimal. The mortality rate from nonketotic hyperosmolar coma has been reported to be 44 percent.[25]

---

*Nabarro[20] has pointed out that serum osmolarity in ketoacidosis may be just as great as in nonketotic hyperosmolar coma. He concludes that cerebral cellular dehydration by itself is not, therefore, a satisfactory explanation for the comatose state seen in the latter condition.

BIBLIOGRAPHY

1. Bradley, R. F.: Treatment of Diabetic Ketoacidosis and Coma, M. Clin. North America, *49*:961, 1965.

1A. Marliss, E. B., Ohman, J. L., Jr., Aoki, T. T., and Kozak, G. P.: Altered Redox State Obscuring Ketoacidosis in Diabetic Patients with Lactic Acidosis, N. Engl. J. Med., *283*:978, 1976.

2. Kirtley, W. R.: Clinical Aspects of Diabetic Coma, J. Indiana M. A., *48*:1408, 1955.

3. Scribner, B. H., and Burnell, J. M.: Diabetic Coma, in Syllabus for the Course on Fluid and Electrolyte Balance, Ed. 5. Seattle: University of Washington School of Medicine, 1960.

4. Nuttall, F. Q.: Metabolic Acidosis—Diabetic, Arch. Int. Med., *116*:709, 1965.

5. Daughaday, W. H.: Diabetic Acidosis, in Diabetes (edited by R. H. Williams), p. 516. New York: Paul B. Hoeber, Inc., 1960.

6. Pines, K. L.: Diabetic Acidosis, in Clinical Diabetes Mellitus (edited by M. Ellenberg and H. Rifkin), p. 340. New York: The Blakiston Division, McGraw-Hill Book Company, Inc., 1962.

7. Frawley, T. F.: Treatment of Diabetic Acidosis, Mod. Treat., *2*:644, 1965.

8. Danowski, T. S.: Acute Problems: Acidosis and Coma, in Diabetes Mellitus: Diagnosis and Treatment (edited by T. S. Danowski), p. 123. New York: American Diabetes Association, Inc., 1964.

9. Shuman, C. B.: Diabetes Mellitus in Adults, in Current Therapy (edited by H. F. Conn), p. 295. Philadelphia: W. B. Saunders Company, 1965.

10. Goodner, C. J.: Newer Concepts in Diabetes Mellitus, Including Management, in Disease-a-Month (edited by H. F. Dowling). Chicago: Year Book Medical Publishers, Inc., September, 1965.

10A. Fisher, J. N., Shahshahani, N., and Kitabchi, A. E.: Diabetic Ketoacidosis: Low Dose Insulin Therapy by Various Routes, N. Engl. J. Med., *297*:238, 1977.

10B. Piters, K. M., Kumar, D., Pei, E., *et al.:* Comparison of Continuous and Intermittent Intravenous Insulin Therapies for Diabetic Ketoacidosis, Diabetologia, *13*:317, 1977.

11. Duncan, G. G., and Gill, R. J.: Clinical Value of a Simple Qualitative Test for Plasma Acetone in Diabetic Coma, Diabetes, *2*:353, 1953.

11A. Alberti, K. G. M., and Hockaday, D. R.: Rapid Blood Ketone Body Estimations in the Diagnosis of Diabetic Ketoacidosis, Br. Med. J., *2*:565, 1972.

12. Posner, J. B., and Plum, F.: Spinal Fluid *p*H and Neurologic Symptoms in Systemic Acidosis, New England J. Med., *277*:605, 1967.

13. Ohman, J. L., Jr., Marliss, E. B., Aoki, T. T., Munichoodappa, C. S., Khanna, V. V., and Kozak, G. P.: The Cerebrospinal Fluid in Diabetic Ketoacidosis, New England J. Med., *284*:283, 1971.

14. Cooke, R. E.: Parenteral Fluid Therapy, in Textbook of Pediatrics, Ed. 8 (edited by W. E. Nelson), p. 190. Philadelphia: W. B. Saunders Company, 1964.

15. Alberti, K. G. M. M., Darley, J. H., Emerson, P. M., and Hockaday, T. D. R.: 2,3-Diphosphoglycerate and Tissue Oxygenation in Uncontrolled Diabetes Mellitus, Lancet, *2*:391, 1972.

16. Young, E., and Bradley, R. F.: Cerebral Edema with Irreversible Coma in Severe Diabetic Ketoacidosis, N. Engl. J. Med., *276*:665, 1967.

17. Bernier, G. M., Miller, M., and Springate, C. S.: Lactic Acidosis and Phenformin Hydrochloride, J.A.M.A., *184*:43, 1963.

18. Tranquada, R. E., Bernstein, S., and Martin, H. E.: Irreversible Lactic Acidosis Associated with Phenformin Therapy. Report of Three Cases, J.A.M.A., *184*:37, 1963.

19. Danowski, T. S., and Nabarro, J. D. N.: Hyperosmolar and Other Types of Nonketoacidotic Coma in Diabetes, Diabetes, *14*:162, 1965.

20. Nabarro, J. D. N.: Diabetic Acidosis: Clinical Aspects, in On the Nature and Treatment of Diabetes (edited by B. S. Leibel and G. A. Wrenshall), p. 545. New York: Excerpta Medica Foundation, 1965.

21. Scribner, B. H., and Burnell, J. M.: Basic Physiology, in Syllabus for the Course on Fluid and Electrolyte Balance, Ed. 5. Seattle: University of Washington School of Medicine, 1960.

22. Umber-Berlin, F.: Stoffwechselkrankheiten. II. Der Diabetes mellitus, München. med. Wchnschr., *71*:1324, 1924.

23. Lucas, C. P., Grant, N., Daily, W. J., and Reaven, G. M.: Diabetic Coma without Ketoacidosis, Lancet, *1*:75, 1963.

24. Dürr, F.: A Case of Hyperosmolar Non-Acidotic Diabetic Coma, German M. Month., *9*:58, 1964.

25. Di Benedetto, R. J., Crocco, J. A., and Soscia, J. L.: Hyperglycemic Nonketotic Coma, Arch. Int. Med., *116*:74, 1965.

Chronic Complications of Diabetes

14

INTRODUCTION

Control of the blood sugar by diet and various forms of antidiabetic therapy is a vital aspect in the care of the diabetic. Equally important is the management of various chronic complications to which the diabetic is subject. It is these complications that account for most diabetic morbidity and mortality. Notable exceptions are disability and death due to trauma, cancer, and other nondiabetic diseases which occur in the diabetic as well as in the general population.

The term "chronic complications of diabetes" ordinarily denotes nephropathy (specifically diabetic glomerulosclerosis, or Kimmelstiel-Wilson disease), retinopathy, and neuropathy. It is important to recognize that numerous other conditions also occur exclusively or with significantly greater frequency in diabetic subjects and often accentuate the severity of diabetes (Table 48). The complications of diabetes include a number of biochemical, structural, and functional abnormalities that tend to increase morbidity and mortality. These abnormalities may be arbitrarily divided into three major categories: (1) large-vessel disease, (2) small-vessel disease, and (3) susceptibility to infection.

Table 48. Manifestations of the Complications of Diabetes

Eyes	Retinopathy, cataract formation, glaucoma, and extraocular muscle palsies
Mouth	Gingivitis, increased incidence of dental caries, periodontal disease, and greater resorption of alveolar bone
Pregnancy	Increased incidence of large babies, stillbirths, miscarriages, neonatal deaths, and congenital defects
Nervous system	Motor, sensory, and autonomic neuropathy
Vascular system	Large-vessel disease and microangiopathy
Skin	Xanthoma diabeticorum, necrobiosis lipoidica diabeticorum, furunculosis, mycosis, and pruritus
Kidneys	Diabetic glomerulosclerosis, arteriolar nephrosclerosis, and pyelonephritis

1. Although large-vessel disease (e.g., atherosclerosis) has a high incidence among nondiabetic subjects, it is thought to occur even more frequently and at an earlier age in diabetic patients. (Evidence to the contrary has been proposed by some authors.[1-3]) In any case, a physician who treats diabetes is often called upon to treat the complications arising from large-vessel disease. These include the vascular syndromes associated with insufficient blood supply to the brain and central nervous system, the kidneys, the lower extremities, and, of special importance, the heart. Bradley and Partamian[4] have described the problem of coronary artery disease in diabetics, particularly its increased incidence in premenopausal normotensive women. Such patients have a greater mortality than nondiabetic women and a shorter life expectancy after an acute attack. *Large-vessel disease*

2. Small-vessel disease includes those disorders which affect the arterioles, venules, and capillaries. The disease of this portion of the vasculature has been one of the focal points of current research in diabetes[5] and is referred to by some investigators as "microangiopathy." However, no definition of microangiopathy at the present time is acceptable to all investigators. Some use the term to encompass all microvascular disease and related pathology in the diabetic (including retinopathy, glomerulosclerosis, thickening of the peripheral capillary basement membrane, and an endothelial proliferative lesion involving arterioles and capillaries). For others, "microangiopathy" denotes the lesion of capillary basement membrane only. In this discussion, the former broad definition will be used. *Small-vessel disease*

The clinical manifestations of arteriole disease are most commonly recognized in the kidney as arteriolar nephrosclerosis and in the lower extremities as dry gangrene. (When there is gangrene, however, large-vessel involvement is usually present also and is severe.) Capillary changes were poorly understood until the advent of the electron microscope, but such investigations have shown that capillary involvement is diffuse. Anatomic areas studied in depth include the eye,[6-8] kidney,[9-11] muscle,[12-14] and skin.[15] Electron microscopy usually reveals a thickening of the capillary

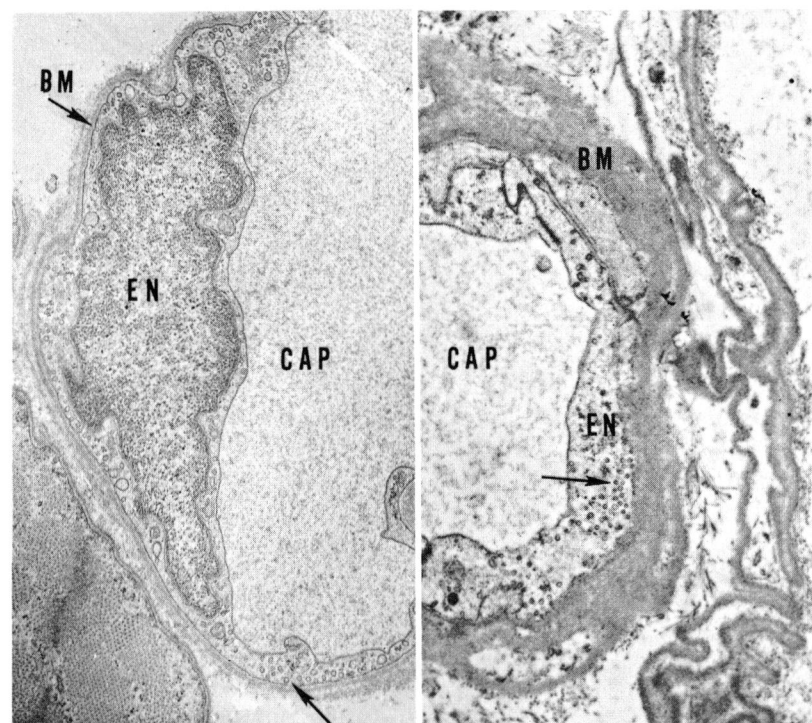

Figure 32. Electron micrographs of muscle capillaries from a nondiabetic (left) and a diabetic patient (right), printed at the same magnification. Each capillary lumen (CAP) is surrounded by an endothelial cell (EN). The nondiabetic capillary contains an endothelial nucleus. The basement membrane (BM) encompassing the endothelial cell is greatly thickened in the diabetic. On the right of the diabetic specimen is a second basement membrane, that of the adjacent muscle. Note the many pinocytic vesicles (arrows) in the endothelial cytoplasm.

(Figures 32, 35, and 36, courtesy of J. M. B. Bloodworth, Jr., M.D., University of Wisconsin)

basement membrane. The typical capillary (such as is in the eye, muscle, etc.) is composed of a lumen surrounded by a thin, but nonfenestrated, layer of endothelial cytoplasm (Figure 32). Occasionally, endothelial nuclei are observed to be completely encompassed by a layer of basement membrane. This basement membrane may split and enclose either an entire cell with its nucleus or portions of a cell. The enclosed cells, which actually cover approximately half the surface of each capillary, are known as pericytes or, in the retina, as mural cells. In the early stages of diabetes, there occurs a reversible venular dilatation in the bulbar conjunctiva.[11]

Increased frequency of infection

3. The increased frequency of infection in the diabetic is well known, but its precise cause has not been discovered. The combination of vascular lesions and infection may constitute a major problem for the diabetic patient.[16]

RELATIONSHIP OF COMPLICATIONS TO BLOOD SUGAR CONTROL

The etiology of diabetic microangiopathy, its development and progression, and its relationship to blood sugar control have been favorite subjects of discussion since the advent of Insulin.[17-21] The view that it is

Table 49. Average Width of Muscle Capillary Basement Membrane and Incidence of Membrane Thickening* in Normal, Diabetic, and Prediabetic Patients (After Siperstein et al.[14])

SUBJECTS	NUMBER OF SUBJECTS	NUMBER OF CAPILLARIES	AVERAGE BASEMENT MEMBRANE WIDTH (A ± SE†)	INCIDENCE OF THICKENING	PERCENT
Normal	50	747	1,080 ± 27‡	4	8
Diabetic	51	765	2,403 ± 119‡	50	98
Prediabetic	30	450	1,373 ± 44‡	16	53

*Average of 15 vessels > 1,325 A
†SE based on number of subjects
‡$p < 0.01$

related to carbohydrate intolerance is supported by the finding that micro-angiopathy occurs in patients who are made diabetic by surgery or disease of the pancreas. The validity of this concept needs further support, however, because the number of such cases is small and some of the individuals might have developed diabetes anyway.

Microangiopathy in the *absence* of demonstrable impairment in carbohydrate tolerance is the principal evidence for considering vascular involvement separately from the carbohydrate aspect of diabetes.

Siperstein et al.,[14] using electron microscopy, examined the normal capillary basement membranes of fifty normal, fifty diabetic, and thirty prediabetic subjects. As indicated in Table 49, basement membrane hypertrophy was found in 98 percent of overt diabetics and 53 percent of prediabetics but in only 8 percent of normal subjects. Basement membrane thickness in diabetic subjects was unrelated to age, weight, or severity or duration of the diabetes. Subjects with severe hyperglycemia due to causes other than genetic diabetes only infrequently showed basement membrane hypertrophy.

Williamson et al.[22] and Kilo et al.[23] measured muscle capillary basement membrane thickening (BMT) in 129 control subjects and 133 diabetics of all degrees of severity. These workers came to the conclusion that BMT increased with age in normal and diabetic subjects but was significantly more evident in diabetics. The latter phenomenon was related to duration and severity of the diabetes.

The controversy over the results of Siperstein et al.[14,24] and of Williamson and Kilo et al.[22,23] is unresolved at present. Kilo and Williamson regard BMT as metabolic in origin, i.e., related to hyperglycemia.[25] Siperstein, on the other hand, considers it a genetic error. He[24] measured 200 to 250 points of the muscle capillary basement membrane and notes that Williamson took only two measurements, at points where the membrane was thinnest. Kilo et al.[23] assert that the high incidence of BMT reported by Siperstein and his failure to correlate BMT with duration of diabetes were due to differences in the criteria for selection of subjects. Since Siperstein's diabetics all had two fasting blood sugars over 140 mg. per 100 ml., the carbohydrate intolerance in this group was of a severe degree

Diabetic microangiopathy

and may have been present in most patients for a considerable period of time.

Recent studies in rats have demonstrated a possible correlation between hyperglycemia and the development of renal lesions characteristic of diabetes. Spiro and Spiro[26] measured kidney glucosyltransferase (an enzyme involved in the synthesis of material found in capillary basement membrane) extracted from the renal cortices of normal and alloxan diabetic rats. The activity of this enzyme was significantly greater in diabetic kidneys than in those of age-matched controls. Moreover, enzyme activity increased with the duration of the diabetes. Whereas short-term treatment with Insulin restored the activity of glucosyltransferase to normal, long-term treatment reduced but did not normalize enzyme activity. The authors attributed this to poorer diabetic control of the long-term diabetic rats.

The effect of blood glucose control on the progression of microangiopathy has been widely studied.[17] However, because there has been a lack of uniformity in the following factors—patient selection, the definition of what constitutes vascular disease, criteria for control, diet treatment, and variables in the degrees of severity and methods of treatment of diabetes—it has not been established that careful control definitely retards the progression of the microangiopathy. On the basis of a prospective study of juvenile diabetics with unmeasured diet over a ten-year period, Knowles et al.[17] concluded that the general course of the patients compared favorably with that of those who were following diets. They also suggested that if diet control does have favorable effects, then either those reported to be following diets are not observing them or factors other than control are more influential in the progression of *juvenile* diabetic vascular disease.

On the other hand, Marble[18], of the Joslin Clinic, stated ". . . that the bulk of the evidence is in favor of the concept that vascular disease probably is related to a deficiency of insulin and/or its effectiveness and that, by careful control of the metabolic defect over the years, the vascular sequelae may be postponed and lessened in severity."

Bressler[27] has reviewed the recent literature concerning blood glucose control and diabetic complications. Citing a number of problems (Table 50) that prevent normalization of the blood glucose, he concludes that the controversy over control and complications is not resolvable at the present time. The American Diabetes Association[28] advises physicians: "Current clinical and experimental data clearly demonstrate that optimal regulation of glucose levels should be achieved in the treatment of diabetes, particularly in young and middle-aged individuals, who are at greatest risk of developing the microvascular complications.

"It can be concluded that current means of therapy are only partly effective at best, and therefore a high priority must be assigned to the development of more physiologic insulin delivery systems or to approaches to the correction of the deficient insulin-producing mechanism itself. Finally, good diabetic management necessitates education and training of both patients and health professionals in the technics involved, and close coordination and cooperation in patient management. Most important is a commitment to the view that better 'control,' when achievable, is beneficial."

Table 50. Problems of Diabetic Control (After Bressler[27])

Patient errs in carrying out prescribed regimens (diet; activity; Insulin dose, type, and timing).
Periodic urine or occasional blood testing is inadequate for proper assessment of blood glucose control.
Insulin schedules are fixed, whereas activity and diet vary. Regimentation is difficult and imperfect (sociopsychologic problem).
Weapons for blood glucose control are inadequate. Insulin delivery systems are insensitive and crude.
Drugs are not available for control of gluconeogenesis (lipolysis, glucagon secretion, growth-hormone levels, proteolysis).
Dangerous hypoglycemia may occur, with the attendant risk of mental deterioration.
Emotional problems may result from the obligatory regimentation necessary for rigid blood glucose control.

NEPHROPATHY

The diabetic patient's predisposition to renal disease is well recognized. In addition to the pathological changes of pyelonephritis, arteriolar nephrosclerosis, and papillary necrosis, the kidney of the patient is subject to other more specific lesions. There are three forms of glomerulosclerosis—nodular, diffuse, and exudative (Figures 33 and 34[29]).

Figure 33. Types of Renal Lesions in Glomerulosclerosis

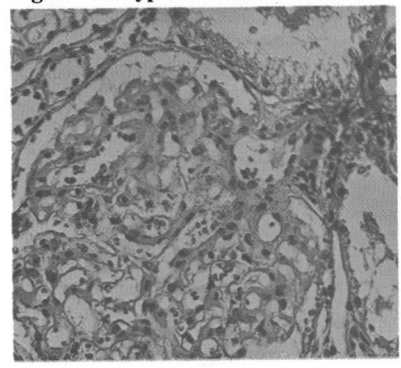

Diffuse Lesion (Early)

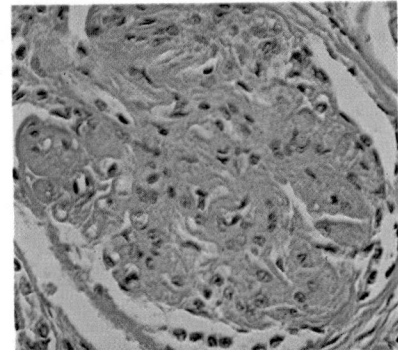

Diffuse Lesion (Advanced)

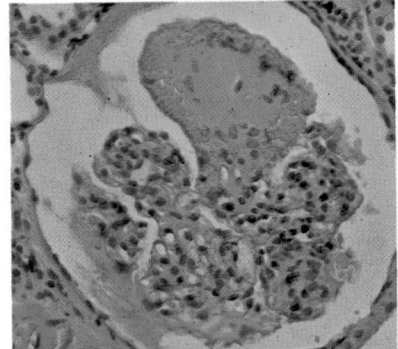

Nodular Lesion

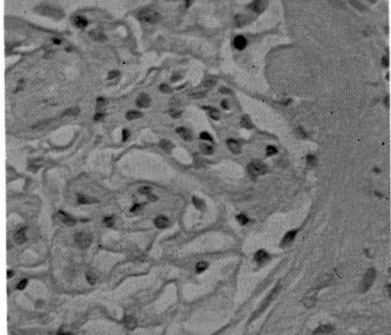

Exudative Lesion

(*Photomicrographs courtesy of Dr. R. M. Kark, Rush Presbyterian-St. Luke's Medical Center, Chicago, Illinois*)

Figure 34. Artist's Interpretation of the Glomerular Lobule in Glomerulosclerosis

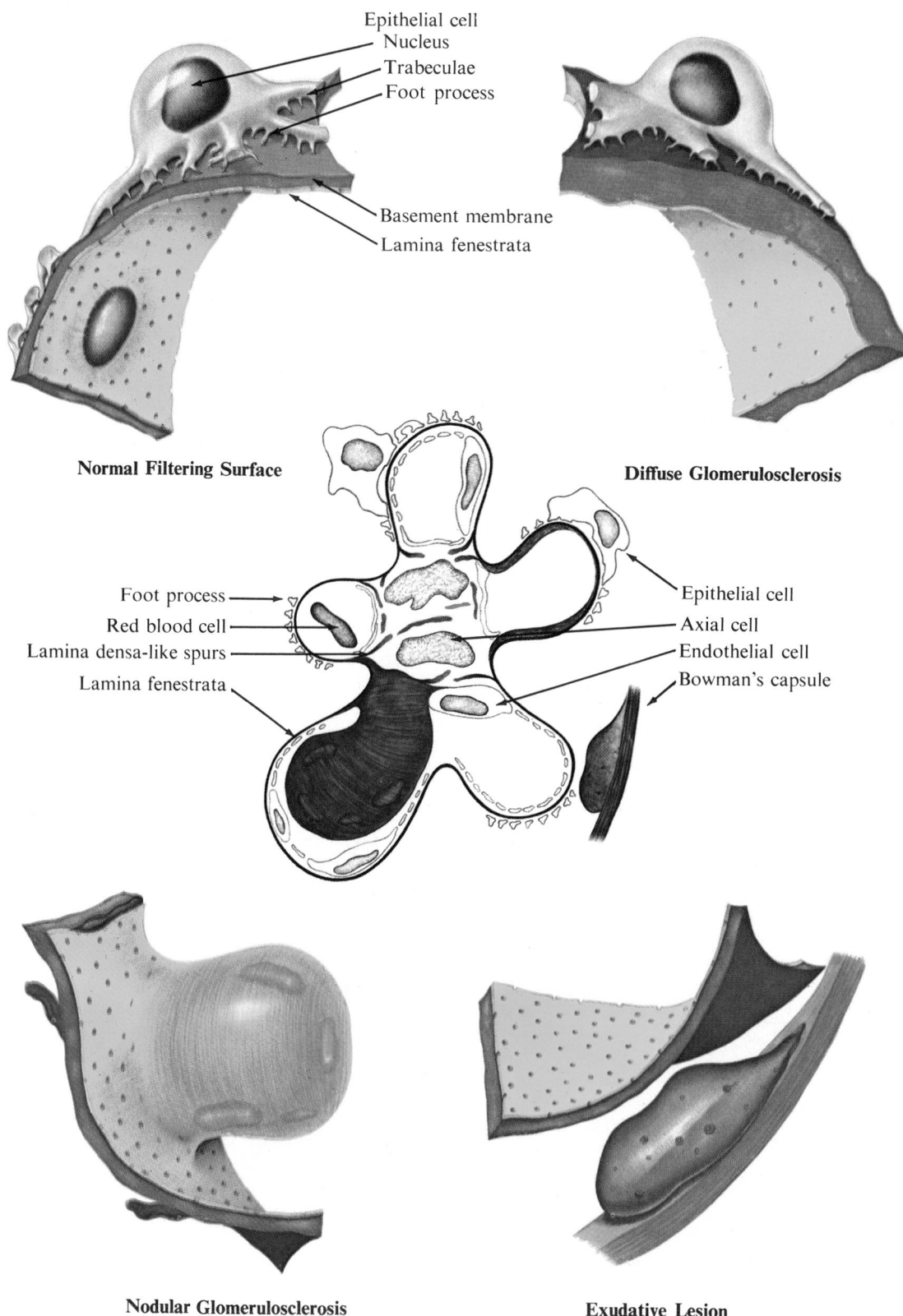

Epithelial cell
Nucleus
Trabeculae
Foot process

Basement membrane
Lamina fenestrata

Normal Filtering Surface

Diffuse Glomerulosclerosis

Foot process
Red blood cell
Lamina densa-like spurs
Lamina fenestrata

Epithelial cell
Axial cell
Endothelial cell
Bowman's capsule

Nodular Glomerulosclerosis

Exudative Lesion

PATHOLOGY AND CLINICAL MANIFESTATIONS

For an understanding of diabetic glomerulosclerosis, the normal architecture of the capillary tuft in the glomerulus must be appreciated. It is usually composed of three or four capillaries whose lumina are surrounded by fenestrated endothelial cells which, in turn, are encompassed by a basement membrane enveloping all of the associated capillary loops in the tuft. Outside the basement membrane are the epithelial cells. Located deep in the tuft are one, two, or more mesangial cells, usually, but not always, separated from the capillary lumina by a thin layer of endothelial cytoplasm and little projections of basement-membrane-like material which appear to be continuous with the membrane at many points and probably represent the same substance (Figure 35).

Normal anatomy of the glomerulus

It sometimes appears that the typical pathology of diabetic glomerulosclerosis is, first, a thickening of the basement membrane and, second, a proliferation of mesangial cells. Simultaneously, an abnormal matrix is formed by an increase in the size, number, and complexity of interlacing pieces of mesangial material between which are found the proliferating mesangial cells (Figure 36). It is important that diabetic glomerulosclerosis begins as a very subtle thickening of the mesangial area; it is associated with basement membrane widening (which is not nodular initially) and is known by the term "diffuse glomerulosclerosis." Although this glomerulosclerosis is specifically due to the diabetes and with time will progress until the diffuse thickening becomes nodular (forming the nodules described by

Glomerulosclerosis

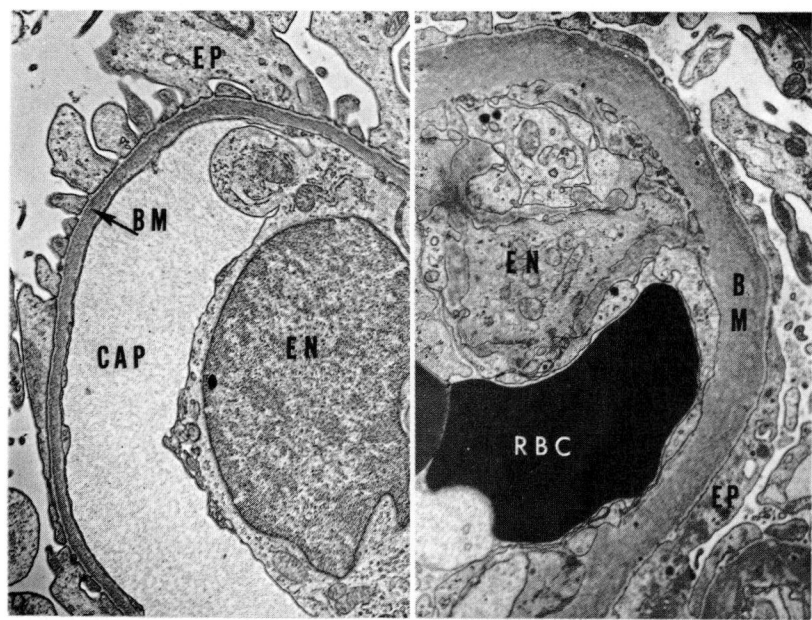

Figure 35. Electron micrographs of portions of glomerular capillary loops from a non-diabetic (left) and a diabetic patient (right), printed at the same magnification. Note the basement membrane (BM) lined internally by a delicate layer of endothelial cytoplasm in the normal capillary loop. An endothelial nucleus (EN) is present. Portions of epithelial cell (EP) showing normal foot-process structure are apposed to the external surface of the basement membrane. The capillary loop from the diabetic shows marked thickening of the basement membrane, swelling of the endothelial cytoplasm, and obliteration of the foot-process structure of the epithelial cell. The lumen is filled by a red blood cell (RBC).

Kimmelstiel and Wilson[30]), it is no different in its early stages from diffuse glomerulosclerosis of chronic glomerulonephritis and other conditions. Therefore, even though diffuse glomerulosclerosis may be specific for diabetes, the fact that its diabetic etiology usually cannot be proved by either light or electron microscopy has led to much confusion regarding its nature and significance. Most but not all authorities agree that the thickened areas of diffuse glomerulosclerosis may gradually enlarge to produce the nodules of Kimmelstiel-Wilson lesions. Kimmelstiel himself believes that nodules occur in the absence of the diffuse lesions.[31] Although the changes which take place within the circumscribing basement membrane are integrated primarily in the mesangial area, the process may also extend into the peripheral capillary areas (Figures 34-36).

The black granular material deposited around the basement membrane in so-called exudative glomerulosclerosis resembles that seen in glomerulonephritis, lupus, and eclampsia of pregnancy. However, the deposits are much larger; they are brightly eosinophilic, glassy, and strongly positive to Periodic-Acid-Schiff (PAS) substance under the light microscope and black and granular under the electron microscope. The exact relationship of these exudative lesions to diabetes is uncertain. Also, they appear quite frequently in ischemic, rapidly advancing renal failure and are not specific for diabetes. The clinical findings in diabetic patients with nephropathy are better correlated with the extent of arteriolar nephrosclerosis, pyelonephritis, and renal arterial atherosclerosis than with diabetic glomerulosclerosis.[32]

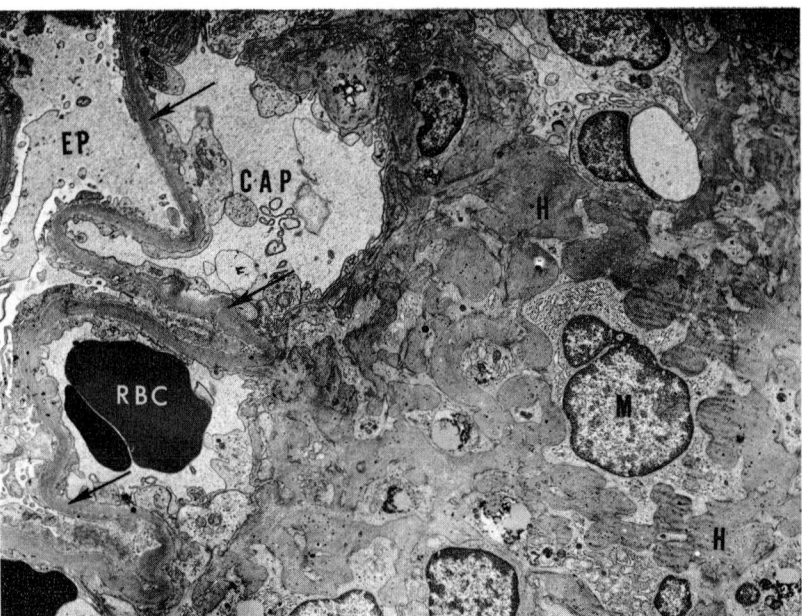

Figure 36. Electron micrograph of a portion of a Kimmelstiel-Wilson nodule in the glomerulus of a diabetic patient. The nodule, on the right of the photograph, is composed of several mesangial nuclei (M). They are surrounded by interdigitating fingers of pale cell cytoplasm containing many intracellular organelles, such as endoplasmic reticulum and mitochondria. The cell cytoplasm is separated by the hyalinoid matrix (H), which is gray and resembles the basement membrane. At the left are two capillaries (CAP) surrounded by a thickened basement membrane (arrows). One contains a red blood cell (RBC). Outside the basement membrane is a portion of an epithelial cell (EP) which has lost its normal foot-process structure.

DIAGNOSIS AND TREATMENT

The problem of diagnosis and treatment of diabetic nephropathy has recently received the attention of several authors.[33-36] It seldom occurs in individuals who have been diabetic for less than five years but may develop occasionally when impairment in carbohydrate tolerance is minimal or absent.[37] In most cases, diabetes has been present for ten to fifteen years.

There is no single clinical manifestation of diabetic nephropathy except that the first sign is protein in the urine. It is different from other systemic disorders associated with glomerular involvement in that hematuria is rarely found. Doubly refractile fat bodies may be seen in the urinary sediment but occur also in the absence of the nephrotic syndrome. Occasionally, a physician will find the total picture of hypertension, azotemia, hypoalbuminemia, edema, and marked proteinuria on the patient's first visit. The two characteristic manifestations of end-stage diabetic glomerulosclerosis are (1) a nephrotic syndrome and (2) azotemia resulting from advanced destruction of the nephrons. The antemortem diagnosis can be made definitively only if renal biopsy shows the nodular lesion.

In diabetic nephropathy, careful attempts must be made to detect and treat coexistent urinary tract infections as well as other manifestations of the disease, e.g., hypertension, edema, heart failure, and encephalopathy.[33,38] If renal failure supervenes, dialysis[38] or renal transplantation is considered.[39]

RETINOPATHY

Diabetic retinopathy is the leading cause of blindness in the United States in adults under age sixty-five.[40-42] The risk of retinopathy increases with age and is the greatest between the ages of thirty and fifty.[41] Although the finding of diabetic retinopathy does not necessarily herald the onset of blindness, the availability of new methods of treatment and the personal and economic impact of blindness justify the careful surveillance of *all* diabetic patients with ocular complications of diabetes.

PATHOLOGY AND CLINICAL MANIFESTATIONS

Since 1943, when Ballantyne and Loewenstein[43] "rediscovered" the capillary microaneurysms originally described in 1877, the histopathology of diabetic retinopathy has received careful attention. Flat preparations of the retina have afforded a unique opportunity for studying the intact retinal vasculature (Figure 37). Both PAS staining of vessel basement membrane[44] and intravascular injection of an opaque substance such as India ink[45] have been utilized to investigate the vasculature in the unstained (transparent) intact retina. More recently, the trypsin digestion technic[46] has permitted isolation of large areas of vascular network after dissolution of the surrounding retina. Conventional stains can then be used to study the cells of the vessel wall.

There is general agreement among workers using such technics that the capillaries are the principal areas involved. These are obliterated in

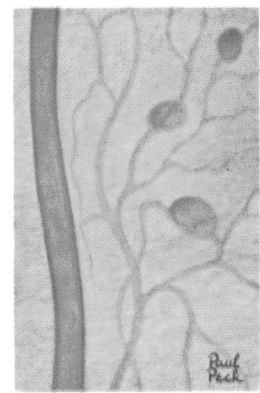

Figure 37. An enlarged view of retinal microaneurysms. In the excised eye, the retinal layer can be separated from the choroid coat and floated flat onto a glass slide. Following appropriate technics designed to create translucency and to stain mucopolysaccharides of the vascular basement membranes, low-power microscopic examination will reveal the appearance shown.

some parts of the retina; in others they are dilated, and some are hypercellular. Microaneurysms occur with greatest frequency in the capillaries that border on areas of occluded capillaries (Figure 38). Most workers have assumed that this obliteration is probably the primary abnormality, with dilatation being a secondary effect.

Figure 38. A three-dimensional reconstruction of a portion of the retina in a diabetic, revealing the capillary network with clusters of aneurysms which occur chiefly in the macular region.

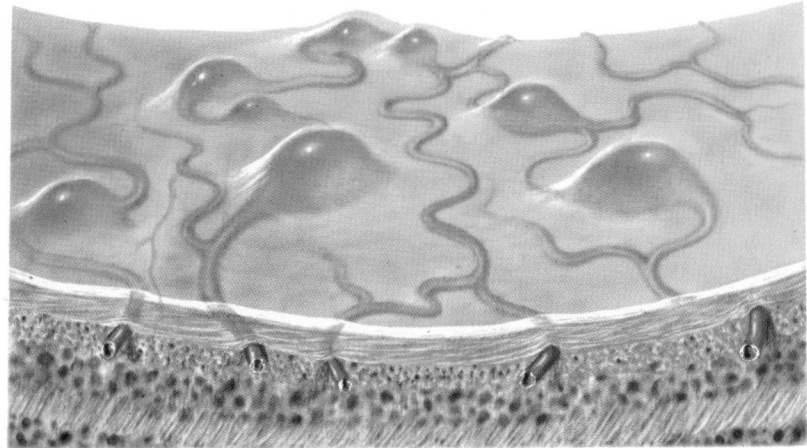

Cogan and Kuwabara,[47] however, have proposed that the dilated channels may represent the primary lesion. They suggest that blood is shunted through these channels from arterioles to venules and thus bypasses parts of the capillary network, which then become atrophic. They base their interpretation on the preferential loss of mural cells (pericytes) of the retinal capillaries in diabetes and, since the function of these cells is similar to that of smooth muscle, their loss leads to impairment of vascular tone.

Many theories have been advanced to explain the occurrence of microaneurysms. Various investigators have proposed that increased intravascular pressure is the cause or have attributed them to loss of external support of the capillary wall resulting from degeneration of neural and glial elements. Other workers have emphasized endothelial proliferation and have suggested that microaneurysms represent a sort of abortive attempt at neovascularization. These and other theories have been reviewed by Ashton,[45] Bloodworth,[6] and Cogan et al.,[46] among others.

Clinical stages of diabetic retinopathy

The clinical evaluation of diabetic retinopathy takes into consideration four characteristics (the O'Hare Classification)[48]: (1) background retinopathy, (2) vitreous hemorrhage, (3) new vessels, and (4) fibrous proliferation extending into the vitreous (Figure 39). The course of the retinopathy is extremely variable. In some cases, a scattering of microaneurysms is the only clinical evidence for many years. Usually, however, fine, deep exudates eventually appear adjacent to the microaneurysms. These apparently result from leakage of plasma proteins and lipids across the excessively permeable walls of microaneurysms and adjacent capillaries. Degeneration of retinal neurons and glial cells may also play a role in the production of exudates. Such recent improvements in clinical examination as stereoscopic fundus photography, slit-lamp biomicroscopy of the retina, and intravenous fluorescein fundus photography have demonstrated that

Figure 39. Ophthalmoscopic Classification of Diabetic Retinopathy*

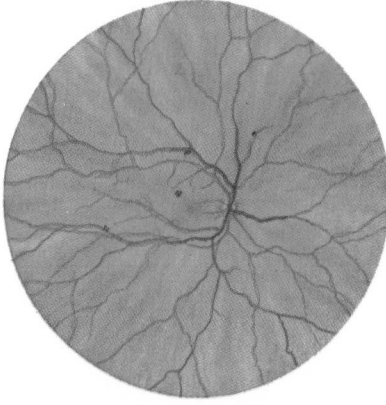

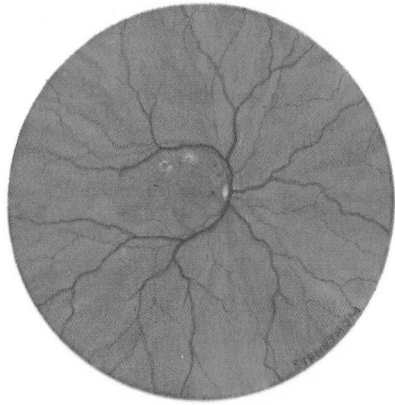

Example A. Microaneurysms and distention of the retinal veins. These changes constitute the first clinically apparent evidence of background retinopathy. They occur in the posterior pole of the fundus.

Example B. The findings depicted in Example A plus deep retinal punctate hemorrhages and waxy exudates. The latter indicate chronic vascular leakage.

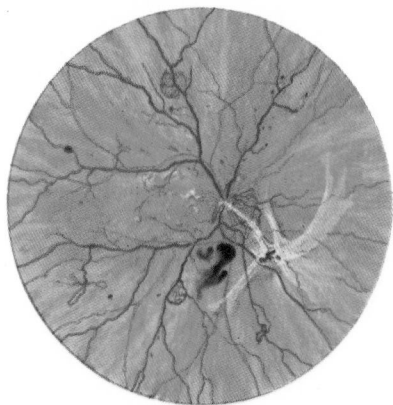

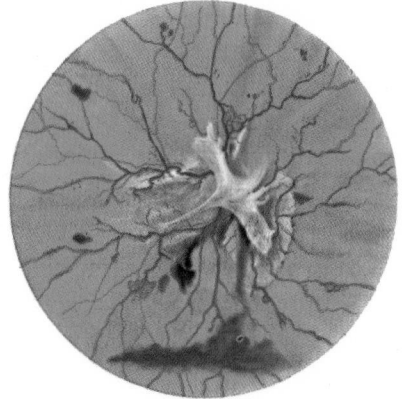

Example C. Example B findings plus superficial retinal hemorrhages, dilatation of existing capillary networks, neovascularization, preretinal hemorrhages, and fibrosis of the surface of the retina.

Example D. Example C findings plus vitreous hemorrhages, proliferating retinopathy with its sequelae—rubeosis iridis diabetica, retinal detachment, secondary glaucoma, and loss of useful vision.

*In combination with these findings, there frequently are changes due to arteriolar sclerosis, hypertension, and renal disease.

some microaneurysms are abnormally permeable.[49,50] A zone of thickened (edematous) retina characteristically surrounds the microaneurysms, and a ring of exudate in turn encloses the edematous area. When such leaky microaneurysms are situated near the macula, resultant edema is often particularly severe and produces moderate to severe impairment of central visual acuity. Patients with this condition, however, usually retain a useful visual field and are able to get about and care for themselves.

More marked visual loss is generally confined to the proliferative phase of diabetic retinopathy. Its neovascular proliferation typically occurs on the anterior surface of the retina and leads to firm vitreoretinal adhesions. Subsequent vitreous contraction—in some cases presumably caused by advancing age but in others perhaps directly due to the new vessels—

then pulls on the new vessels and underlying retina and leads to vitreous hemorrhage and retinal detachment.[50] The new vessels themselves characteristically follow a cycle of proliferation and regression; and if vitreous contraction does not occur, good vision may be retained indefinitely.

A puzzling aspect of diabetic retinopathy is that, although the thickening of the capillary basement membrane is generalized, the above-mentioned changes are focal. Bloodworth[51] points out that when the ophthalmoscope is used, more lesions may be observed around the nerve head, but even here large areas are spared. Because of this patchy distribution, he and Ashton[52] postulate that some local changes must occur which predispose the affected areas to the lesions.

TREATMENT

There is no satisfactory therapy for diabetic retinopathy. Treatment of all patients with retinopathy begins with an attempt to bring about strict control of the diabetes. This procedure occasionally has been reported to produce marked improvement in the ocular lesions.[53]

Specific dietary alterations have been utilized with various degrees of success in patients with early retinopathy. A low-fat, high-carbohydrate diet and the Kempner rice diet have brought about a reduction in the retinopathic changes in a significant number of patients.[54,55]

Photocoagulation and other methods

For the advanced and rapidly progressive forms of diabetic retinopathy (including new vessel formation, vitreous hemorrhage, and the production of connective tissue with or without retinal detachment), more aggressive therapies are considered.[41] These are photocoagulation, vitrectomy and vitreolysis, and pituitary ablation. Photocoagulation involves directing a beam of light from either an incandescent or a laser source through the dilated pupil onto the retina. The light energy impinging on the retina is converted to heat and coagulates the tissue it strikes. Although photocoagulation is of limited value in patients with macular involvement, this modality has been demonstrated to be significantly efficacious in two randomized, controlled trials in patients with neovascularization.[56,57] The usefulness of this therapy highlights the need for the early recognition and treatment of proliferative lesions, particularly those of a severe nature. Less-marked proliferative lesions ordinarily are treated only if there is evidence of fresh bleeding from them.[41]

Vitrectomy is utilized in eyes that have been rendered blind by vitreous hemorrhage.[41] The procedure consists in aspirating the blood, membranes, and fibrin through a special device and replacing them with clear Ringer's solution. This does not restore vision if the retina is severely damaged.

Pituitary ablation currently is reserved for patients with rapidly progressive florid retinopathy. Enthusiasm for this procedure formerly was based on a study[58] which reported that well-established diabetic retinopathy cleared completely after the development of postpartum pituitary necrosis. The method has been widely investigated.[58-63] The decision to carry out a procedure as serious as pituitary ablation must take two facts into consideration. First, proliferative retinopathy often progresses to blindness. Second, the majority of patients with vision-threatening retinopathy are in their middle years and the most productive time of their lives.[62]

Two other ocular conditions occurring in the diabetic deserve special mention. These are hemorrhagic glaucoma and cataracts.

The retinal neovascularization so characteristic of diabetic retinopathy has its counterpart on the anterior surface of the iris and on the trabecular meshwork at the anterior chamber angle. Such neovascularization is most often observed in advanced retinopathy but occasionally occurs with relatively mild involvement. The vessels remain asymptomatic until anterior synechiae form; they occlude the outflow channels and lead to marked elevation of intraocular pressure. This type of glaucoma is notoriously resistant to treatment and often progresses rapidly to total blindness.

Glaucoma and cataracts

There is an increased incidence of cataracts in diabetics. The majority of cataracts are of the senile type observed in nondiabetic elderly patients. However, like large-vessel disease, cataracts may appear at an earlier age and progress more rapidly in the diabetic subject. In another lesion which is unique among diabetic patients, multiple white snowflake dots develop over a network of vacuoles. This type of cataract is found under both the anterior and the posterior lens capsule and is particularly prevalent in the young, although it also occurs in older patients.

NEUROPATHY

PATHOLOGY AND CLINICAL MANIFESTATIONS

Neurological disturbances are common in association with diabetes (Figure 40). Authorities disagree as to whether neuropathy is a metabolic or a vascular problem. Many, however, believe that neurological dysfunction due to large-vessel disease has a vascular basis. Fagerberg[64] noted the histological appearance of intraneural vessels from diabetics with and without clinical neuropathy. The lesions were found to be more marked in those with neuropathy. One abnormality was the patchy noninflammatory degeneration of the medullary sheath. The walls of the intraneural vessels showed thickening, there was deposition of PAS substance, and the lumina were constricted.

Evidence favoring a metabolic etiology for diabetic neuropathy was presented by Pirart.[65] In a large series of unselected diabetic subjects, severity of neuropathy was related to poor control and to duration of the diabetes. Another argument favoring the metabolic basis for neuropathy is that it is too patchy and reversible to be due to a diffuse and progressive disorder such as diabetic microangiopathy. Moreover, the vascular lesions do not improve but actually progress, whereas the neuropathy frequently shows remission. Unfortunately, the exact site(s) of primary injury in diabetic neuropathy has not yet been identified.[66]

The neurological abnormality associated with diabetes mellitus and its treatment (or lack of it) may be expressed as the result of dysfunction in the nervous system at any level and possibly in the muscles proper. The manifestations of neuropathy may be caused by disease of the large vessels and their secondary branches which supply the brain and/or by diabetic

Peripheral neuritis

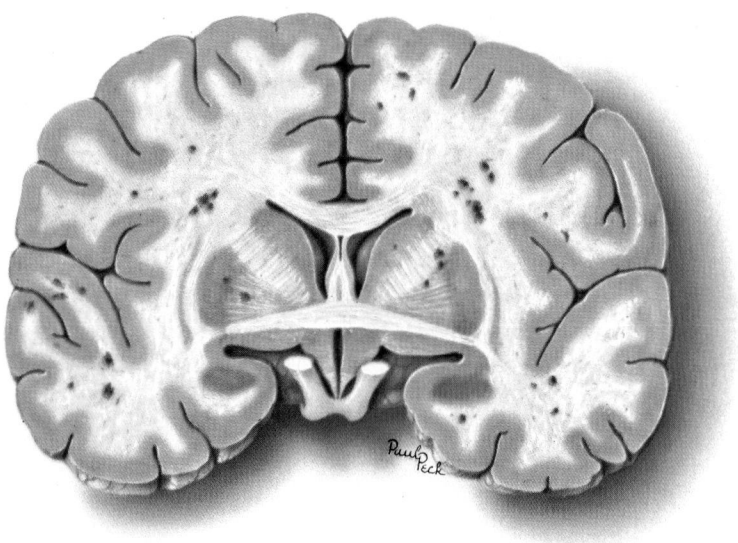

Figure 40. Focal, flame-shaped hemorrhages in the brain may occur in diabetic coma. Their appearance and distribution are not unique.

acidosis with coma or hypoglycemia. Aside from these conditions, the commonest disorders are those related to dysfunction of the somatic and visceral nerves. Somatic neuropathy, also known as peripheral neuritis, may occur with no evidence of visceral involvement, but the visceral form is rarely found without somatic signs and symptoms.

The most frequent manifestations of somatic neuropathy are pain and paresthesia in the lower extremities. The symptoms may be so mild that a history of pain may not be obtained except by direct questioning, or they may be very severe and a source of extreme discomfort to the patient. Neurological examination reveals absence of knee and ankle jerks, and vibratory sensation frequently is impaired. When these findings are elicited, motor-nerve conduction velocity is reduced in the affected part. Occasionally, the presenting sign is weakness of the extremity.

Visceral neuropathy includes those deficiencies in function related to diabetes which affect the various organs and the autonomic nervous system. The areas of involvement have been catalogued in Table 51.[67]

Diabetic amyotrophy

Another neurological syndrome which deserves mention is diabetic amyotrophy.[68] It occurs principally in middle-aged or elderly men with mild diabetes and is associated with pain, weakness, and wasting in the proximal portions of the lower extremities. This syndrome includes reduction of the patellar tendon reflex and marked myalgia. There may be fasciculations in the involved muscles. Fine extensor plantar responses occur. Although this condition may be unilateral in its initial phases, eventually it becomes bilateral. Diabetic amyotrophy may be associated with such severe weakness, weight loss, and debility that it is difficult to differentiate it from carcinoma. The lesion consists of patchy degeneration and atrophy of muscle fibers, and these changes are subject to exacerbations and remissions. Involvement of single fibers suggests that the fundamental lesion is related primarily to a biochemical defect rather than to anatomic abnormalities in the nerve endings or their blood supply.

Table 51. Manifestations of Visceral Neuropathy

SITE AND TYPE OF ALTERATION	CLINICAL FINDINGS
Eyes	Extraocular muscle palsies, preceded by pain on affected side; usually 3d or 6th nerve involved. Prognosis good.
	Pupillary reflex may be abnormal, but Argyll Robertson pupil rarely occurs.
Ears	Decreased hearing acuity.
Gastro-intestinal tract	Delayed gastric emptying, with marked retention.
	Intermittent attacks of nocturnal or postprandial diarrhea, occasionally nocturnal fecal incontinence; deficiency pattern in small bowel on x-ray; associated autonomic and peripheral neuropathy; normal exocrine pancreatic function.
Genito-urinary tract	Bladder involvement may result in same clinical picture as cord bladder. Prompt recognition is essential to avoid urinary infection and renal damage.
	Impotence frequent in the male diabetic. Prognosis poor. Retrograde ejaculation may occur.
Neurotrophic arthropathy	Clinical picture comparable to that of Charcot's joint of tabes. Differs from tabes in that tarsal and ankle joints are most frequently involved. X-ray shows extensive destruction and dissolution of bone which is unrelated to osteoporosis or osteomyelitis.
Neurotrophic ulcer	Ulcer usually on foot, painless at pressure point. Attention called to it by pus or serous drainage.
Autonomic nervous system	Involvement may be so extensive as to simulate lumbar sympathectomy. Postural or orthostatic hypotension from failure of peripheral vascular bed to constrict. Other autonomic disorders include anhidrosis, vasomotor instability, tachycardia, dependent edema, trophic skin disturbances, facial sweating after eating, and abnormal responses to the Valsalva maneuver.

DIAGNOSIS AND TREATMENT

Since they may simulate a number of disorders, these various conditions may often pose a difficult diagnostic problem. A family history of diabetes or other findings suggestive of diabetes and an abnormal glucose tolerance test provide valuable information in establishing a diagnosis.

In all forms of diabetic neuropathy, there must be proper nutrition and control of the diabetes. Since concurrent vitamin deficiencies may be present, administration of a multivitamin may be useful. Vitamin B_{12} is frequently given parenterally to patients with neuropathy; however, there are no objective data to show that this is efficacious in patients who are not deficient. Cholinesterase inhibitors have been used in bladder atony and may be beneficial.

The prognosis varies according to the type of the deficiency and the condition of the patient. Somatic neuropathies generally respond within four to six weeks after control of the diabetes has been established. The autonomic neuropathies are usually more resistant to treatment, and their prognosis is poor. The type of involvement determines what supportive therapy is given.

BIBLIOGRAPHY

1. Colwell, A. R., Sr.: Vascular Disease in Diabetes, Diabetes, *14:*110, 1965.

2. Wilens, S. L.: The Nature of Diffuse Intimal Thickening of Arteries, Am. J. Path., *27:*825, 1951.

3. Dible, J. H.: Some Pathological Adaptations in the Peripheral Circulation, Lancet, *1:*1031, 1958.

4. Bradley, R. F., and Partamian, J. O.: Coronary Heart Disease in the Diabetic Patient, M. Clin. North America, *49:*1093, 1965.

5. Siperstein, M. D., Colwell, A. R., Sr., and Meyer, K.: Small Blood Vessel Involvement in Diabetes Mellitus. Washington, D. C.: American Institute of Biological Sciences, 1964.

6. Bloodworth, J. M. B., Jr.: Diabetic Retinopathy, Diabetes, *11:*1, 1962.

7. Cogan, D. G.: Diabetic Retinopathy, New England J. Med., *270:*787, 1964.

8. Leopold, I. H. (Editor): Diabetic Retinopathy, Surv. Ophthal., *6:*483, 1961.

9. Bloodworth, J. M. B., Jr.: Diabetic Microangiopathy, Diabetes, *12:*99, 1963.

10. MacDonald, M. K., and Ireland, J. T.: The Glomerular Lesion in Idiopathic and Secondary Diabetes, in Aetiology of Diabetes Mellitus and Its Complications, Ciba Foundation Colloquia on Endocrinology, *15:*301, 1964.

11. Rees, S. B., Camerini-Dávalos, R. A., Caulfield, J. B., Lozano-Castaneda, O., Cervantes-Amezcus, A., Taton, J., Pometta, D., Krauthammer, J. P., and Marble, A.: Pathophysiology of Microangiopathy in Diabetes Mellitus, in Aetiology of Diabetes Mellitus and Its Complications, Ciba Foundation Colloquia on Endocrinology, *15:*315, 1964.

12. Sims, E. A. H., MacKay, B. R., and Shirai, T.: The Relation of Capillary Angiopathy and Diabetes Mellitus to Idiopathic Edema, Ann. Int. Med., *63:*972, 1965.

13. Bencosme, S. A., West, R. O., Kerr, J. W., and Wilson, D. L.: Diabetic Capillary Angiopathy in Human Skeletal Muscles, Am. J. Med., *40:*67, 1966.

14. Siperstein, M. D., Unger, R. H., and Madison, L. L.: Studies of Muscle Capillary Basement Membranes in Normal Subjects, Diabetic, and Prediabetic Patients, J. Clin. Invest., *47:*1973, 1968.

15. Binkley, G. W.: Dermopathy in the Diabetic Syndrome, Arch. Dermat., *92:*625, 1965.

16. Younger, D.: Infections and Diabetes, M. Clin. North America, *49:*1005, 1965.

17. Knowles, H. C., Jr., Guest, G. M., Lampe, J., Kessler, M., and Skillman, T. G.: The Course of Juvenile Diabetes Treated with Unmeasured Diet, Diabetes, *14:*239, 1965.

18. Marble, A.: Relation of Control of Diabetes to Vascular Sequelae, M. Clin. North America, *49:*1137, 1965.

19. Berson, S. A., and Yalow, R. S.: Some Current Controversies in Diabetes Research, Diabetes, *14:*549, 1965.

20. Rifkin, H., and Leiter, L.: Diabetic Microangiopathy, in Clinical Diabetes Mellitus (edited by M. Ellenberg and H. Rifkin), p. 360. New York: The Blakiston Division, McGraw-Hill Book Company, Inc., 1962.

21. Ricketts, H. T.: The Influence of Diabetic Control on Angiopathy, in On the Nature and Treatment of Diabetes (edited by B. S. Leibel and G. A. Wrenshall), p. 588. New York: Excerpta Medica Foundation, 1965.

22. Williamson, J. R., Vogler, N. J., and Kilo, C.: Estimation of Vascular Membrane Thickness, Theoretical and Practical Considerations, Diabetes, *18:*567, 1969.

23. Kilo, C., Vogler, N. J., and Williamson, J. R.: Basement Membrane Thickening in Diabetes, in Diabetes Mellitus: Diagnosis and Treatment (edited by S. S. Fajans and K. E. Sussman), III:289. New York: American Diabetes Association, Inc., 1971.

24. Siperstein, M. D.: Capillary Basement Membranes in Diabetes, in Diabetes Mellitus: Diagnosis and Treatment (edited by S. S. Fajans and K. E. Sussman), III:281. New York: American Diabetes Association, Inc., 1971.

25. Kilo, C., Vogler, N., and Williamson, J. R.: Muscle Capillary Basement Membrane Changes Related to Aging and to Diabetes Mellitus, Diabetes, *21:*881, 1972.

26. Spiro, R. G., and Spiro, M. J.: Effect of Diabetes on the Biosynthesis of the Renal Glomerular Basement Membrane. Studies on the Glucosyltransferase, Diabetes, *20:*641, 1971.

27. Bressler, R.: The Controversy over Blood Glucose Control, Drug Therapy, *8:*24, 1978.

28. Cahill, G. F., Jr., Etzwiler, D. D., and Freinkel, N.: Blood Glucose Control in Diabetes, Diabetes, *25:*237, 1976.

29. Latta, H., Maunsbach, A. B., and Madden, S. C.: The Centrolobular Region of the Renal Glomerulus Studied by Electron Microscopy, J. Ultrastructure Res., *4:*455, 1960.

30. Kimmelstiel, P., and Wilson, C.: Intercapillary Lesions in the Glomeruli of the Kidney, Am. J. Path., *12:*83, 1936.

31. Kimmelstiel, P.: Basement Membrane in Diabetic Glomerulosclerosis, Diabetes, *15:*61, 1966.

32. Bell, E. T.: Renal Vascular Disease in Diabetes Mellitus, Diabetes, *2:*376, 1953.

33. Garrett, J. J.: Treatment of the Diabetic with Renal Disease, Mod. Treat., *2:*660, 1965.

34. LeCompte, P. M.: Long-Term Problems: Glomerulosclerosis, in Diabetes Mellitus: Diagnosis and Treatment (edited by T. S. Danowski), p. 167. New York: American Diabetes Association, Inc., 1964.

35. Ellenberg, M.: Diabetic Nephropathy, Texas J. Med., 60:823, 1964.

36. Bricker, N. S., and Slatopolsky, E.: Glomerulonephritis and Other Glomerulopathies, in Disease-a-Month (edited by H. F. Dowling). Chicago: Year Book Medical Publishers, Inc., October, 1965.

37. Ellenberg, M.: Diabetic Nephropathy without Manifest Diabetes, Diabetes, 11:197, 1962.

38. Balodimos, M. C.: Diabetic Nephropathy, in Joslin's Diabetes Mellitus, Ed. 11 (edited by A. Marble, P. White, R. F. Bradley, and L. P. Krall), p. 526. Philadelphia: Lea & Febiger, 1973.

39. Zincke, H., Woods, J. E., Palumbo, P. J., Leary, F. J., and Johnson, W. J.: Renal Transplantation in Patients with Insulin-Dependent Diabetes Mellitus, J.A.M.A., 237:1101, 1977.

40. Blankenship, G. W., and Skyler, J. S.: Diabetic Retinopathy: A General Survey, Diabetes Care, 1:127, 1978.

41. L'Esperance, F. A., Jr.: Diabetic Retinopathy, Med. Clin. North Am., 62:767, 1978.

42. Morse, P. H., and Duncan, T. G.: Ophthalmologic Management of Diabetic Retinopathy, N. Engl. J. Med., 295:87, 1976.

43. Ballantyne, A. J., and Loewenstein, A.: The Pathology of Diabetic Retinopathy, Tr. Ophth. Soc. U. Kingdom, 63:95, 1944.

44. Friedenwald, J. S.: A New Approach to Some Problems of Retinal Vascular Disease, Am. J. Ophth., 32:487, 1949.

45. Ashton, N.: Studies of the Retinal Capillaries in Relation to Diabetic and Other Retinopathies, Brit. J. Ophth., 47:521, 1963.

46. Cogan, D. G., Toussaint, D., and Kuwabara, T.: Retinal Vascular Patterns. IV. Diabetic Retinopathy, Arch. Ophth., 66:366, 1961.

47. Cogan, D. G., and Kuwabara, T.: Capillary Shunts in the Pathogenesis of Diabetic Retinopathy, Diabetes, 12:293, 1963.

48. Symposium on the Treatment of Diabetic Retinopathy (edited by M. F. Goldberg and S. L. Fine), p. XXI. Washington, D.C.: Public Health Service Publication No. 1890, 1968.

49. Norton, E. W. D., and Gutman, F.: Diabetic Retinopathy Studied by Fluorescein Angiography, Ophthalmologica, 150:5, 1965.

50. Davis, M. D.: Vitreous Contraction in Proliferative Diabetic Retinopathy, Arch. Ophth., 74:741, 1965.

51. Bloodworth, J. M. B., Jr.: The Present Status of Degenerative Vascular Disease in Diabetes Mellitus, Clin. Med., 72:1267, 1965.

52. Ashton, N.: Diabetic Retinopathy. A New Approach, Lancet, 2:625, 1959.

53. Dollery, C. T., and Oakley, N. W.: Reversal of Retinal Vascular Changes in Diabetes, Diabetes, 14:121, 1965.

54. Van Eck, W. F.: The Effect of a Low Fat Diet on the Serum Lipids in Diabetes and Its Significance in Diabetic Retinopathy, Am. J. Med., 27:196, 1959.

55. Kempner, W., Peschel, R. L., and Schlayer, C.: Effect of Rice Diet on Diabetes Mellitus Associated with Vascular Disease, Postgrad. Med., 24:359, 1958.

56. Proliferative Diabetic Retinopathy: Treatment with Xenon-Arc Photocoagulation, Br. Med. J., 1:739, 1977.

57. Preliminary Report on Effects of Photocoagulation Therapy, Am. J. Ophthalmol., 81:383, 1976.

58. Poulsen, J. E.: Recovery from Retinopathy in a Case of Diabetes with Simmonds' Disease, Diabetes, 2:7, 1953.

59. Born, J. L., Lawrence, J. H., Linfoot, J. A., Tobias, C. A., Manougian, E., and Snyder, N. J.: Hypophyseal Suppression with Heavy Particles in Diabetic Retinopathy, in On the Nature and Treatment of Diabetes (edited by B. S. Leibel and G. A. Wrenshall), p. 475. New York: Excerpta Medica Foundation, 1965.

60. Field, R. A.: Approaches to Treatment of Retinopathy by Modifying Pituitary Function, in On the Nature and Treatment of Diabetes (edited by B. S. Leibel and G. A. Wrenshall), p. 487. New York: Excerpta Medica Foundation, 1965.

61. Fraser, R.: Pituitary Ablation by Needle Implantation of Yttrium-90 for Diabetic Retinopathy, in On the Nature and Treatment of Diabetes (edited by B. S. Leibel and G. A. Wrenshall), p. 491. New York: Excerpta Medica Foundation, 1965.

62. Bradley, R. F., Rees, S. B., and Fager, C. A.: Pituitary Ablation in the Treatment of Diabetic Retinopathy, M. Clin. North America, 49:1105, 1965.

63. International Diabetes Federation Convention Report, Appl. Therap., 6:822, 1964.

64. Fagerberg, S.-E.: Diabetic Neuropathy. A Clinical and Histological Study on the Significance of Vascular Affections, Acta med. scandinav., 164 (Supplement No. 345):1, 1959.

65. Pirart, J.: Diabetic Neuropathy: A Metabolic or a Vascular Disease?, Diabetes, 14:1, 1965.

66. Spritz, N.: Nerve Disease in Diabetes Mellitus, Med. Clin. North Am., 62:787, 1978.

67. Ellenberg, M.: Long-Term Problems: Diabetic Neuropathy, in Diabetes Mellitus: Diagnosis and Treatment (edited by T. S. Danowski), p. 171. New York: American Diabetes Association, Inc., 1964.

68. Locke, S.: Diabetes and the Nervous System, M. Clin. North America, 49:1081, 1965.

Index

ence, the disease appears to me to have got the name "diabetes" as if from the Greek word διαβήτης (which signifies a siphon), because the fluid does not remain in the body, but uses the man's body as a ladder (διαβάθρη), whereby to leave it. They stand out for a certain time, but not very long, for they pass urine with pain, and the emaciation is dreadful; nor does any great portion of flesh pass out along with the urine.

The cause of it may be, that some of the acute diseases may have terminated in this: and during the crisis the diseases may have left some malignity lurking in the part. It is not improbable, also, that something pernicious, derived from the other diseases which attack the bladder and kidneys, may sometimes prove the cause of this affection.

ARETAEUS THE CAPPADOCIAN, A.D. 81-138

60-PJ-2110-5 PRINTED IN U.S.A. 000119-28095 JANUARY, 1980